Advances in Postoperative Pain Management and Chronic Postoperative Pain

Advances in Postoperative Pain Management and Chronic Postoperative Pain

Editor

Marco Cascella

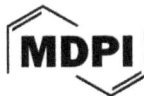

Basel • Beijing • Wuhan • Barcelona • Belgrade • Novi Sad • Cluj • Manchester

Editor
Marco Cascella
University of Salerno
Baronissi
Italy

Editorial Office
MDPI
St. Alban-Anlage 66
4052 Basel, Switzerland

This is a reprint of articles from the Special Issue published online in the open access journal *Journal of Clinical Medicine* (ISSN 2077-0383) (available at: https://www.mdpi.com/journal/jcm/special_issues/chronic_postoperative_pain).

For citation purposes, cite each article independently as indicated on the article page online and as indicated below:

Lastname, A.A.; Lastname, B.B. Article Title. *Journal Name* **Year**, *Volume Number*, Page Range.

ISBN 978-3-0365-9272-5 (Hbk)
ISBN 978-3-0365-9273-2 (PDF)
doi.org/10.3390/books978-3-0365-9273-2

© 2023 by the authors. Articles in this book are Open Access and distributed under the Creative Commons Attribution (CC BY) license. The book as a whole is distributed by MDPI under the terms and conditions of the Creative Commons Attribution-NonCommercial-NoDerivs (CC BY-NC-ND) license.

Contents

Marco Cascella
Editorial for the Special Issue: "Advances in Postoperative Pain Management and Chronic Postoperative Pain"
Reprinted from: *J. Clin. Med.* **2022**, *11*, 6667, doi:10.3390/jcm11226667 1

Emiliano Petrucci, Franco Marinangeli, Barbara Pizzi, Francesco Sciorio, Gioele Marrocco, Massimo Antonio Innamorato, et al.
A Modified Approach for Ultrasound-Guided Thoracic Paravertebral Block via Thoracic Intervertebral Foramen in an Adolescent Patient: A Case Report
Reprinted from: *J. Clin. Med.* **2022**, *11*, 2646, doi:10.3390/jcm11092646 5

Abdalkarem Fedgash Alsharari, Faud Hamdi Abuadas, Yaser Salman Alnassrallah and Dauda Salihu
Transversus Abdominis Plane Block as a Strategy for Effective Pain Management in Patients with Pain during Laparoscopic Cholecystectomy: A Systematic Review
Reprinted from: *J. Clin. Med.* **2022**, *11*, 6896, doi:10.3390/jcm11236896 15

Xiaoshen Liang, Xin Yang, Shuang Liang, Yu Zhang, Zhuofeng Ding, Qulian Guo and Changsheng Huang
Effect of Intravenous Ketamine on Hypocranial Pressure Symptoms in Patients with Spinal Anesthetic Cesarean Sections: A Systematic Review and Meta-Analysis
Reprinted from: *J. Clin. Med.* **2022**, *11*, 4129, doi:10.3390/jcm11144129 57

Christa K. Raak, Thomas Ostermann, Anna-Li Schönenberg-Tu, Oliver Fricke, David D. Martin, Sibylle Robens and Wolfram Scharbrodt
No Gender Differences in Pain Perception and Medication after Lumbar Spine Sequestrectomy —A Reanalysis of a Randomized Controlled Clinical Trial
Reprinted from: *J. Clin. Med.* **2022**, *11*, 2333, doi:10.3390/jcm11092333 69

Hyean Yeo, Ji Won Choi, Seungwon Lee, Woo Seog Sim, Soo Jung Park, Heejoon Jeong, et al.
The Lack of Analgesic Efficacy of Nefopam after Video-Assisted Thoracoscopic Surgery for Lung Cancer: A Randomized, Single-Blinded, Controlled Trial
Reprinted from: *J. Clin. Med.* **2022**, *11*, 4849, doi:10.3390/jcm11164849 79

Uri Hochberg, Silviu Brill, Dror Ofir, Khalil Salame, Zvi Lidar, Gilad Regev and Morsi Khashan
Is the Erector Spinae Plane Block Effective for More than Perioperative Pain? A Retrospective Analysis
Reprinted from: *J. Clin. Med.* **2022**, *11*, 4902, doi:10.3390/jcm11164902 89

Pascaline Dorges, Mireille Michel-Cherqui, Julien Fessler, Barbara Székély, Edouard Sage, Matthieu Glorion, et al.
Early Postoperative Pain Trajectories after Posterolateral and Axillary Approaches to Thoracic Surgery: A Prospective Monocentric Observational Study
Reprinted from: *J. Clin. Med.* **2022**, *11*, 5152, doi:10.3390/jcm11175152 99

Sujin Kim, Seung Woo Song, Hyejin Do, Jinwon Hong, Chun Sung Byun and Ji-Hyoung Park
The Analgesic Efficacy of the Single Erector Spinae Plane Block with Intercostal Nerve Block Is Not Inferior to That of the Thoracic Paravertebral Block with Intercostal Nerve Block in Video-Assisted Thoracic Surgery
Reprinted from: *J. Clin. Med.* **2022**, *11*, 5452, doi:10.3390/jcm11185452 113

Marco Cascella, Sergio Coluccia, Federica Monaco, Daniela Schiavo, Davide Nocerino, Mariacinzia Grizzuti, et al.
Different Machine Learning Approaches for Implementing Telehealth-Based Cancer Pain Management Strategies
Reprinted from: *J. Clin. Med.* **2022**, *11*, 5484, doi:10.3390/jcm11185484 . . . . **123**

Marcin Wiech, Sławomir Żurek, Arkadiusz Kurowicki, Beata Horeczy, Mirosław Czuczwar, Paweł Piwowarczyk, et al.
Erector Spinae Plane Block Decreases Chronic Postoperative Pain Severity in Patients Undergoing Coronary Artery Bypass Grafting
Reprinted from: *J. Clin. Med.* **2022**, *11*, 5949, doi:10.3390/jcm11195949 . . . . **139**

Yuexin Huang, Tingting Li, Tianhong Wang, Yanhuan Wei, Liulin Xiong, Tinghua Wang and Fei Liu
Real Time Ultrasound-Guided Thoracic Epidural Catheterization with Patients in the Lateral Decubitus Position without Flexion of Knees and Neck: A Preliminary Investigation
Reprinted from: *J. Clin. Med.* **2022**, *11*, 6459, doi:10.3390/jcm11216459 . . . . **147**

Andrea Angelini, Gian Mario Parise, Mariachiara Cerchiaro, Francesco Ambrosio, Paolo Navalesi and Pietro Ruggieri
Sublingual Sufentanil Tablet System (SSTS-Zalviso®) for Postoperative Analgesia after Orthopedic Surgery: A Retrospective Study
Reprinted from: *J. Clin. Med.* **2022**, *11*, 6864, doi:10.3390/jcm11226864 . . . . **159**

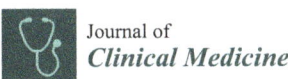

Editorial

Editorial for the Special Issue: "Advances in Postoperative Pain Management and Chronic Postoperative Pain"

Marco Cascella

Division of Anesthesia and Pain Medicine, Istituto Nazionale dei Tumori, IRCCS Fondazione G. Pascale, 80100 Napoli, Italy; m.cascella@istitutotumori.na.it

Citation: Cascella, M. Editorial for the Special Issue: "Advances in Postoperative Pain Management and Chronic Postoperative Pain". *J. Clin. Med.* **2022**, *11*, 6667. https://doi.org/10.3390/jcm11226667

Received: 12 October 2022
Accepted: 7 November 2022
Published: 10 November 2022

Publisher's Note: MDPI stays neutral with regard to jurisdictional claims in published maps and institutional affiliations.

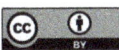

Copyright: © 2022 by the author. Licensee MDPI, Basel, Switzerland. This article is an open access article distributed under the terms and conditions of the Creative Commons Attribution (CC BY) license (https://creativecommons.org/licenses/by/4.0/).

Acute and chronic pain are two completely distinct universes. The clinical aspects underlying their physiopathology, epidemiology, and therapeutic problems are different. Acute pain is generally caused by a definite illness or trauma, and is usually limited to the period of time required to repair the damage. By contrast, chronic pain is not just a symptom and becomes a disease itself, affecting different aspects of the patient's health-related quality of life [1]. In this context, the biological injury is no longer the main actor. Chronic pain is not a linear experience directly induced by sensory inputs that are evoked by the stimulation of nociceptors ("nociception") [2]. It is a multidimensional experience induced by the activation of a diffuse brain network (pain matrix) and involving a widely distributed neural network. A complex series of biopsychosocial phenomena paint clinical pictures that often highlight a cause (secondary chronic pain), although some subtypes of chronic pain are not directly related to a disease (primary chronic pain) [1]. Consequently, the management of this leading source of suffering can be very challenging [3].

Pain occurring after surgery is called postoperative pain (POP). This type of acute pain is usually predictable and is characterized by a high intensity and short duration (usually 2 to 5 days). The clinical aspects of POP may vary from patient to patient and for the same individual over time. They depend on the pre-existing pathology and anatomy as well as on the type and invasiveness of the surgical approach. Distinct variables such as psychological factors, as well as cultural, religious, and socioeconomic aspects, and other components may impact the clinical features of the pain.

Clinically, POP involves various troublesome sensory and emotional experiences that may or may not be combined with autonomic and behavioral changes. When excessive and prolonged, these complicated humoral responses, which are originally aimed at maintaining homeostasis, can provoke organic, psychological, and behavioral changes such as anxiety, insomnia, and depression. If not accurately managed, POP can develop into a composite chronic pain problem [4]. In this context, chronic postsurgical pain (CPSP) is characterized by painful symptoms at the site of the surgical wound or in related areas. This pain lasts for more than 3 months and is not due to surgical complications [1]. Although the magnitude of the phenomenon varies according to the type of surgery, approximately one patient in four suffers from mildly severe CPSP, and one in six suffers from very severe symptoms [5].

CPSP is associated with significant discomfort, distress, and disability. Given the clinical and social impacts of CPSP, its prevention is of paramount importance. Regional anesthesia techniques can represent a favorable approach to addressing this issue [6]. In a prospective cohort study, Wiech et al. [7] assessed the effects of bilateral erector spinae plane block (ESPB) on the severity and incidence of CPSP in patients undergoing coronary artery bypass grafting via sternotomy. They administered 0.375% ropivacaine under ultrasound guidance before the induction of general anesthesia and proved that, compared with that in the control group ($n = 24$), the CPSP intensity was lower in patients treated with the block ($n = 27$). The result was significant at 1, 3, and 6 months after surgery ($p < 0.001$). Significant differences in favor of the ESPB group were also reported for the opioid intake, mechanical ventilation time, and hospital length of stay.

Regional anesthesia techniques have also been investigated for evaluating the short-term effects of preventive analgesic strategies on POP. In a single-blinded, randomized controlled trial, Kim et al. [8] evaluated the analgesic efficacy of ESPB combined with intercostal nerve block (ICNB). In particular, they compared this combination with a strategy focused on the association of thoracic paravertebral block (PVB) and ICNB in patients (n = 52) who underwent video-assisted thoracic surgery (VATS). The results showed that ESPB was not inferior to PVB when combined with ICNB for addressing pain at 24 and 48 h after the operation.

Thoracic ESPB is a simple and secure procedure. It can provide effective postoperative analgesia [9] and reduce the opioid consumption and length of stay after surgery [10]. Hochberg et al. [11] conducted a retrospective analysis to evaluate the efficacy of ESPB (10 mL of 1% lidocaine plus 10 mg of dexamethasone for a unilateral technique; 15–20 mL of 1% lidocaine and the same dose of the synthetic glucocorticoid for a bilateral approach) in patients suffering from pain related to chronic thoracic cancer (n = 44) and non-cancer-related pain (n = 66). Their results showed a mean reduction in pain scores (NRSs) of 2.4 points (p > 0.001) compared to the pre-procedure values. Prospective trials should be conducted to better define the operative modalities in different clinical settings.

Divergences between women and men in pain concern both sex and gender, where the word "sex" applies to human anatomy and physiology, and the word "gender" is related to psychosocial relationships [12]. Raak et al. [13] conducted a secondary analysis of a randomized controlled clinical trial for studying gender differences after lumbar spinal sequestrectomy due to degenerative diseases of the lumbar spine. The outcomes included the pain intensity (VAS), affective and sensory pain perception, and morphine equivalent doses of opioid painkillers used. The authors found no significant differences in any of the outcomes between men (n = 46) and women (n = 42). Since previous investigations found worse pain, disability, and quality of life in women than in men [14], further studies are warranted to clarify the gender differences in this clinical setting [15].

Several innovative and interesting mathematical approaches can be applied to the study of POP. For example, pain can be viewed as a trajectory rather than as one or more simple point estimates of its degree [16]. In a prospective monocentric cohort study, Dorges et al. [17] studied the pain trajectories in patients who underwent posterolateral (n = 92) or axillary thoracotomies (n = 89). They recognized four trajectories of postoperative pain, including a "worst" trajectory (30%) with constantly high pain; a trajectory with constantly low pain (32.6%); another trajectory with a steep decrease in pain (22.7%); and, finally, a trajectory featuring a steep increase (15%). Notably, the risk factors for chronic pain were the occurrence of preoperative pain (OR = 6.94; CI 95% (1.54–31.27)) and scar length (OR = 1.20 (1.05–1.38)). On the contrary, ASA class III seemed to be a protective factor for the worst pain group (OR = 0.02 (0.001–0.52)).

As highlighted in other articles collected in this Special Issue, regional anesthesia techniques are an interesting field of study. Researchers are seeking innovative approaches that are easy and safe. In a case report, Petrucci et al. [18] described an adjusted technique for ultrasound-guided thoracic PVB via the thoracic intervertebral foramen in a patient who underwent emergent laparotomy due to a small intestinal volvulus. They used two continuous catheters for a bilateral extended block (levobupivacaine 0.25% at a rate of 5–8 mL/h) and conducted clinical observations and virtual dissections to demonstrate the effective spread of the injection. The "Petrucci's block" is a fascinating perspective, but a cadaver study is necessary to refine the technique and proceed with its clinical validation.

In pregnant women, cerebrospinal fluid outflow after spinal anesthesia for a cesarean section can cause headaches, vomiting, and nausea. Since ketamine increases intracranial pressure, it could prevent postpuncture symptoms due to perioperative hypocranial pressure. Liang and collaborators [19] conducted a systematic review and meta-analysis on the topic. The search strategy yielded 12 randomized trials (n = 2099), and, interestingly, there was no significant association between intravenous ketamine and the improvement of symptoms due to hypocranial pressure.

Chronic cancer pain is a subset of chronic secondary pain produced by a primary cancer itself, its metastases, or its therapy [1]. Its management requires a complex and multimodal approach. Telemedicine-based strategies can be adopted for this aim [20]. Nevertheless, there is a need for establishing the correct model of care by combining remote consultations and in-person visits for emergencies or for diagnostic or clinical aims. Predictive models are a meaningful opportunity in medicine, and machine learning (ML) approaches can probably be used for designing careful telemedicine processes. In a study conducted at the Istituto Tumori Fondazione Pascale (Italy), the authors implemented different ML models including random forest, gradient boosting machine, a single layer artificial neural network, and the LASSO–RIDGE algorithm to define the variable(s) that can influence the number of remote consultations. The ML-based simulations demonstrated that this parameter can be influenced by selected variables, mostly the patient's age, the cancer type, and the occurrence of bone metastases [21].

Multimodal analgesia is fundamental for acute and chronic pain management. Nefopam is a centrally acting, non-opioid, non-steroidal analgesic drug. Several studies have demonstrated its efficacy for multimodal analgesia [22]. In a randomized, single-blinded, controlled trial reported in this Special Issue, the authors evaluated the analgesic efficacy of the intraoperative administration of nefopam (20 mg after induction and 15 min before the end of surgery) [23]. The patients of the nefopam group ($n = 50$) and control ($n = 49$) underwent VATS for lung cancer. The results indicated that the pain intensity at 72 h after the operation and after 3 months (chronic pain) and the total opioid consumption did not vary between the groups. Since nefopam has not been assessed in this setting, the results have important value in this research field.

In conclusion, the articles in this Special Issue should be helpful for identifying gaps in the prevention, diagnosis, and management of acute and chronic pain issues.

Funding: This research received no external funding.

Conflicts of Interest: The author declares no conflict of interest.

References

1. Treede, R.-D.; Rief, W.; Barke, A.; Aziz, Q.; Bennett, M.I.; Benoliel, R.; Cohen, M.; Evers, S.; Finnerup, N.B.; First, M.B.; et al. Chronic pain as a symptom or a disease: The IASP Classification of Chronic Pain for the International Classification of Diseases (ICD-11). *Pain* **2019**, *160*, 19–27. [CrossRef] [PubMed]
2. Cascella, M.; Muzio, M.R.; Monaco, F.; Nocerino, D.; Ottaiano, A.; Perri, F.; Innamorato, M.A. Pathophysiology of Nociception and Rare Genetic Disorders with Increased Pain Threshold or Pain Insensitivity. *Pathophysiology* **2022**, *29*, 35. [CrossRef] [PubMed]
3. Raja, S.N.; Carr, D.B.; Cohen, M.; Finnerup, N.B.; Flor, H.; Gibson, S.; Keefe, F.J.; Mogil, J.S.; Ringkamp, M.; Sluka, K.A.; et al. The revised International Association for the Study of Pain definition of pain: Concepts, challenges, and compromises. *Pain* **2020**, *161*, 1976–1982. [CrossRef] [PubMed]
4. Glare, P.; Aubrey, K.R.; Myles, P.S. Transition from acute to chronic pain after surgery. *Lancet* **2019**, *393*, 1537–1546. [CrossRef]
5. Fletcher, D.; Stamer, U.M.; Pogatzki-Zahn, E.; Zaslansky, R.; Tanase, N.V.; Perruchoud, C.; Kranke, P.; Komann, M.; Lehman, T.; Meissner, W.; et al. Chronic postsurgical pain in Europe. *Eur. J. Anaesthesiol.* **2015**, *32*, 725–734. [CrossRef] [PubMed]
6. Weinstein, E.; Levene, J.; Cohen, M.; Andreae, D.; Chao, J.; Johnson, M.; Hall, C.; Andreae, M. Local anaesthetics and regional anaesthesia versus conventional analgesia for preventing persistent postoperative pain in adults and children. *Cochrane Database Syst. Rev.* **2018**, *4*, CD007105. [CrossRef]
7. Wiech, M.; Żurek, S.; Kurowicki, A.; Horeczy, B.; Czuczwar, M.; Piwowarczyk, P.; Widenka, K.; Borys, M. Erector Spinae Plane Block Decreases Chronic Postoperative Pain Severity in Patients Undergoing Coronary Artery Bypass Grafting. *J. Clin. Med.* **2022**, *11*, 5949. [CrossRef]
8. Kim, S.; Song, S.W.; Do, H.; Hong, J.; Byun, C.S.; Park, J.-H. The Analgesic Efficacy of the Single Erector Spinae Plane Block with Intercostal Nerve Block Is Not Inferior to That of the Thoracic Paravertebral Block with Intercostal Nerve Block in Video-Assisted Thoracic Surgery. *J. Clin. Med.* **2022**, *11*, 5452. [CrossRef]
9. Koo, C.-H.; Hwang, J.-Y.; Shin, H.-J.; Ryu, J.-H. The Effects of Erector Spinae Plane Block in Terms of Postoperative Analgesia in Patients Undergoing Laparoscopic Cholecystectomy: A Meta-Analysis of Randomized Controlled Trials. *J. Clin. Med.* **2020**, *9*, 2928. [CrossRef]
10. Vaughan, B.N.; Bartone, C.L.; McCarthy, C.M.; Answini, G.A.; Hurford, W.E. Ultrasound-Guided Continuous Bilateral Erector Spinae Plane Blocks Are Associated with Reduced Opioid Consumption and Length of Stay for Open Cardiac Surgery: A Retrospective Cohort Study. *J. Clin. Med.* **2021**, *10*, 5022. [CrossRef]

11. Hochberg, U.; Brill, S.; Ofir, D.; Salame, K.; Lidar, Z.; Regev, G.; Khashan, M. Is the Erector Spinae Plane Block Effective for More than Perioperative Pain? A Retrospective Analysis. *J. Clin. Med.* **2022**, *11*, 4902. [CrossRef]
12. Templeton, K.J. Sex and Gender Issues in Pain Management. *J. Bone Jt. Surg.* **2020**, *102*, 32–35. [CrossRef]
13. Raak, C.K.; Ostermann, T.; Schönenberg-Tu, A.-L.; Fricke, O.; Martin, D.D.; Robens, S.; Scharbrodt, W. No Gender Differences in Pain Perception and Medication after Lumbar Spine Sequestrectomy—A Reanalysis of a Randomized Controlled Clinical Trial. *J. Clin. Med.* **2022**, *11*, 2333. [CrossRef]
14. MacLean, M.A.; Touchette, C.J.; Han, J.H.; Christie, S.D.; Pickett, G.E. Gender differences in the surgical management of lumbar degenerative disease: A scoping review. *J. Neurosurg. Spine* **2020**, *32*, 799–816. [CrossRef]
15. Gigliotti, S.; Cascella, M.; Santè, G.; De Marinis, P.; Cuomo, A.; ASON Study Group. Lumbar spinal stenosis as a model for the multimodal and multiprofessional treatment of mixed non-cancer pain. Survey response from a panel of experts of the Italian National Association of Osteoarticular Specialists (ASON). *Anaesthesiol. Intensive Ther.* **2021**, *53*, 252–264. [CrossRef]
16. Bayman, E.O.; Oleson, J.J.; Rabbitts, J.A. AAAPT: Assessment of the Acute Pain Trajectory. *Pain Med.* **2021**, *22*, 533–547. [CrossRef]
17. Dorges, P.; Michel-Cherqui, M.; Fessler, J.; Székély, B.; Sage, E.; Glorion, M.; Kennel, T.; Fischler, M.; Martinez, V.; Vallée, A.; et al. Early Postoperative Pain Trajectories after Posterolateral and Axillary Approaches to Thoracic Surgery: A Prospective Monocentric Observational Study. *J. Clin. Med.* **2022**, *11*, 5152. [CrossRef]
18. Petrucci, E.; Marinangeli, F.; Pizzi, B.; Sciorio, F.; Marrocco, G.; Innamorato, M.A.; Cascella, M.; Vittori, A. A Modified Approach for Ultrasound-Guided Thoracic Paravertebral Block via Thoracic Intervertebral Foramen in an Adolescent Patient: A Case Report. *J. Clin. Med.* **2022**, *11*, 2646. [CrossRef]
19. Liang, X.; Yang, X.; Liang, S.; Zhang, Y.; Ding, Z.; Guo, Q.; Huang, C. Effect of Intravenous Ketamine on Hypocranial Pressure Symptoms in Patients with Spinal Anesthetic Cesarean Sections: A Systematic Review and Meta-Analysis. *J. Clin. Med.* **2022**, *11*, 4129. [CrossRef]
20. Cascella, M.; Coluccia, S.; Grizzuti, M.; Romano, M.C.; Esposito, G.; Crispo, A.; Cuomo, A. Satisfaction with Telemedicine for Cancer Pain Management: A Model of Care and Cross-Sectional Patient Satisfaction Study. *Curr. Oncol.* **2022**, *29*, 80439. [CrossRef]
21. Cascella, M.; Coluccia, S.; Monaco, F.; Schiavo, D.; Nocerino, D.; Grizzuti, M.; Romano, M.C.; Cuomo, A. Different Machine Learning Approaches for Implementing Telehealth-Based Cancer Pain Management Strategies. *J. Clin. Med.* **2022**, *11*, 5484. [CrossRef] [PubMed]
22. Tiglis, M.; Neagu, T.P.; Elfara, M.; Diaconu, C.C.; Bratu, O.G.; Vacaroiu, I.A.; Grintescu, I.M. Nefopam and its role in modulating acute and chronic pain. *Rev. Chim.* **2018**, *69*, 2877–2880. [CrossRef]
23. Yeo, H.; Choi, J.W.; Lee, S.; Sim, W.S.; Park, S.J.; Jeong, H.; Yang, M.; Ahn, H.J.; Kim, J.A.; Lee, E.J. The Lack of Analgesic Efficacy of Nefopam after Video-Assisted Thoracoscopic Surgery for Lung Cancer: A Randomized, Single-Blinded, Controlled Trial. *J. Clin. Med.* **2022**, *11*, 4849. [CrossRef] [PubMed]

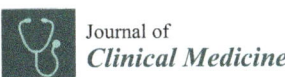

Case Report

A Modified Approach for Ultrasound-Guided Thoracic Paravertebral Block via Thoracic Intervertebral Foramen in an Adolescent Patient: A Case Report

Emiliano Petrucci [1,*], Franco Marinangeli [2], Barbara Pizzi [3], Francesco Sciorio [2], Gioele Marrocco [2], Massimo Antonio Innamorato [4], Marco Cascella [5] and Alessandro Vittori [6]

1. Department of Anesthesia and Intensive Care Unit, San Salvatore Academic Hospital of L'Aquila, Via Vetoio 48, 67100 L'Aquila, Italy
2. Department of Anesthesiology, Intensive Care and Pain Treatment, University of L'Aquila, Piazzale Salvatore Tommasi 1, Coppito, 67100 L'Aquila, Italy; francomarinangeli@gmail.com (F.M.); francesco.sciorio@gmail.com (F.S.); gioelemarrocco9@gmail.com (G.M.)
3. Department of Anesthesia and Intensive Care Unit, SS Filippo and Nicola Academic Hospital of Avezzano, Avezzano, 67051 L'Aquila, Italy; bpizzi@hotmail.it
4. Department of Neuroscience, Pain Unit, Santa Maria delle Croci Hospital, AUSL Romagna, Viale Vincenzo Randi 5, 48121 Ravenna, Italy; massimo.innamorato@auslromagna.it
5. Department of Anesthesia and Critical Care, Istituto Nazionale Tumori—IRCCS, Fondazione Pascale, Via Mariano Semmola 53, 80131 Naples, Italy; m.cascella@istitutotumori.na.it
6. Department of Anesthesia and Critical Care, ARCO ROMA, Ospedale Pediatrico Bambino Gesù IRCCS, Piazza S. Onofrio 4, 00165 Rome, Italy; alexvittori@libero.it
* Correspondence: petrucciemiliano@gmail.com

Abstract: This case report describes a modified approach for a thoracic paravertebral block by performing a bilateral ultrasound-assisted injection of 12 mL of 0.5% levobupivacaine near the thoracic intervertebral foramen, combined with general anesthesia, in a patient who underwent emergent laparotomy for small intestinal volvulus. Two continuous catheter sets were used for a bilateral continuous block with levobupivacaine 0.25% at a rate of 5–8 mL/h. No complications during the execution of the block were recorded. No supplemental opioids were administered and the patient was hemodynamically stable, requiring no pharmacological cardiovascular support during surgery. At the end of the surgical procedure, the patient received a continuous flow of 0.2% levobupivacaine as postoperative analgesia, at a basal flow of 4 mL/h per each side, a bolus of 4 mL, and a lockout time of 60 min was used. The postoperative pain on the Numeric Rating Scale was 2 at rest and it was 4 in motion, without neurological or respiratory sequelae due to block in the first 72 h after surgery.

Keywords: anesthesia; regional anesthesia; pediatric anesthesia; adolescent; paravertebral block; epidural anesthesia; pain; postoperative pain; anesthetic absorption; local anesthetic

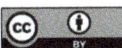

1. Introduction

Regional anesthetic techniques provide anesthesia during surgery followed by effective long-acting postoperative analgesia [1,2]. International literature underlines the role of regional anesthesia in the improvement of perioperative pain control, reducing the request for opioids and related side effects [3,4]. Epidural analgesia (EA) and thoracic paravertebral block (TPVB) are considered useful techniques for the control of postoperative pain of thoracic and visceral abdominal surgery, as well as from the opioid sparing point of view [5]. The current literature on ultrasound-guided TPVB describes a wide range of techniques for use on patients and cadavers, but it is currently not possible to provide an evidence-based recommendation on the choice between techniques. Many factors can influence the weighing of procedure choice, because of individual preferences per individual physician, skills, and experience with other ultrasound-guided regional anesthesia techniques and with landmark-guided blockades [6]. Thus, we hypothesized an alternative way to perform this block, attempting to minimize the relative disadvantages of the various described techniques and the risk of iatrogenic damage [7,8].

During an alternative approach for the TPVB, the local anesthetic (LA) spreads into the thoracic paravertebral space through the needle tip, which is placed over and behind the transverse process (TP) of vertebra, via the thoracic intervertebral foramen (TIF). We found that injecting into this site was successful in clinical terms. This technique was named the TIF block.

Based on our clinical observations and virtual dissections, we hypothesized that injection at this site would result in an effective injection spread, presumably because the thoracic paravertebral space (TPVS) and epidural space (ES) could be reached by TIF [9].

In this case report, we performed a bilateral continuous TIF block, providing opioid-free anesthesia and postoperative analgesia for emergent laparotomy (EL) due to a small intestinal volvulus.

2. Case Presentation

On 12 October 2021, at the San Salvatore Academic Hospital of L'Aquila (Italy), the alternative approach to thoracic paravertebral block (TPVB) was performed on a 17-year-old male who had EL for a small intestinal volvulus associated with bowel obstruction and ischemia. The patient was 165 cm tall and weighed 70 kg (BMI was 25.71). He was taking bronchodilators and inhaled corticosteroids because of asthma. The American Society of Anesthesiologists (ASA) status was II. A consent form, signed by a legal surrogate of the patient, was obtained for the execution of the anesthesia, while the consent for publication was subsequently signed by the patient, who, in the meantime, had reached the age of majority according to Italian law.

Peripheral venous access was obtained and 2.5 mg of midazolam and 0.1 mcg·kg^{-1} sufentanil were administered intravenously before execution of the block. The patient was placed in the left and then right lateral position to perform the bilateral block. Ultrasonography was performed from the seventh cervical spinous process (SP) to the tenth thoracic SP vertebra. The tip of the spinous process (SP) of the tenth thoracic vertebra (T$_{10}$) was identified using a high-frequency linear array ultrasound (US) transducer (EDAN, Acclarix AX4, Rome, Italy), which was transversally placed. We began ultrasound scanning in the transverse plane, visualizing the tip of spinous processes as hyperechoic, round shapes with acoustic shadowing beneath it. A protective plastic sheath was used for the US procedure. The transducer was slightly moved from the medial to the lateral direction, while maintaining a transverse orientation and was observed at the angle between the SP and TP. This was visualized as a caved structure that lay deep on the fascial plane of the erector spinae muscle (ESM). The skin site of injection was anesthetized with 2 mL of lidocaine 1%. A Tuohy needle (18 gauge, 90 mm, Contiplex, BBraun, Bethlehem, PA, USA) was gently inserted, in-plane to the US beam in a lateral-to-medial direction to contact the SP, into the skeletal muscle plane of the erector spinae muscle (ESM). Then, the needle tip was moved from the cephalic to the caudal direction, tilting the probe in the same direction when the angle between the TP and SP was reached (Figure 1). Subsequently, the needle tip was gently inserted and advanced 2 mm along the superior limit of the vertebral pedicle, until losing contact with the bone. Six milliliters of levobupivacaine 0.5% were subsequently injected. Similarly, the same anesthetic solution was injected from the caudal in the cephalic direction, overcoming the inferior articular process, 2 mm along the inferior limit of the vertebral pedicle (Figures 1 and 2). Injection pressure monitoring was provided by using the half-the-air technique through a three-way stopcock, which was used to keep the injection pressure below 15 psi [10,11]. The anesthetic procedure was performed bilaterally. Two continuous catheter sets were used and threaded 1 cm from the needle tip for a bilateral continuous block. The catheters were inserted from the caudal in the cephalic direction (Figure 2) and were secured using a cyanoacrylate tissue adhesive (Dermabond, Ethicon,

Somerville, NJ, USA) and two layers of a transparent adhesive dressing (Tegaderm™, 3M, Maplewood, MN, USA) to prevent retrograde leakage. Cold tests and touch tests were performed bilaterally every 2 min and the patient was judged operable when a loss of cold and touch sensations was observed for the T_7 to T_{12} dermatomes, in a 4 cm lateral line to the thoracic spine and to the parasternal line.

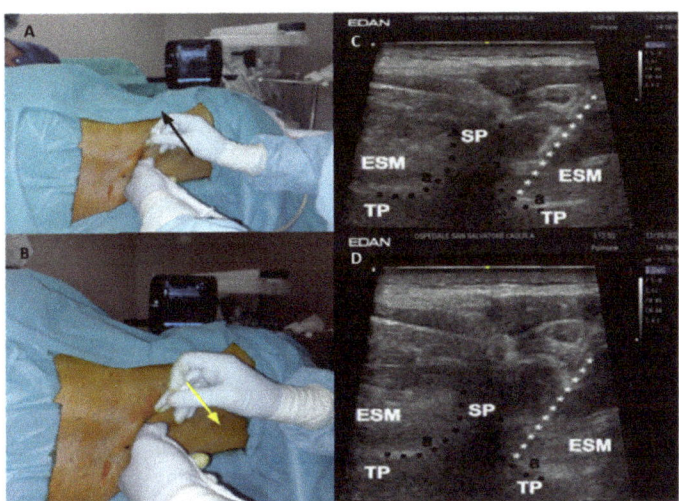

Figure 1. Ultrasound-assisted thoracic intervertebral block. The anesthesiologist injected local anesthetic by overcoming the angle (a, black points) between the spinous (SP) and transverse process (TP) of vertebra. (**A**) The needle back was moved upwards (black arrow), directing the tip from the cephalic to caudal position; (**B**) the needle back was moved down (yellow arrow), directing the tip from the caudal to cephalic position. The transducer was slightly moved from the medial to lateral direction, while maintaining a transverse orientation and observing the angle (a) between SP and TP. This was visualized as a caved structure (black points) that lay deep on the fascial plane of the erector spinae muscle (ESM). The needle (white stars) was inserted and advanced along the inferior (**C**) and the superior (**D**) limit of the angle between TP and SP, until losing contact with the bone.

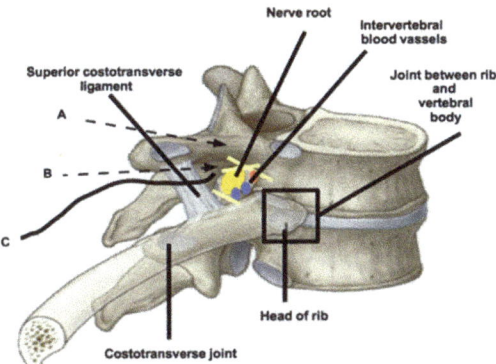

Figure 2. Needle direction and catheter position. Black arrow A indicates the needle tip position in the cephalic to caudal direction; black arrow B indicates the needle tip in the caudal to cephalic direction. Black line C is the catheter position, inserted from the caudal to the cephalic direction. Yellow lines represent the transforaminal ligaments.

General anesthesia was induced with propofol 2 mg·kg^{-1}. Rocuronium 0.6 mg·kg^{-1} was administered to facilitate the intubation with an endotracheal tube. Anesthesia was maintained with sevoflurane 1.5–2% in oxygen with positive pressure ventilation in a circle system. A bolus of 5 mL levobupivacaine 0.5% was injected through the catheter, followed by a continuous infusion of levobupivacaine 0.25% at a rate of 5–8 mL/h (2.5–4 mL/h for side, titrated to patient weight and clinical effect) using an infusion pump (CADD-Solis, Smiths Medical, Dublin, OH, USA), before surgical incision. ASA guidelines for anesthetic monitoring were respected [12].

No complications due to the execution of the block were recorded. No supplemental opioids were administered and the patient was hemodynamically stable, requiring no pharmacological cardiovascular support during surgery. At the end of surgical procedure, the patient was admitted into the post-anesthesia care unit (PACU) phase 1 and then into the PACU phase 2, before going to the ward [13]. The patient received a continuous flow of 0.2% levobupivacaine as postoperative analgesia, with a basal flow of 8 mL/h (4 mL/h for side), bolus of 4 mL, and a lockout time of 60 min. No pharmacological cardiovascular support was required to the patient's hemodynamic stability during his stay in the PACU. Acute pain at rest (on laying position), and in motion (during a deep breath) were recorded at 36, 48, and 72 h after surgery. The Numeric Rating Scale for pain (NRS, an 11-point numeric scale, from "0" ("no pain") to "10" ("worst pain imaginable")) was used. No patient discomfort, infections, side effects of local anesthetic (LA), nor other complications were observed. Postoperative pain was 2 at rest, and it was 4 in motion, without neurological or respiratory sequelae in the first 72 h after surgery due to execution of the block. Bowel function recovery was recorded after 8 h from surgery. The infusion of analgesic solution was interrupted 76 h after surgery and the catheters were removed. The patient required a mean of 4 bolus per day administered using a PCA pump. Acetaminophen 2000 mg per day was systematically administered in the first 96 h after surgery, without the use of supplemental opioids or non-steroidal anti-inflammatory drugs.

Before catheter removal, a second-look ultrasound scan of thoracic paravertebral space (TPVS) was performed, documenting anechoic fluid in the TPVS at a level of T_8 and presumably indicating the LA spread (Figure 3).

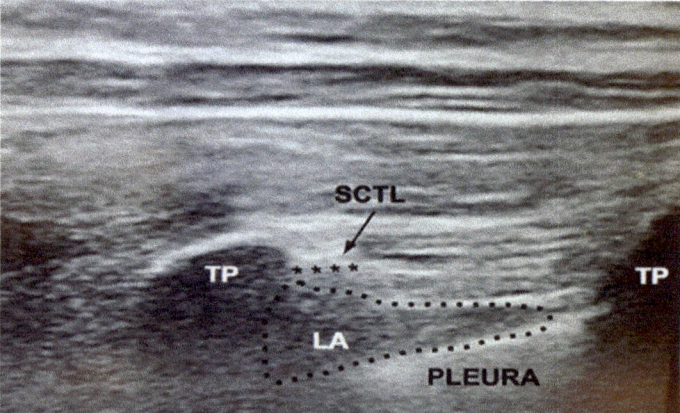

Figure 3. Second-look ultrasound scan. The transducer was placed in the sagittal plane, between transverse processes (TPs) of the eighth (T_8) and ninth (T_9) vertebra. Anechoic fluid in the thoracic paravertebral space (TPVS, black points), (T_8) presumably indicating the local anesthetic (LA) spread. TP, transverse process of T_8 and T_9. The TPVS was located between the hyperechoic lines of the superior costotransverse ligament (SCTL, black arrow and stars) and the pleura.

3. Discussion

Epidural anesthesia (EA) and thoracic paravertebral block (TPVB) are considered useful for anesthesia and postoperative analgesia in thoracic and visceral abdominal surgery, achieving useful pain relief and avoiding the side effects of opioids. However, it should be emphasized that these regional anesthesia techniques can be burdened by possible intrinsic side effects, especially in the pediatric population, which has some important peculiarities [7,8,14]. This case description demonstrates that an injection point 2 mm over and behind the angle between the TP and SP achieved spread of dye into the thoracic paravertebral space (TVPS) via thoracic intervertebral foramen (TIF) at the level of injection, and to adjacent levels, providing thoracic and visceral abdominal anesthesia and analgesia.

We performed this anesthetic procedure, presuming that it was an alternative approach for TPVB. Surprisingly, we believe to have found an alternative way to also perform EA under US assistance.

Recently, the erector spinae plane block has been described as more effective at reducing postoperative opioid consumption and pain scores for a broad spectrum of surgeries involving incisions from T_1 to L_4 [15]. The hypothesis is that, by injecting anesthetics in this block, they may centrally reach the ventral and posterior branches of the thoracic and thoracolumbar spinal nerves, communicating branches, and sympathetic trunk, and also spread into the ES [16].

Although the anatomical boundaries of the TPVS are well described, there is still controversy regarding the injection point of a local anesthetic (LA) because of the complex thoracic paravertebral anatomy. This indeed underlines the hypothesis of the anatomical space of the TPVS. The TPVS is commonly described as triangular-shaped, located bilaterally alongside the whole length of the thoracic vertebral column, filled with fat, and traversed by the dorsal branches and ventral branches of spinal nerves, communicating branches, intercostal nerves and blood vessels, hemiazygos vein, thoracic duct, and sympathetic trunk [17]. The vertebral column forms the base, and the intercostal space is the apex of the TPVS. The parietal pleura represents the anterolateral boundary and the transverse processes of the vertebrae; the head and neck of the ribs form the posterior boundary. The psoas muscle at L_1 is considered the caudal boundary of the TPVS but the cranial boundary remains undescribed [17]. It is important to underline that, medially, the TIF were found as TPVS boundaries. The TPVS appeared to communicate with the ES and with the contralateral paravertebral space through the intervertebral foramen (IVF) [17]. The TIF is an oval area, laterally faced. Medially, there is the dural sleeve with its emerging nerve root. Laterally, there is a fascial sheet that is part of the anterior layer of the thoracolumbar fascia. Usually, there are two separate oval perforations in this fascia: a posterior perforation for the nerve root ("*nerve root compartment*") and a smaller anterior perforation for the intervertebral blood vessels ("blood vessels compartment") [18]. Various foraminal ligaments limit the posterior compartment of the fascia, closely related to the exiting nerve root. Anteriorly, the superior corporopedicular ligament extends from the superior pedicle traversing to the posterolateral vertebral body. Superiorly, the superior transforaminal ligament extends from the arches of the superior and inferior vertebral notches to the articular capsule of the superior pedicle. Inferiorly, the mid-transforaminal ligament runs from the annulus fibrosus and superior and inferior corporopedicular ligaments to the articular capsule. The inferior transforaminal ligament extends from the junction of the annulus fibrosus and the posterior vertebral body to the superior articular facet, limiting the nerve to the vascular compartment (Figures 2 and 4). The number of dorsal rootlets that emerge to give rise to a dorsal root varies at each spinal segment; Bozkurt et al. [19] found that T_1 segment contained the largest number of thoracic nerve rootlets, in contrast to the T_6, T_7, and T_{10} segments which contained the fewest. The central and dorsal rootlets form the segmental spinal nerve, converging in the TIF area. Two layers of pia mater, the arachnoid, and the dura mater surround the rootlets until they advance toward the IVF, then the pial and arachnoidian layers are fused with the dura mater of the thecal sac. A thin connective tissue sheath loosely surrounds the dorsal and ventral roots when they exit through separate perforations in the dura. It has been estimated that the mean foraminal width is 0.8 cm, while the widths of thoracic TP are between 1.2 and 1.3 cm [20,21]. With this premise, we speculated that the *"nerve root compartment"* of TIF is presumably 1.5 cm from the anterior limit of TP of vertebra. Thus, it can be filled with anesthetic solution by gently locating the needle 2 mm over and behind the angle between TP and SP, providing an effective block without the necessity of approaching the pleura from TPVS or the ES directly, and avoiding the attendant risks. The catheter placement should not exceed 1.5 cm from the tip of the needle, avoiding iatrogenic damages for the vulnerable structures of TIF. Shibata et al. described the costotransverse foramen block. This technique aims to posteriorly reach the TPVS via the costotransverse foramen [22]. They focused the US beam to identify the superior costotransverse ligament (SCTL) above the paravertebral space. The SCTL is a part of the interconnecting musculoaponeurotic system which forms the posterior boundary of TPVS together with the TP of vertebrae and the head and neck of the ribs [23]. The musculoaponeurotic system is also formed by the aponeurosis of the internal intercostal muscle (ICM) [24]. On the contrary, our procedure can be considered a modified approach to TPVB without penetrating into the TPVS through its boundaries. We aimed to place LA over and behind the transverse process (TP) of vertebra, by placing the needle tip along the superior limit of the vertebral pedicle until losing contact with the bone, to overcome the articular processes. While it is important to underline that, medially, TIF were found as TPVS boundaries; during our procedure, the needle tip was outside the TPVS (Figure 4).

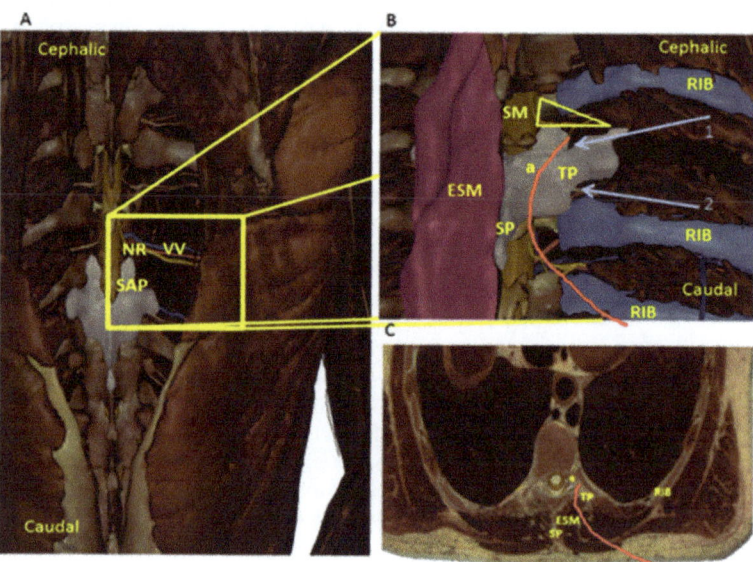

Figure 4. Virtual dissection. (**A**) Virtual dissection of thorax: posterior wall; skin, subcutaneous tissue, and all muscle plane were dissected, reaching the spine. Eighth and ninth vertebrae were removed to identify nerve root (NR) and intervertebral blood vessels (VV). The tenth thoracic vertebra is represented in white. SAP: superior articular process. (**B**) The red line identifies the catheter position inserted in the caudal to the cephalic direction, outside the boundaries of the thoracic paravertebral space (yellow triangle). a, angle between spinous (SP) and transverse process (TP). 1. Light blue arrow indicates the needle tip position from the cephalic to the caudal direction; 2. light blue arrow indicates the needle tip in the caudal to the cephalic direction. (**C**) Transverse plane virtual dissection: the red line identifies the catheter position lying on the ESM plane, over and behind the TP, from the angle between SP and TP, close to the thoracic intervertebral foramen (yellow star).

Our study has limitations that should be underlined. The first limitation of our findings may be due to the width of TP of T_{10}, which we estimated to be 1.1–1.2 cm. The second limitation may be due to the fact that the US beam cannot identify the TIF content and the needle tip behind the acoustic shadow from the TP and the vertebral articular processes (Figure 1). Nevertheless, iatrogenic damage was avoided by carefully advancing the needle tip along the vertebral pedicle no more than 2 mm until contact with bone ended. However, concerns about damaging a nerve root or blood vessel remain. It possible to speculate that the transforaminal ligaments and connective tissue sheath presumably protect the content of the TIF, maybe minimizing the risk for neural and vascular damages. We identified virtual dissection as a potentially useful option to allow the emulation of anatomical dissection as close as possible to reality, notwithstanding the physical absence of a corpse (Figure 4) [9]. Thus, we believe our findings might demonstrate the necessary safety of the procedure regarding this approach, as Figure 4 shows. However, cadaveric studies are requested to provide exact evidence of LA placement and spread and the exact location of the catheters.

In effect, the second-look ultrasound scan of TPVS was performed, documenting anechoic fluid in the TPVS at a level of T_8 and presumably indicating the LA spread (Figure 3). This might indirectly demonstrate that the catheter tip location was in the correct position near the TIF area, although the US beam cannot clearly identify it. We designed a cadaveric study to demonstrate the anatomical implications of our findings. In addition, another limit of this report is that two cases or more should be described to demonstrate the efficacy and reproducibility of a new technique. However, we intend to perform clinical trials after the cadaver dissection study to confirm our speculations.

We are confident that our procedure is quite fast to perform. The US beam allows us to quickly identify the needle while the angle between SP and TP is reached. The needle tip is inserted into the skeletal muscle plane of the ESM by maintaining the contact with SP of vertebra. The US guidance and the contact with bone allows us to quickly place the needle and the catheters onto the anesthetic target, without delay for surgical operation, as the emergent laparotomy. The flow diagram depicts the main steps for a safe and quick procedure of the block, as shown in Figure 5.

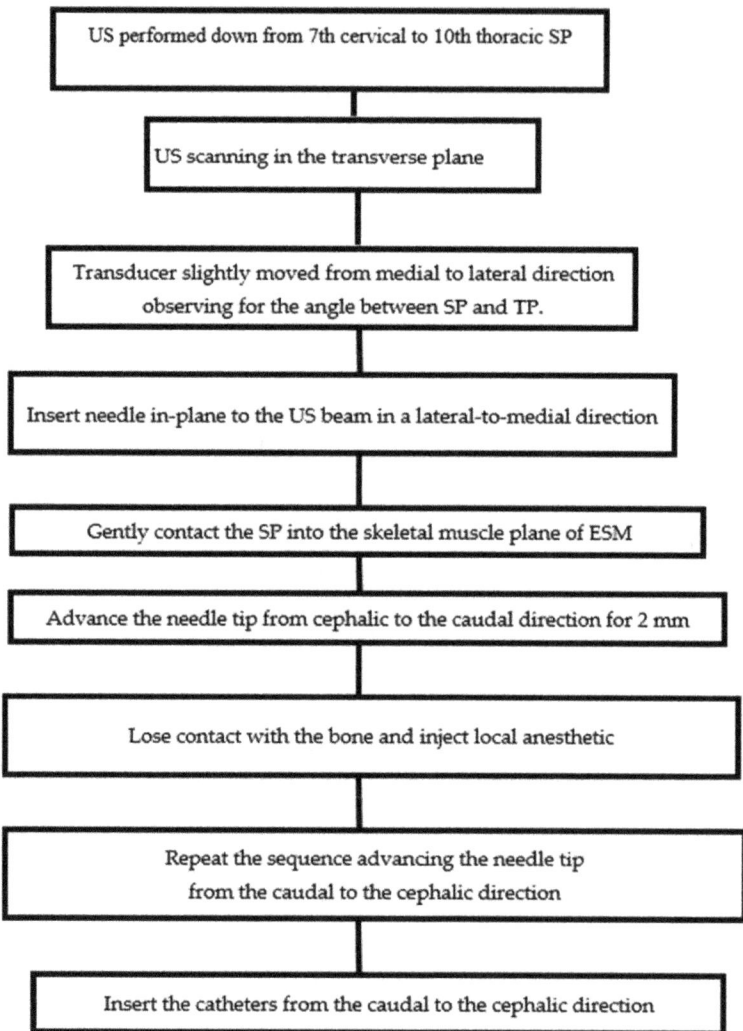

Figure 5. Flow diagram of the thoracic intervertebral foramen block. The main steps of the block are shown.

4. Conclusions

In conclusion, based on our clinical observations, we are confident that use of the thoracic intervertebral foramen (TIF) block could be considered an effective alternative to thoracic paravertebral block (TPVB) and to other paraspinal anesthetic procedures, as an opioid-sparing strategy, for fast-track recovery after pediatric abdominal surgeries. Our case report provides important evidence for future randomized clinical trials.

Author Contributions: Conceptualization, E.P., F.M. and A.V.; methodology, E.P., B.P., F.S. and G.M.; validation, E.P., B.P., M.A.I. and F.M.; formal analysis, E.P., F.M., M.C., M.A.I. and A.V.; investigation, E.P., F.M., B.P., F.S. and G.M.; resources, E.P., F.M. and A.V.; data curation, E.P., F.M., M.A.I., M.C. and A.V.; writing—original draft preparation, E.P., F.M., B.P. and A.V.; writing—review and editing, E.P., F.M., M.A.I., M.C. and A.V.; visualization, E.P., F.S. and G.M.; supervision, E.P., F.M. and A.V.; project administration, E.P. and A.V. All authors have read and agreed to the published version of the manuscript.

Funding: This research received no external funding.

Institutional Review Board Statement: Not applicable.

Informed Consent Statement: Written informed consent has been obtained from the patient.

Data Availability Statement: Not applicable.

Acknowledgments: The authors thank the patient for his cooperation.

Conflicts of Interest: The authors declare no conflict of interest.

References

1. Andreae, M.H.; Andreae, D.A. Regional anaesthesia to prevent chronic pain after surgery: A cochrane systematic review and meta-analysis. *Br. J. Anaesth.* **2013**, *111*, 711–720. [CrossRef] [PubMed]
2. Cuomo, A.; Bimonte, S.; Forte, C.A.; Botti, G.; Cascella, M. Multimodal approaches and tailored therapies for pain management: The trolley analgesic model. *J. Pain Res.* **2019**, *12*, 711–714. [CrossRef] [PubMed]
3. Chia, P.A.; Cannesson, M.; Bui, C.C.M. Opioid free anesthesia: Feasible? *Curr. Opin. Anaesthesiol.* **2020**, *33*, 512–517. [CrossRef] [PubMed]
4. Chitnis, S.S.; Tang, R.; Mariano, E.R. The role of regional analgesia in personalized postoperative pain management. *Korean J. Anesthesiol.* **2020**, *73*, 363–371. [CrossRef]
5. Kehlet, H.; Rung, G.W.; Callesen, T. Postoperative opioid analgesia: Time for a reconsideration? *J. Clin. Anesth.* **1996**, *8*, 441–445. [CrossRef]
6. Krediet, A.C.; Moayeri, N.; van Geffen, G.-J.; Bruhn, J.; Renes, S.; Bigeleisen, P.E.; Groen, G.J. Different approaches to ultrasound-guided thoracic paravertebral block: An illustrated review. *Anesthesiology* **2015**, *123*, 459–474. [CrossRef]
7. Petrucci, E.; Vittori, A.; Cascella, M.; Vergallo, A.; Fiore, G.; Luciani, A.; Pizzi, B.; Degan, G.; Fineschi, V.; Marinangeli, F. Litigation in anesthesia and intensive care units: An Italian retrospective study. *Healthcare* **2021**, *9*, 1012. [CrossRef]
8. Madafferi, S.; Accinni, A.; Martucci, C.; Voglino, V.; Frediani, S.; Picardo, S.; Inserra, A. Paraplegia after thoracotomy: A single center experience with pediatric patients and a review of the literature. *Ann. Ital. Chir.* **2022**, *92*, 27–32.
9. Boscolo-Berto, R.; Tortorella, C.; Porzionato, A.; Stecco, C.; Picardi, E.E.E.; Macchi, V.; De Caro, R. The additional role of virtual to traditional dissection in teaching anatomy: A randomised controlled trial. *Surg. Radiol. Anat.* **2021**, *43*, 469–479. [CrossRef]
10. Lin, J.-A.; Blanco, R.; Shibata, Y.; Nakamoto, T.; Lin, K.-H. Corrigendum to "advances of techniques in deep regional blocks". *Biomed. Res. Int.* **2018**, *2018*, 5151645. [CrossRef]
11. Tsui, B.C.H.; Li, L.X.Y.; Pillay, J.J. Compressed air injection technique to standardize block injection pressures. *Can. J. Anaesth.* **2006**, *53*, 1098–1102. [CrossRef]
12. Standards for Basic Anesthetic Monitoring. Available online: https://www.asahq.org/standards-and-guidelines/standards-for-basic-anesthetic-monitoring (accessed on 2 April 2022).
13. Aldrete, J.A. The post-anesthesia recovery score revisited. *J. Clin. Anesth.* **1995**, *7*, 89–91. [CrossRef]
14. Wolfler, A.M.; De Silvestri, A.; Camporesi, A.; Ivani, G.; Vittori, A.; Zadra, N.; Pasini, L.; Astuto, M.; Locatelli, B.G.; Cortegiani, A.; et al. Pediatric anesthesia practice in Italy: A multicenter national prospective observational study derived from the apricot trial. *Minerva Anestesiol.* **2020**, *86*, 295–303. [CrossRef] [PubMed]
15. Holland, E.L.; Bosenberg, A.T. Early experience with erector spinae plane blocks in children. *Paediatr. Anaesth.* **2020**, *30*, 96–107. [CrossRef] [PubMed]
16. Nielsen, M.V.; Moriggl, B.; Hoermann, R.; Nielsen, T.D.; Bendtsen, T.F.; Børglum, J. Are single-injection erector spinae plane block and multiple-injection costotransverse block equivalent to thoracic paravertebral block? *Acta Anaesthesiol. Scand.* **2019**, *63*, 1231–1238. [CrossRef] [PubMed]
17. Bouman, E.A.C.; Sieben, J.M.; Balthasar, A.J.R.; Joosten, E.A.; Gramke, H.-F.; van Kleef, M.; Lataster, A. Boundaries of the thoracic paravertebral space: Potential risks and benefits of the thoracic paravertebral block from an anatomical perspective. *Surg. Radiol. Anat.* **2017**, *39*, 1117–1125. [CrossRef]
18. Gkasdaris, G.; Tripsianis, G.; Kotopoulos, K.; Kapetanakis, S. Clinical anatomy and significance of the thoracic intervertebral foramen: A cadaveric study and review of the literature. *J. Craniovertebral Junction Spine* **2016**, *7*, 228–235. [CrossRef]
19. Bozkurt, M.; Canbay, S.; Neves, G.F.; Aktüre, E.; Fidan, E.; Salamat, M.S.; Başkaya, M.K. Microsurgical anatomy of the dorsal thoracic rootlets and dorsal root entry zones. *Acta Neurochir.* **2012**, *154*, 1235–1239. [CrossRef]
20. Cui, X.; Cai, J.; Sun, J.; Jiang, Z. Morphology study of thoracic transverse processes and its significance in pedicle-rib unit screw fixation. *J. Spinal Disord. Tech.* **2015**, *28*, E74–E77. [CrossRef]
21. Chen, F.; Liu, X.; Wang, G.; Sun, J.; Cui, X. Anatomic relationship of bony structures in pedicle-rib unit and its significance. *World Neurosurg.* **2020**, *139*, e691–e699. [CrossRef]
22. Shibata, Y.; Kampitak, W.; Tansatit, T. The novel costotransverse foramen block technique: Distribution characteristics of injectate compared with erector spinae plane block. *Pain Physician* **2020**, *23*, E305–E314. [PubMed]

23. Cowie, B.; McGlade, D.; Ivanusic, J.; Barrington, M.J. Ultrasound-guided thoracic paravertebral blockade: A cadaveric study. *Anesth. Analg.* **2010**, *110*, 1735–1739. [CrossRef] [PubMed]
24. Vallières, E. The costovertebral angle. *Thorac. Surg. Clin.* **2007**, *17*, 503–510. [CrossRef] [PubMed]

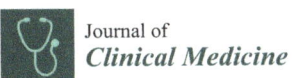

Systematic Review

Transversus Abdominis Plane Block as a Strategy for Effective Pain Management in Patients with Pain during Laparoscopic Cholecystectomy: A Systematic Review

Abdalkarem Fedgash Alsharari [1,*], Faud Hamdi Abuadas [1], Yaser Salman Alnassrallah [2] and Dauda Salihu [1]

1 College of Nursing, Jouf University, Sakaka 72388, Saudi Arabia
2 Ministry of Health, Riyadh 12613, Saudi Arabia
* Correspondence: afalsharari@ju.edu.sa; Tel.: +966-557-470-077

Abstract: Laparoscopic cholecystectomy (LC), unlike laparotomy, is an invasive surgical procedure, and some patients report mild to moderate pain after surgery. Transversus abdominis plane (TAP) block has been shown to be an appropriate method for postoperative analgesia in patients undergoing abdominal surgery. However, there have been few studies on the efficacy of TAP block after LC surgery, with unclear information on the optimal dose, long-term effects, and clinical significance, and the analgesic efficacy of various procedures, hence the need for this review. Five electronic databases (PubMed, Academic Search Premier, Web of Science, CINAHL, and Cochrane Library) were searched for eligible studies published from inception to the present. Post-mean and standard deviation values for pain assessed were extracted, and mean changes per group were calculated. Clinical significance was determined using the distribution-based approach. Four different local anesthetics (Bupivacaine, Ropivacaine, Lidocaine, and Levobupivacaine) were used at varying concentrations from 0.2% to 0.375%. Ten different drug solutions (i.e., esmolol, Dexamethasone, Magnesium Sulfate, Ketorolac, Oxycodone, Epinephrine, Sufentanil, Tropisetron, normal saline, and Dexmedetomidine) were used as adjuvants. The optimal dose of local anesthetics for LC could be 20 mL with 0.4 mL/kg for port infiltration. Various TAP procedures such as ultrasound-guided transversus abdominis plane (US-TAP) block and other strategies have been shown to be used for pain management in LC; however, TAP blockade procedures were reported to be the most effective method for analgesia compared with general anesthesia and port infiltration. Instead of 0.25% Bupivacaine, 1% Pethidine could be used for the TAP block procedures. Multimodal analgesia could be another strategy for pain management. Analgesia with TAP blockade decreases opioid consumption significantly and provides effective analgesia. Further studies should identify the long-term effects of different TAP block procedures.

Keywords: cholecystectomy; laparoscopy; pain management; postoperative; anesthesia

1. Introduction

Laparoscopic cholecystectomy (LC) is a minimally invasive technique that causes mild postoperative discomfort in the parietal, visceral, incisional, and referred regions [1]. In these patients, multimodal approaches [2], epidural analgesia, and intraperitoneal injection of local anesthetics (LA) are often used in conjunction with patient-controlled intravenous analgesia. Transversus abdominal plane (TAP) block is a well-known procedure for postoperative analgesia during laparoscopic abdominal surgery as part of this approach [3]. TAP block is safe; it reduces or eliminates the need for analgesics and has fewer side effects such as postoperative nausea and vomiting (PONV) [4]. In addition, several physicians are actively improving the precision of LA absorption by ultrasound [5–8]. Thus, this innovative approach has demonstrated the analgesic efficacy of laparotomy and laparoscopic procedures [9].

Rafi [10] pioneered the TAP block in 2001 as a historically guided practice for achieving a field block through the petit triangle. In this procedure, a solution (LA) is injected further

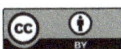

into the plane between the obliquus internus and transversus abdominis muscles. The thoracolumbar nerves travel through this plane after exiting the T6 to L1 spinal roots, directing sensory nerves to the anterolateral abdominal wall [11]. The propagation of LA in this plane blocks neurological afferents and provides analgesia to the anterolateral abdominal cavity. TAP blockades are becoming technically easier and more feasible as ultrasound technology advances. As a result, curiosity about TAP blocks as a clinical tool for analgesia after abdominal surgical treatment has increased. The most commonly reported pain during laparoscopic cholecystectomy was of moderate to severe intensity [12].

TAP blocks are effective for a number of abdominal practices, including hysterectomy, cesarean section, cholecystectomy, colectomy, hernia repair, and prostatectomy [10,13–15]. Since the analgesic effect is limited to somatic pain and has a short life span [16], a single TAP blockade is efficient in multimodal analgesia. TAP blockades could solve the problem of limited duration by continuous infusion [17,18] or prolonged release of liposome's LA [19]. In contrast, clinical studies on TAP block yielded negative results [20,21]. Consequently, analgesic consistency, duration of analgesia, patient comfort, and different corporate strategies need further analysis. Numerous regional anesthetic adjutants such as Dexmedetomidine, Clonidine, Epinephrine, and Dexamethasone are usually combined with enhancement of analgesic efficacy and length chains [22,23].

Most patients undergoing laparoscopic cholecystectomy experience pain in the first 24 h after surgery, with port sites being the most painful. After laparoscopic surgery, pain is mainly felt as visceral pain due to the trauma of gallbladder resection and parietal pain due to skin incision [24]. However, the frequency and intensity of incisional pain were higher than visceral pain after laparoscopic cholecystectomy. Therefore, to optimize postoperative pain control in these patients, analgesic studies should focus on reducing incisional pain.

A number of reviews have been conducted on postoperative pain management, some of which include ultrasound-guided transversus abdominis pain block, with some exploring the best anesthetic technique [25–28] and abdominal surgeries [3,29–34]. Other reviews focused on specific conditions, such as colorectal surgery [35,36], wound infiltration [33,37], caesarean delivery [38], bariatric surgery [39,40], lower abdominal incisions [16], breast reconstruction [41], and minimally invasive surgery [42]. Notably, few studies investigated laparoscopic cholecystectomy. Koo, Hwang, Shin, and Ryu [43] investigated the use of an erector spinae block in patients undergoing laparoscopic cholecystectomy. Ni, Zhao, Li, Li, and Liu [44] and Zhao et al. [45] studied the effects of transversus abdominis block on laparoscopic cholecystectomy, while Peng et al. [28] studied the efficacy of ultrasound-guided laparoscopic cholecystectomy. Specifically, some studies examined the clinical safety and efficacy results of the TAP block across clinical domains [3,46–49] or identifying the best evidence [50]. There appears to be a paucity of data on the optimal dose of TAP block anesthesia for laparoscopic cholecystectomy and the procedure's long-term effects [28]. Again, there seems to be no attempt to comprehensively compare the analgesic efficacy of different TAP strategies for laparoscopic cholecystectomy. Furthermore, the clinical significance of TAP remains unclear and no study compares the types of anesthetic agents used and their dosages, hence the need for this study.

2. Objectives

This review should therefore achieve the following objectives:

1. Explore the optimal dose of TAP block anesthesia for laparoscopic cholecystectomy.
2. Identify the types and concentrations of local anesthetics and other supportive agents commonly used for laparoscopic cholecystectomy.
3. Compare the analgesic efficacy of different types of TAP block procedures and their long-term effects.
4. Examine the clinical significance of TAP.

3. Methods

This review was prepared in accordance with the 2020 PRISMA (Preferred Reporting Items for Systematic Review and Meta-analysis) guidelines [51].

4. Eligibility Criteria

Inclusion Criteria

5. Population: Adult patients undergoing LC.
6. Intervention: Postoperative pain management using TAP block or in combination with adjutants.
7. Comparators: Active placebo or adjunct treatment.
8. Outcomes: Postoperative use of analgesia use if they reported a visual analogue scale (VAS) or numeric rating scale (NRS) outcome of postoperative pain after 24 h.
9. Design: Randomized trials published in peer-reviewed journals.

5. Exclusion Criteria

Articles were considered ineligible if they were letters to the editor, commentary, not peer-reviewed papers (e.g., dissertations), case studies, were not published in full text (e.g., conference proceedings), or were non-experimental studies (e.g., qualitative studies). Furthermore, studies that did not include an active control group were also excluded.

6. Information Sources

The five electronic databases of PubMed, Academic Search Premier, Web of Science, CINAHL, and Cochrane Library were searched for randomized trials. The search was conducted primarily between 12 and 13 August 2022. A supplemental search was conducted in Google Scholar and trial registries (http://clinicaltrials.gov/, accessed on 15 August 2022). All registries and conclusions with the keywords "TAP block laparoscopic cholecystectomy", "postoperative pain in laparoscopic cholecystectomy", and "postoperative pain management in hospitalized patients undergoing laparoscopic cholecystectomy" were explored.

7. Search

We employed the keywords (search terms) transversus abdominis block OR transversus abdominal plane OR transversus abdominis plane AND laparoscopic cholecystectomy OR laparotomy. We limited the search to published articles from the beginning to the present. We considered articles that were published in English and had an abstract. The publication period ranged from inception to the present day. We also manually searched the reference lists for eligible studies.

8. Study Selection

Studies were selected using the PRISMA framework [51]. Results from the five databases were exported to Endnote Reference Manager, and duplicates were removed. The titles and abstracts were screened according to the eligibility criteria. Eligible studies for inclusion were identified after the full-text screening. Two independent reviewers (A.F.A. and D.S.) performed the screening independently, and a third reviewer (F.H.A.) was asked to clarify any discrepancies identified during the process.

9. Data Collection Process

Data were extracted from eligible studies and entered into a spreadsheet in Microsoft Excel. Two independent reviewers performed this task. A third reviewer was asked to clarify any discrepancies. The authors of the papers under consideration were contacted for queries or clarifications.

10. Data Items

Information on the study profile included participant demographics (i.e., gender and age), study design, population characteristics, sample size, study groups (intervention and control), and duration of follow-up. Components of the intervention include the setting in which it was delivered, the dose (frequency, duration, and course) of TAP, the total exposure in minutes to TAP, and the associated theories underlying the therapeutic effects of TAP as reported. For the outcomes, we extracted the mean (M) and standard deviation (SD) for VAS, NRS, and postoperative pain for all groups (i.e., intervention and control) at baseline, post-intervention, and follow-up. For accuracy, two reviewers (A.F.A. and D.S.) performed this task.

11. Risk of Bias in Individual Studies

Appraisals of the eligible studies were conducted using the Physiotherapy Evidence Database scale (PEDro scale). Because of its high construct validity, the PEDro scale was selected for evaluation in randomized controlled trials [52]. To obtain a PEDro total score, items 2–11 were summed. The Internal Validity subscale is scored with items 2–9, and the Statistical Reporting subscale is scored with items 10 and 11 [53,54]. The study is classified as moderate if it scores 4–5, good if it scores 6–8, and excellent if it scores 9–10 [55].

12. Summary of Measure and Synthesis of Results

The Cochrane Handbook for Systematic Reviews of Interventions was used as a guide for data processing [56]. A meta-analysis would be conducted in cases where more than two studies were eligible and measured the same outcomes at which data might be collected: T0 (baseline), T1 (immediately after intervention), and T2 (follow-up). We used a standardized approach in reporting results because different studies measured the same outcome differently. Given the differences in group means and variance within the study population, we determined the minimum clinically significant difference (MCID) using the distribution-based approach [57]. A small effect was described as 0.2, a medium effect as 0.5, and a large effect as 0.8, based on Cohen's d [58].

13. Results

As shown in Figure 1, a total of 758 results were generated from the five databases: CINAHL (n = 37), PubMed (n = 154), Web of Science (n = 183), Cochrane (n = 196), and Academic Search Premier (n = 183). Manual searches yielded five results (n = 5). After deduplicating 231 papers with endnotes and manual search, 527 papers were used for the title and/or abstract screening. After title and/or abstract screening, 77 records were selected for full-text screening. Twenty-nine records were removed after full-text screening for failure to meet the criteria. Forty-eight articles were included in the qualitative and quantitative synthesis.

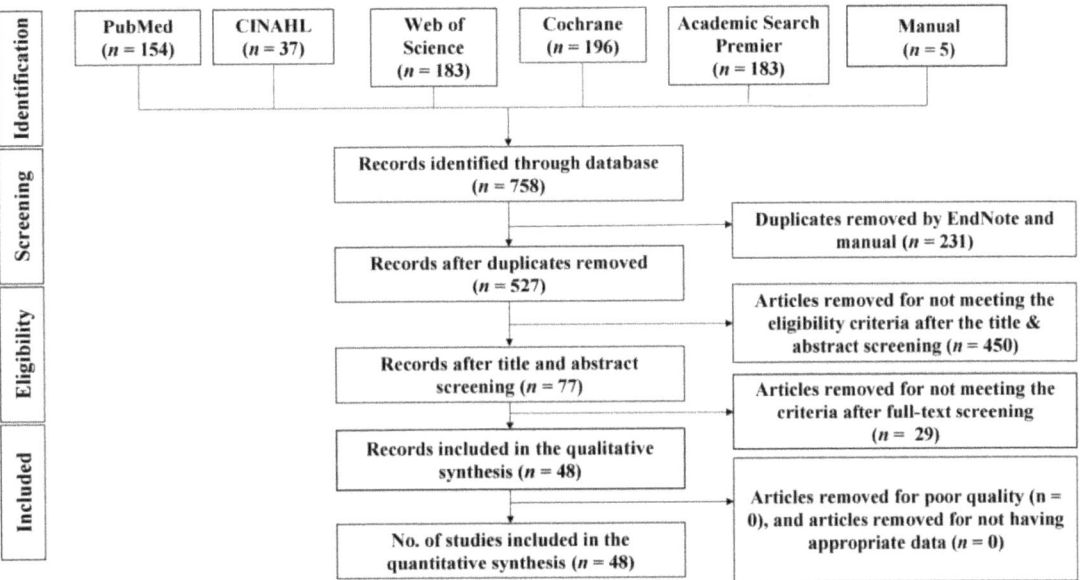

Figure 1. PRISMA flow chart.

14. Risk of Bias within Studies

As shown in Table 1, nineteen (39.6%) did not conceal the assignment of participants. Thirteen (27.1%), twenty-nine (60.52%), and thirty-one (64.58%) studies did not blind assessors, participants, and therapists, respectively. Twenty-six studies underwent an intention-to-treat analysis. In all studies, the dropout rate was less than 15%. All studies reported between-group statistical comparisons, point measures, and variability data. Overall PEDro ratings ranged from 4 to 10, with only one study rated as excellent and three as moderate, while the rest were of good quality.

Table 1. Quality appraisal using PEDro scale.

Author	Year	Eligibility	Randomized Allocation	Concealed Allocation	Similarity at Baseline	Blinding of Participants	Blinding of Therapist	Blinding of Assessor	Dropout	Intention to Treat	Group Comparison	PMVD	Total Score (10)	Internal Validity (8)	Sub Scale (2)	Interpretation
El-Dawlatly [59]	2009	Yes	Yes	Yes	Yes	No	Yes	No	Yes	Yes	Yes	Yes	8	6	2	Good
Ra [7]	2010	Yes	Yes	Yes	Yes	No	No	Yes	Yes	Yes	Yes	Yes	8	6	2	Good
Ortiz [20]	2012	Yes	Yes	Yes	Yes	Yes	No	Yes	Yes	No	Yes	Yes	8	6	2	Good
Petersen [21]	2012	Yes	Yes	Yes	Yes	Yes	Yes	No	Yes	Yes	Yes	Yes	9	7	2	Good
Tolchard [60]	2012	Yes	Yes	Yes	Yes	Yes	No	Yes	Yes	Yes	Yes	Yes	9	7	2	Good
Bhatia [6]	2014	Yes	Yes	Yes	Yes	No	No	Yes	Yes	No	Yes	Yes	8	6	2	Good
Shin [61]	2014	Yes	Yes	Yes	Yes	No	No	Yes	Yes	No	Yes	Yes	7	5	2	Good
Basaran [62]	2015	Yes	Yes	Yes	Yes	No	Yes	Yes	Yes	No	Yes	Yes	8	6	2	Good
Elamin [63]	2015	Yes	Yes	Yes	Yes	Yes	No	Yes	Yes	No	Yes	Yes	8	6	2	Good
Saliminia [64]	2015	Yes	Yes	Yes	Yes	Yes	No	Yes	Yes	Yes	Yes	Yes	9	7	2	Good
Al-refaey [65]	2016	Yes	Yes	Yes	Yes	No	No	No	Yes	Yes	Yes	Yes	7	5	2	Good
Bava [66]	2016	Yes	Yes	Yes	Yes	Yes	Yes	Yes	Yes	No	Yes	Yes	9	7	2	Good
Huang [67]	2016	Yes	Yes	No	Yes	Yes	Yes	Yes	Yes	No	Yes	Yes	8	6	2	Good
Oksar [68]	2016	Yes	Yes	No	Yes	No	Yes	No	Yes	No	Yes	Yes	6	4	2	Good
Sinha [69]	2016	Yes	Yes	Yes	Yes	No	Yes	Yes	Yes	No	Yes	Yes	8	6	2	Good
Breazu [70]	2017	Yes	Yes	No	Yes	No	No	Yes	Yes	Yes	Yes	Yes	6	4	2	Good
Choi [71]	2017	Yes	Yes	Yes	Yes	Yes	No	Yes	Yes	Yes	Yes	Yes	8	6	2	Good
Sahin [72]	2017	Yes	Yes	Yes	Yes	No	No	Yes	Yes	No	Yes	Yes	8	6	2	Good
Baral [73]	2018	Yes	Yes	No	Yes	No	No	No	Yes	No	Yes	Yes	6	4	2	Good
Bhalekar [74]	2018	Yes	Yes	Yes	Yes	Yes	No	Yes	Yes	Yes	Yes	Yes	9	7	2	Good
Sarvesh [75]	2018	Yes	Yes	No	Yes	No	No	No	Yes	No	Yes	Yes	5	3	2	Moderate
Suseela [76]	2018	Yes	Yes	No	Yes	Yes	No	Yes	Yes	Yes	Yes	Yes	8	6	2	Good
Altiparmak [77]	2019	Yes	Yes	Yes	Yes	Yes	No	Yes	Yes	No	Yes	Yes	8	6	2	Good
Bayrar [78]	2019	Yes	Yes	Yes	Yes	Yes	No	Yes	Yes	No	Yes	Yes	8	6	2	Good
Houben [79]	2019	Yes	Yes	No	Yes	No	Yes	Yes	Yes	No	Yes	Yes	7	5	2	Good
Janjua [80]	2019	Yes	Yes	No	Yes	Yes	No	Yes	Yes	Yes	Yes	Yes	8	6	2	Good

Table 1. Cont.

Author	Year	Eligibility	Randomized Allocation	Concealed Allocation	Similarity at Baseline	Blinding of Participants	Blinding of Therapist	Blinding of Assessor	Dropout	Intention to Treat	Group Comparison	PMVD	Total Score (10)	Internal Validity (8)	Sub Scale (2)	Interpretation
Karnik [81]	2019	Yes	Yes	Yes	Yes	Yes	No	Yes	Yes	Yes	Yes	Yes	9	7	2	Good
Khandelwal [82]	2019	Yes	Yes	No	Yes	No	No	Yes	Yes	No	Yes	Yes	6	4	2	Good
Ribeiro [83]	2019	Yes	Yes	Yes	Yes	No	Yes	No	Yes	Yes	Yes	Yes	8	6	2	Good
Siriwardana [84]	2019	Yes	Yes	No	Yes	No	No	Yes	Yes	No	Yes	Yes	7	5	2	Good
Wu [85]	2019	Yes	Yes	Yes	Yes	No	No	Yes	Yes	Yes	Yes	Yes	8	6	2	Good
Arik [86]	2020	Yes	Yes	No	Yes	No	No	Yes	Yes	Yes	Yes	Yes	7	5	2	Good
Kharbuja [87]	2020	Yes	Yes	Yes	Yes	No	No	Yes	Yes	Yes	Yes	Yes	8	6	2	Good
Liang [88]	2020	Yes	Yes	Yes	Yes	No	Yes	Yes	Yes	No	Yes	Yes	8	6	2	Good
Abdelfatah [89]	2021	Yes	Yes	Yes	Yes	Yes	No	Yes	Yes	Yes	Yes	Yes	9	7	2	Good
Ergin [90]	2021	Yes	Yes	Yes	Yes	Yes	Yes	Yes	Yes	No	Yes	Yes	9	7	2	Good
Jung [91]	2021	Yes	Yes	Yes	Yes	Yes	Yes	Yes	Yes	Yes	Yes	Yes	10	8	2	Excellent
Sahu [92]	2021	Yes	Yes	Yes	Yes	No	Yes	Yes	Yes	No	Yes	Yes	8	6	2	Good
Saravanan [93]	2021	Yes	Yes	Yes	Yes	No	Yes	No	Yes	No	Yes	Yes	7	5	2	Good
Vindal [94]	2021	Yes	Yes	No	Yes	Yes	Yes	No	Yes	Yes	Yes	Yes	8	6	2	Good
Priyanka [95]	2022	Yes	Yes	No	Yes	No	No	No	Yes	No	Yes	Yes	4	2	2	Moderate
Emile [96]	2022	Yes	Yes	Yes	Yes	No	Yes	Yes	Yes	No	Yes	Yes	8	6	2	Good
Fargaly [97]	2022	Yes	Yes	Yes	Yes	Yes	No	Yes	Yes	Yes	Yes	Yes	9	7	2	Good
Han [98]	2022	Yes	Yes	No	Yes	No	No	No	Yes	Yes	Yes	Yes	6	4	2	Good
Lee [99]	2022	Yes	Yes	No	Yes	No	No	No	Yes	No	Yes	Yes	5	3	2	Moderate
Ozcifci [100]	2022	Yes	Yes	No	Yes	No	No	No	Yes	Yes	Yes	Yes	6	4	2	Good
Paudel [101]	2022	Yes	Yes	No	Yes	No	No	Yes	Yes	No	Yes	Yes	6	4	2	Good
Rahimzadeh [102]	2022	Yes	Yes	No	Yes	No	No	Yes	Yes	Yes	Yes	Yes	7	5	2	Good

PMVD = point measures and variability data. Note: Each item was scored either Yes = 1 or No = 0. Items 2–11 are summed for a PEDro total score. The sum of items 2–9 yields the internal validity subscale score, while the sum of items 10 and 11 yields the statistical reporting subscale score. The PEDro total score was rated 0–3 = poor, 4–5 = moderate, 6–8 = good, and 9–10 = excellent.

15. Study Characteristics

As shown in Table 2, a total of 3651 subjects participated in the study, with the majority being female (n = 1822, 49.9%) and ages ranging from 18 to 80 years. The TAP block techniques ranges from ultrasound-guided transversus abdominis plane block, oblique subcostal transversus abdominis plane, posterior transversus abdominis plane block, erector spinae plane, subcostal Transversus abdominis, and transversus abdominis plane block. Other approaches were transversus abdominis plane block, oblique subcostal transversus abdominis, subcostal transversus abdominis, subcostal block, subcostal transversus abdominis plane block, quadratus lumborum, laparoscopic transversus abdominis plane, rectus sheath block, blocking the branches of intercostal nerves at the level of mid-axillary line, and laparoscopic subcostal TAP. Infiltration of the surgical site was 10 mL, 15 mL, 16 mL, 20 mL, 30 mL, 40 mL, and 100 mLand either unilateral or bilateral or to the respective or conventional port sites using local anesthetics or other relevant agents. Eighteen (37.5%) of the studies reported the use of patient-controlled analgesia (PCA) or patient-controlled intravenous analgesia (PCIA). The Visual Analogue Scale is the most commonly used outcome measure (n = 30, 62.5%).

As shown in Table 2, seven classes of drugs were used as premedication before induction of anesthesia: benzodiazepines (Lorazepam 2 mg; Midazolam 0.12 mg/kg, 1–2 mg, 0.01–0.02 mg/kg, 0.03 mg, 0.05 mg/kg, 0.5 mg and 7.5 mg; Diazepam 10 mg; Alprazolam 0.25 mg/kg), analgesics (Paracetamol 15–20 mg/kg; Diclofenac 0.5 mg/kg; Fentanyl 20 mcg, 2 mcg/kg; Etocoxib 120 mg), prokinetic agents (Metoclopramide 10 mg), anticholinergics agents (Glycopyrrolate 0.003 mg/kg, 0.05 mg/kg, 0.2 mg), 5-HT3 antagonists (Ondansetron 4 mg), H2 receptor blockers (Ranitidine 150 mg), and alkalizing agents (Ringer lactate solution 500 mL).

15.1. Objective #1. The Optimal Dose of TAP Block Anesthesia for Laparoscopic Cholecystectomy

As already shown in Table 2, the minimum dose of local anesthetic for transversus abdominis plane blockade could be 20 mL for US-TAP and US-OSTAP and 0.4 mg/kg for port infiltration. However, the agents and their concentration may vary.

15.2. Objective #2. Types and Concentrations of Local Anesthetics and Other Supportive Agents Commonly Used for Laparoscopic Cholecystectomy

As shown in Table 2, the most commonly used solutions were Ropivacaine (0.2%, 0.25%, 0.4%, 0.5%, 0.75%, 0.365%, and 0.375%), Bupivacaine (0.25%, 0.5%, and 0.375%), Levobupivacaine (0.25%, 0.5%, and 0.375%), and Lidocaine (2%, 5 mg). Other supportive agents that can be used alone or in addition to the above anesthetics are 0.9% Normal saline (1 mL,2 mL, 10 mL, 20 mL, 32 mL, 40 mL, 100 mL), Dexamethasone (2 mL,1 mcg/kg, 4 mg), Magnesium Sulfate (0.5 mg), Oxycodone (40 mg), Ketorolac (180 mg), Dexmedetomidine (0.5 mcg/2 mL), Epinephrine (5 mcg/mL), Esmolol 0.05 mg/kg, Tropisetron (10 mg), and Sufentanil (2 mg/kg). The most commonly used local anesthetic is Bupivacaine (n = 27, 5.3%), followed by Ropivacaine (n = 17, 35.4) in different concentrations. From this review, US-TAP block is the most commonly used procedure (n = 31), followed by port infiltration (n = 13), general anesthesia only (n = 13), and US-OSTAP blocks (n = 7).

15.3. Objective #3. Effects of TAP Block Anesthesia

a. Comparison of different approaches to ultrasound-guided blockade of the transversus abdominis plane

Table 2. Demographic and clinical characteristics of the participants.

No	Author (Year)	Sample Size	Gender, Age (Mean Age and/or Range, Ratio)	Pre-Medication	TAP Block Technique	Anesthetics Used for Surgical Infiltrations	Analgesia Used (Intra-Operative and Postoperative)	Use of PCA or PCIA	Outcomes	Outcome Measures
1	El-Dawlatly (2009) [59]	42	Gender (male n = 7, 16.7%; female n = 35, 83.3%); Age: TAP = 22–77 years; Control 34–65 years.	Lorazepam 2 mg, Ringers lactate 500 mL	1. US-TAP Block, bilateral 2. Control (No TAP)	1. 30 mL of Bupivacaine (5 mg/mL) 15 mL on each side (i.e., right and left).	Intra-operative: Sufentanil 0.1 mcg/kg. Postoperative: Morphine 1.5 mg bolus, and total Morphine consumed in 24 h via PCIA were recorded.	Yes	Pain	NA
2	Ra (2010) [7]	54	Gender (male n = 28, 51.9%; female n = 26, 48.1%); Age: Control = 43.4 ± 12.4; US-TAP Block 0.25 = 48.2 ± 10.7; and US-TAP Block 0.5 = 45.0 ± 11.1.	None	1. US-TAP Block 1, bilateral 2. US-TAP Block 2, bilateral 3. Control (No TAP)	1. 30 mL of Levobupivacaine 0.25%, 15 mL on each side (i.e., left and right). 2. 30 mL of Levobupivacaine 0.5%, 15 mL on each side (i.e., left and right).	Intra-operative: Remifentanil. Postoperative: Ketorolac 30 mg tds by 24 h, and Fentanyl 20 mcg for those with un-relieved pain.	Yes	Pain	VNRS
3	Ortiz (2012) [20]	74	Gender (male n = 14, 18.9%; female n = 60, 81.0%); Age: US-TAP Block = 37 (11); Control = 36 (11).	Midazolam 1–2 mg	1. US-TAP Block, bilateral 2. Control (Port sites infiltration)	1. 30 mL Ropivacaine 0.5%, 15 mL on each side (i.e., left and right). 2. 20 mL to the port sites 7 mL for each of the 10 mm trocar sites, and 3 mL for each of the 5 mm trocar sites.	Intra-operative: Fentanyl 2 mcg/kg, additional 50 mg bolus were added, and Morphine was given as needed at the end of the procedure. Postoperative: Ketorolac 30 mg.	No	Pain	NAS
4	Petersen (2012) [21]	74	Gender (male n = 53, 71.6%; female n = 21, 28.4%); Age: US-Posterior TAP (Ropivacaine) = 42 (13.5); US-Posterior TAP (saline) = 43 (17.0).	None	1. US-Posterior TAP Block, bilateral (Ropivacaine) 2. US-Posterior TAP Block, bilateral (saline)	1. 20 mL of Ropivacaine 0.5%, 10 mL on each side (i.e., left and right) + 2 mL saline. 2. 20 mL of Normal saline, 10 mL on each side (i.e., left and right).	Preoperative: Remifentanil 0.4 mL/kg/h. Postoperative: Acetaminophen 1000 mg by 4, Ibuprofen 400 mg by 3, Ketobemidone 2–24 h, and IV Morphine 0–2 h.	No	Pain	VAS
5	Tolchard (2012) [60]	43	Gender (male/female 2.0/5:16) Age: Intervention = 52 ± 3; Control = 48 ± 3.	Paracetamol 15–20 mg/Kg; Diclofenac 0.5 mg/kg, Fentanyl 20 mg	1. US-STA Block, bilateral, 2. Control (Port site local infiltration)	Standardized dose of 1 mg/kg Bupivacaine	Intra-operative: Fentanyl 3 mcg/kg, Diclofenac 0.5 mg/kg, and Paracetamol 15–20 mg/kg. Postoperative: Fentanyl 20 mcg bolus.	No	Pain	VPAS

Table 2. *Cont.*

No	Author (Year)	Sample Size	Gender, Age (Mean Age and/or Range, Ratio)	Pre-Medication	TAP Block Technique	Anesthetics Used for Surgical Infiltrations	Analgesia Used (Intra-Operative and Postoperative)	Use of PCA or PCIA	Outcomes	Outcome Measures
6	Bhatia (2014) [6]	64	Gender = NA; Age: Control = 35.4 ± 7.16; TAP Posterior = 36.4 ± 10.4; TAP Subcostal = 36.4 ± 10.4.	Alprazolam 0.25 mg, Ranitidine 150 mg	1. US-guided posterior TAP Block 2. Subcostal US-TAP block 3. Control (Standard GA).	1. 30 mL of Ropivacaine 0.375%, 15 mL on each side (i.e., left and right). 2. 30 mL of Ropivacaine 0.375%, 15 mL on each side (i.e., left and right). 3. General anesthesia only.	Intra-operative: Morphine 0.1 mg/kg Postoperative: Paracetamol 1000 mg every 6 h; IV Tramadol 2 mg/kg were given as an initial dose for those with VAS scores >4, with a subsequent dose of 1 mg/kg.	NA	Pain	VAS
7	Shin (2014) [61]	45	Gender (male n = 25, 53.2%; female n = 22, 46.8%); Age: Control = 44.7 ± 11.1; US-TAP group = 43.9 ± 9.5, and OSTAP group = 43.0 ± 9.6.	NA	1. US-OSTAP Block, bilateral 2. US-TAP block, bilateral 3. Control (GA only)	1. 40 mL of 0.375% Ropivacaine. 20 mL on each side (i.e., left and right). 2. 40 mL of 0.375% Ropivacaine. 20 mL on each side (i.e., left and right).	Intra-operative: Fentanyl 1 mcg/kg, Ketorolac 30 mg/kg (pre-emptive analgesia). Postoperative: Fentanyl 25 mcg for pain score >6, Ketorolac 30 mg for pain score 4–6, and Nalbuphine 10 mg for those needing analgesia at ward.	NA	Pain	VNRS
8	Basaran (2015) [62]	76	Gender (male n = 11, 14.5%; female n = 65, 85.5%); age: Control = 44.89 ± 14.2; Intervention = 43.2 ± 12.2.	Diazepam 10 mg	1. US-OSTAP Block, bilateral 2. Control (GA only)	1. 20 cc of 0.25% Bupivacaine on each side (i.e., left and right). 2. General anesthesia only.	Intra-operative: Fentanyl 2 mcg/kg, 1 mcg/kg given (bolus) if heart rate or mean arterial pressure increased by 20% of initial values, Remifentanil 0.1 mcg/kg (maintenance), and 0.5 mg/kg Meperidine prior to the cessation of Remifentanil. Ephedrine 5 mg was given to reduce mean arterial pressure with an additional dose permitted after 2 min. IV Tenoxicam 20 mg after induction. Postoperative: Tramadol 50 mg IV on request with minimum of 20 min between doses, and a maximum dose was capped at 500 mg at 24 h.	NA	Pain	VAS

Table 2. Cont.

No	Author (Year)	Sample Size	Gender, Age (Mean Age and/or Range, Ratio)	Pre-Medication	TAP Block Technique	Anesthetics Used for Surgical Infiltrations	Analgesia Used (Intra-Operative and Postoperative)	Use of PCA or PCIA	Outcomes	Outcome Measures
9	Elamin (2015) [63]	80	Gender (male n = 10, 12.5%, female 70, 87.5%); Age = 49.5 years versus 52.1 years.	None	1. LAP-TAP Block (Bupivacaine), bilateral, subcostal plus (Periportal saline injection) 2. LAP-TAP (saline), bilateral, subcostal plus (Periportal Bupivacaine injection)	1. TAP (50 mL of 0.25% Bupivacaine), Periportal (20 mL Normal saline), and intraperitoneal (10 mL of 0.25% Bupivacaine. 10 mL each to anterior axillary and mid-clavicular lines; bilateral infiltration in the petite triangle 15 mL each. 2. TAP (50 mL of Normal saline), Periportal (20 mL of 0.25% Bupivacaine), intraperitoneal (10 mL of 0.25% Bupivacaine).	Intra-operative: NA Postoperative: Paracetamol 1 g q6h, Diclofenac sodium 75 mg.	Yes	Pain	NRS
10	Saliminia (2015) [64]	54	Gender (male n = 24, 24.4%; female n = 30, 54.6%); Age = 28–61 years.	None	1. US-TAP Block, bilateral, Bupivacaine + normal saline 2. US-TAP Block, (Bupivacaine + Sufentanil) 3. US-TAP Block, bilateral, (normal saline only)	1. 32 mL (Bupivacaine 30 mL + 2 mL of Sufentanil). 16 mL on each side (i.e., left and right). 2. 30 mL of Bupivacaine + 2 mL of normal saline. 16 mL on each side (i.e., left and right). 3. 32 mL of Normal saline. 16 mL of 0.9% Normal saline on each side.	Intra-operative: Fentanyl 3 mcg/kg, with 1 mcg/kg as maintenance dose. Postoperative: 50 mL of Fentanyl bolus with a lockout time of 8 min.	Yes	Pain	VAS
11	Al-refaey (2016) [65]	90	Gender (NA); Years = Control = 32 ± 6; US-TAP Block B= 37 ± 8; US-TAP Block M = 34 ± 8.	None	1. US-TAP Block, bilateral subcostal. 2. US-TAP Block, bilateral subcostal 3. GA only.	1. 20 mL Bupivacaine 0.25%. 2. 20 mL of Bupivacaine 0.25% + 0.3 g of magnesium sulphate. 3. Anesthesia only.	Intra-operative: Fentanyl 1 mcg/kg Postoperative: Morphine 0.02 mg/kg bolus	No	Pain	VAS

Table 2. Cont.

No	Author (Year)	Sample Size	Gender, Age (Mean Age and/or Range, Ratio)	Pre-Medication	TAP Block Technique	Anesthetics Used for Surgical Infiltrations	Analgesia Used (Intra-Operative and Postoperative)	Use of PCA or PCIA	Outcomes	Outcome Measures
12	Bava (2016) [66]	42	Gender (male n = 3, 7.1%; female n = 39, 92.3%); Age: TAP group = 33.7 ± 10.5, Control = 33.5 ± 6.5.	None	1. US-TAP Block, bilateral 2. Control (port site infiltration)	1. 30 mL 0.365% Ropivacaine. 15 mL on each side (i.e., left and right). 2. 10 mL of 0.25% Bupivacaine.	Intra-operative: Fentanyl 2 mcg/kg and 0.5 mg was used as supplemental. Postoperative: Morphine 0.5 mg/kg with a maximum dose of 20 mg in 4 h.	Yes	Pain	VAS
13	Huang (2016) [67]	60	Gender: NA Age: Control I: 38.5 ± 7.7; Group II: 39.7 ± 5.5; Group III: 38.6 ± 8.9.	None	1. General anesthesia; 2. US-TAP Block, bilateral; 3. US-TAP Block, bilateral + 2 mL Dexamethasone	1. GA only 2. 30 mL of 0.375% Ropivacaine 7.5 mL/kg. 15 mL on each side (i.e., left and right). 3. 32 mL (30 mL of 0.375% Ropivacaine + 2 mL Dexamethasone. 16 mL on each side (i.e., left and right).	Intra-operative: Remifentanil until its plasma concentration reaches 2.5 mcg./mL. Postoperative: Sufentanil 5–10 mcg.	No	Pain	NRS
14	Oksar (2016) [68]	60	Gender (male = 17, 28.3%; female 43, 71.7%); Age: 18–74.	Midazolam 2 mg IV, Ringers' lactate solution 500 mL	1. Intercostal-iliac US-TAP block, bilateral + PCA. 2. US-OSTAP + PCA, bilateral; 3. GA + PCA alone	1. 40 mL Lidocaine (5 mg/mL), 20 each to the left and right 2. 40 mL Lidocaine (5 mg/mL), 20 each to the left and right.	Intra-operative: Remifentanil Postoperative: Paracetamol 1 g, and Diclofenac 75 mg. Pain relief using PCA was by 200 mg Tramadol (7 mL, 2 mg/kg bolus) with a 15 min lockout time.	Yes	Pain	VAS
15	Sinha (2016) [69]	60	Gender: (NA); Age: >40 years.	Oral Ranitidine 150 mg and alprazolam 0.25 mg	1. US-TAP block (Bupivacaine), bilateral 2. US-TAP block (Ropivacaine), bilateral	1. 40 mL of 0.25% Bupivacaine. 20 mL each to the right and left. 2. 40 mL of 0.375% Ropivacaine. 20 mL each to the right and left.	Intra-operative: Fentanyl 2 mcg/kg. Postoperative: Diclofenac sodium 75 mg.	No	Pain	VAS
16	Breazu (2017) [70]	74	Gender (male 29, 39.2%; female 45, 60.8%); Age: 42–65 years OSTAP-placebo; 38–67 years OSTAP-Bupivacaine; 40–65 OSTAP-Pethidine.	7.5 mg Midazolam	1. US-OSTAP-placebo, bilateral; 2. OSTAP-Bupivacaine, bilateral; 3. OSTAP-Pethidine, bilateral.	1. 40 mL of sterile saline (20 mL on each side). 2. 40 mL of 0.25% Bupivacaine. 20 mL for each of the right and left. 3. 20 mL of 1% Pethidine 10 mL on each side.	Intra-operative: Fentanyl 2 mcg/kg Postoperative: Pethidine 25–50 mg, at the ward level, Acetaminophen 1 g 8-hourly; however, those with moderate to severe pain continue to receive 25–50 mg of Pethidine until the VAS score is lower than 3.	Yes	Pain	VAS

Table 2. Cont.

No	Author (Year)	Sample Size	Gender, Age (Mean Age and/or Range, Ratio)	Pre-Medication	TAP Block Technique	Anesthetics Used for Surgical Infiltrations	Analgesia Used (Intra-Operative and Postoperative)	Use of PCA or PCIA	Outcomes	Outcome Measures
17	Choi (2017) [71]	103	Gender: (male n = 48, 46.6%; female n = 55, 53.4%); Age: IV-PCA + GA (Control): 50.4 ± 15.9; US-TAP block: 49.1 ± 14.2; TAP block: 52.2 ± 11.8.	Midazolam 0.05 mg/kg, Glycopyrrolate 0.003 mg/kg	1. PCA + GA 2. US-TAP block (indwelling catheter) 3. US-TAP block+ PCA	1. 100 mL of Normal saline + 40 mg Oxycodone and 180 mg of Ketorolac via IV-PCA pump. 2. 20 mL of 0.2% Ropivacaine 3. 20 mL of 0.2% Ropivacaine.	Intra-operative: Remifentanil 1 mcg/kg and 0.5–1 mcg was used for maintenance. Postoperative: Morphine 3–5 mg was given for unrelieved pain.	Yes	Pain	NRS
18	Sahin (2017) [72]	60	Gender: (male n = 33, 55%; female n = 27, 45%); Age: Group 1: 47.2 ± 13.0; Group 2: 64.5 ± 11.5.	No	1. Group 1. US-TAP block, unilateral (right sided) 2. Group 2. US-TAP block, unilateral	1. 30 mL (20 mL: 50 mg of Bupivacaine 0.5% + 10 mL of normal saline). 2. 30 mL of 50 mg Bupivacaine plus 20 mL of normal saline.	Intra-operative: Fentanyl 2 mcg/kg. Postoperative: Diclofenac 25 mg when the VAS is < 7.	No	Pain	VAS
19	Baral (2018) [73]	60	Gender: (male n = 19, 31.7%; female n = 41, 68.3%); Age Subcostal TAP block 42.47 ± 14.41; Control: 45.93 ± 14.34.	No	1. US-TAP block, Subcostal 2. Control (Port site infiltration).	1. 20 mL of Bupivacaine. 10 mL on each side (i.e., left and right). 2. 20 mL of 0.25% Bupivacaine. 5 mL to each of the 4 port sites).	Intra-operative: Fentanyl 2 mcg/kg. Postoperative: Pethidine 0.5 mg/kg if the VAS score is less than equal to 4.	No	Yes	VAS
20	Bhalekar (2018) [74]	50	Gender: US-TAP (saline): (male = 11(44); female = 14(56.00); US-TAP block: male 14(56.00); female 11(44.00). Age: Subcostal TAP block = 44.1 ± 13.1; Control: 44.1 ± 13.3.	0.2 mg glycopyrrolate, Ranitidine 50 mg and Ondansetron 4 mg.	1. US-TAP block, Subcostal, bilateral 2. US-TAP block (saline)	1. 40 mL of Bupivacaine 0.25%. 20 mL on each side (i.e., left and right). 2. 40 mL of 0.9% normal saline. 20 mL on each side (i.e., left and right).	Intra-operative: Fentanyl 2 mcg/kg; Diclofenac 75 mg administered after induction. Postoperative: Nalbuphine 10 mg/70 kg with a further dose of 5 mg/kg when required.	No	Pain	VAS
21	Sarvesh (2018) [75]	60	Gender: (NA); Age > 50 years.	Midazolam 0.03 mg/kg.	1. US-TAP Block 1, Subcostal, bilateral, 2. US-TAP Block 2, Subcostal, bilateral.	1. 18 mL of 0.375% Ropivacaine+ 2 mL of normal saline. 20 mL on each side (i.e., left and right). 2. 18 mL of 0.375% Ropivacaine with 2 mL of 0.5 μg/kg Dexmedetomidine 2 mL. 20 mL on each side (i.e, left and right).	Intra-operative: Fentanyl 2 mcg/kg Postoperative: Morphine 1 mg loading dose with a lockout time of 10 min. and 0.25 mg/kg 4 h limit.	Yes	Pain	NRS

Table 2. Cont.

No	Author (Year)	Sample Size	Gender, Age (Mean Age and/or Range, Ratio)	Pre-Medication	TAP Block Technique	Anesthetics Used for Surgical Infiltrations	Analgesia Used (Intra-Operative and Postoperative)	Use of PCA or PCIA	Outcomes	Outcome Measures
22	Suseela (2018) [76]	80	Gender: (NA); Age: US-TAP Block = 42.25 ± 11.91; Control (Port site infiltration) = 41.00 ± 11.34.	Metoclopramide 10 mg and Ranitidine 150 mg and midazolam 0.5 mg.	1. US-TAP Block, Subcostal, bilateral, 2. Control (Port site infiltration).	1. 40 mL of 0.25% Bupivacaine. 20 mL on each side (i.e., left and right). 2. 20 mL (0.5% Bupivacaine 5 mL each at 4 ports). 5 mL to each of the 4 ports.	Intra-operative: Fentanyl 2 mcg/kg and Paracetamol 1 g. Postoperative: Paracetamol 1 g 8-hourly, Tramadol 1 mg/kg bolus, Diclofenac 1 mg/kg.	No	Pain	NRS
23	Altiparmak (2019) [77]	68	Gender: (male 25, 36.8%; female $n = 43$, 63.2%); Age: US-OSTAP Block = 53.1 ± 14.7; US-ESP Block = 51.1 ± 12.3.	No	1. US-OSTAP Block, bilateral 2. US-ESP Block bilateral	1. 40 mL (0.375% Bupivacaine). 20 mL on each side (i.e., left and right). 2. 40 mL of 0.375% Bupivacaine). 20 mL on each side (i.e., left and right).	Intra-operative: Fentanyl 1 mcg/kg Postoperative: Trometamol 50 mg, Tramadol 10 mg bolus with 20 min lockout time.	Yes	Pain	NRS
24	Baytar (2019) [78]	107	Gender: (male $n = 26$, 24.3%; female $n = 81$, 75.7%); Age QL Block: 46.42 ± 16.57; US-TAP Block: 48.12 ± 12.42.	Midazolam 0.01–0.02 mg/kg	1. US-TAP Block, subcostal, bilateral 2. US-TAP quadratus lumborum block, bilateral	1. 40 mL of 0.25% Bupivacaine. 20 mL for each side. 2. 40 mL of 0.25% Bupivacaine. 20 mL for each side.	Intra-operative: Fentanyl 1–2 mcg Postoperative: Tenoxicam 20 mg, 54 mL normal saline + Tramadol 300 mg (6 mL).	Yes	Pain	VAS
25	Houben (2019) [79]	52	Gender: male $n = 17$, 32.7%; female $n = 35$, 67.3%; Age: US-TAP Block = 50.6 ± 12.9; Control (saline) = 47.5 ± 16.0.	Oral Etoricoxib 120 mg	1. US-TAP Block, subcostal, bilateral (Levobupivacaine) 2. US-TAP Block, subcostal, bilateral, (saline)	1. 40 mL Levobupivacaine 0.375% + Epinephrine 5 mcg/mL. 20 mL for each side. 2. 40 mL 0.9% saline + Epinephrine 5 mcg/mL. 20 mL for each side.	Intra-operative: Sufentanil 0.1 mcg/kg Postoperative: Ketamine, Paracetamol 2 g (1 g for those with weight < 60 kg, and Morphine 2 mg bolus.	No	Pain	VAS
26	Janjua (2019) [80]	100	Gender: (male-female ratio = US-TAP Block 1.8: 2.6; Control (Port Site Infiltration): 1.7:2.8); Age: US-TAP Block = 48.70 ± 12.25; Port Site Infiltration = 48.35 ± 13.89.	No	1. US-TAP Block, unilateral 2. Control (Port Site Infiltration)	1. 0.25% Bupivacaine 0.4 mL/kg (1/3 to the fascial plane). 2. 0.25% Bupivacaine 0.4 mL/kg. 1/3 intraperitoneally before the closure of the port sites.	Intra-operative: Nalbuphine 0.15 mg/kg, and Ketorolac 0.45 mg/kg Postoperative: Ketorolac 0.45 mg/kg by 2 8-hourly.	No	Pain	VAS

Table 2. *Cont.*

No	Author (Year)	Sample Size	Gender, Age (Mean Age and/or Range, Ratio)	Pre-Medication	TAP Block Technique	Anesthetics Used for Surgical Infiltrations	Analgesia Used (Intra-Operative and Postoperative)	Use of PCA or PCIA	Outcomes	Outcome Measures
27	Karnik (2019) [81]	80	Gender: (male = 63, 78.8%; female 17, 21.2%); Age: US-TAP Block = 6.3 ± 3.8, Local infiltration = 5.5 ± 2.9.	Midazolam 0.05 mg/kg	1. US-TAP Block, bilateral 2. Control (port sites local infiltration)	1. 40 mL of 0.25% Bupivacaine. 20 mL for each side. 2. 0.25% Bupivacaine. 0.4 mL/kg.	**Intra-operative:** Fentanyl 2 mcg/kg, 1 mcg/kg as maintenance, and Paracetamol 15 mg/kg. **Postoperative:** Diclofenac 1 mg/kg.	No	Pain	VAS
28	Khandelwal (2019) [82]	80	Gender (male = 25, 31.25%; female = 55, 68.75%); Age: US-STA Block = 42 ± 9.4; Control (intraperitoneal infiltration) = 44 ± 8.6.	No	1. US-STA Block, subcostal, bilateral 2. Control (intraperitoneal infiltration)	1. 40 mL of 0.25% Levobupivacaine. 20 mL on each side (i.e., left and right). 2. 40 mL of 0.25% Levobupivacaine diluted with normal saline. 40 mL intraperitoneally.	**Intra-operative:** Fentanyl 2 mcg/kg. **Postoperative:** Tramadol 1 mg/kg.	No	Pain	NRS
29	Ribeiro (2019) [83]	42	Gender: (male = 27, 64.3%; female = 15, 35.7%); Age: US-OSTAP Block (Ropivacaine) = 45.45 ± 14.12; US-OSTAP Block (Normal saline) = 40.05 ± 11.91.	No	1. US-OSTAP Block (Ropivacaine), bilateral 2. US-OSTAP Block (Normal saline), bilateral	1. 40 mL of 0.35% Ropivacaine. 20 mL on each side (i.e., left and right). 2. 40 mL of sterile normal saline. 20 mL on each side (i.e., left and right).	**Intra-operative:** Paracetamol 1 g **Postoperative:** Paracetamol 1 g 8-hourly, and Tramadol 1 mg/kg when pain threshold exceeds 4.	No	Pain	VAS
30	Siriwardana (2019) [84]	90	Gender: male-female ratio LAP-TAP = 0.214; Control = 0.333; (females: 72.2%; Age: 19–80 years).	No	1. LAP-TAP Block, subcostal + Port Site Infiltration 2. Control (Port Site Infiltration).	1. 40 mL of 0.25% Bupivacaine 20 mL on each side (i.e., left and right) + 3–5 mL of standard port site infiltration. 2. 3–5 mL of 0.25% Bupivacaine standard port site infiltration.	**Postoperative:** Morphine 0.1 mg/kg.	Yes	Pain	Unspecified

Table 2. Cont.

No	Author (Year)	Sample Size	Gender, Age (Mean Age and/or Range, Ratio)	Pre-Medication	TAP Block Technique	Anesthetics Used for Surgical Infiltrations	Analgesia Used (Intra-Operative and Postoperative)	Use of PCA or PCIA	Outcomes	Outcome Measures
31	Wu (2019) [85]	160	Gender: (male = 124, 77.5%; female 56, 22.5%); Age: LAI = 48.0 ± 11.4; TL = 47.6 ± 10.1; TR = 48.6 ± 12.1.	No	1. LAI –Group 2. TL-Group (US-TAPB + LAI) 3. TR-Group (US-TAPB + RSB)	1. 30 mL of 0.5% of Ropivacaine + 1 mcg/kg of Dexamethasone. 2. 30 mL of 0.25% Ropivacaine (i.e., 15 mL left and right) + 1 mcg of Dexamethasone. 3. Pre-incisional infiltration: 30 mL 0.25% of Ropivacaine + 1 mcg of Dexamethasone. Plus 40 mL (20 mL to the left and right each), and 20 mL to the bilateral rectus sheath.	Intra-operative: Flurbiprofen Axetil 1.5 mg/kg, and Remifentanil 1 mcg/kg. Postoperative: Flurbiprofen Axetil 1.5 mg/kg 6-hourly.	No	Pain	VAS
32	Arik (2020) [86]	72	Gender: (Male = 16, 23.6%; female = 56, 76.4%); Age: TAP Block = 42.8 ± 9.2; Local Anesthetic infiltration = 42.9 ± 11.2; IV-PCA = 46.6 ± 13.8.	No	1. TAP Block, Unilateral Subcostal 2. Port site local infiltration 3. IV-PCA only	1. 22 mL (0.25% Bupivacaine, and 2 mL saline). 2. 20 mL of 0.25% of Bupivacaine.	Intra-operative: Remifentanil infusion Postoperative: Tramadol 5 mg/mL, 20 mg bolus with 20 min lockout time with a maximum of 200 mg per 4 h.	Yes	Pain	NRS
33	Kharbuja (2020) [87]	60	Gender: (male = 16, 26.7%; female 44, 73.3%); Age: Subcostal TAP = 40.27 ± 12.57; Control (Port Site Infiltration) = 38.77 ± 9.95.	Ranitidine 150 mg.	1. US-TAP Block, subcostal, bilateral 2. Control (Port Site Infiltration)	1. 40 mL of Bupivacaine 0.25% 20 mL to each side. 2. 20 mL of 0.5% Bupivacaine 5 mL at each port.	Intra-operative: Fentanyl 2 mcg/kg and Paracetamol 1 g. Postoperative: Fentanyl 20 mcg/kg, and Paracetamol 1 g 8-hourly.	No	Pain	VAS
34	Liang (2020) [88]	120	Gender: (male 43, 35.8%; female 77, 64.2%); Age: Group H = 49.5 ± 12.1; Group M 50.0 ± 13.0; Group L = 47.2 ± 13.9; Group C = 51.5 ± 12.8.	No	1. Group H wound infiltration port 2. Group M wound infiltration port 3. Group L wound infiltration port 4. Group C (Control)	1. 20 mL of 0.75% Ropivacaine 2. 20 mL of 0.5% Ropivacaine 3. 20 mL of 0.2% Ropivacaine 4. 20 mL of 0.9% Normal saline.	Intra-operative: Fentanyl 3 mcg/Kg), and maintenance using Remifentanil, at a dose of 0.1 mg/kg/hour. Postoperative: Parecoxib 40 mg, Morphine 2.5 mg (rescue) for those at PACU, and 100 mg (rescue) for those at ward.	No	Pain	NRS

Table 2. Cont.

No	Author (Year)	Sample Size	Gender, Age (Mean Age and/or Range, Ratio)	Pre-Medication	TAP Block Technique	Anesthetics Used for Surgical Infiltrations	Analgesia Used (Intra-Operative and Postoperative)	Use of PCA or PCIA	Outcomes	Outcome Measures
35	Abdelfatah (2021) [89]	60	Gender: (female 51, 85%; male 9, 15%); Age: US-TAP Block 1 = 32.66 ± 10; US-TAP Block 2 = 31.67 ± 10.7.	No	1. US-TAP Block 1 (0.25% Bupivacaine + Esmolol); 2. US-TAP Block 2 (0.25% Bupivacaine + Isotonic Saline)	1. 40 mL Bupivacaine (i.e., 20 mL on each side) + Esmolol 0.5 mg/kg. 2. 40 mL Bupivacaine + 30 mL isotonic saline (loading dose), and 0.05 mg/kg/min (maintenance dose).	Intra-operative: Fentanyl 1–2 mcg/kg. Postoperative: Fixed dose of Acetaminophen 500 mg/6 h, Morphine 5 mg.	No	Pain	VAS
36	Ergin (2021) [90]	160	Gender: (male 41, 25.62%; female 119, 74.38%); Age = 18–74 years.	No	1. TAI-Group (administered percutaneously and subcutaneously) 2. TAPB-Group (solutions administered to the left in between two muscles i.e., internal oblique and transversus abdominis. 3. IPLA-Group (administer to the sub-diaphragmatic and pericholecystic areas). 4. Control (no local anesthetic)	1. 20 cc of 0.5% Bupivacaine + 20 cc of physiological saline. 2. 20 cc of 0.5% Bupivacaine solution. 10 cc on each side (i.e., left and right). 3. 20 cc of 0.5% Bupivacaine. 4. No local anesthetics	Intra-operative: Paracetamol 1 g Postoperative: Tramadol 50 mg, and 100 mg for those with ongoing pain, and tabs Tenoxicam 20 mg 8-hourly.	No	Pain	VAS
37	Jung (2021) [91]	76	Gender: (male = 32, 42.1%; female 44, 57.9%): Age: BD-TAP = 48.9 ± 8.3; Control 47.5 ± 8.7.	No	1. BD-TAP Block, bilateral 2. Control (Sham Block), bilateral	1. 60 mL, >50 kg, 15 mL of 0.25% Ropivacaine; < 50 kg more diluted 3 mg/kg, 30 mL on each side (i.e., left and right). 2. 60 mL of 0.9% Normal Saline. 30 mL on each side (i.e., left and right).	Intra-operative: Remifentanil 2–6 μg/mL, Paracetamol 1 g, and Ibuprofen 400 mg. Postoperative: Oxycodone 3 mg (rescue), Ketorolac 30 mg (Day 0–1), and Tramadol 50 mg 8-hourly (from Day 1).	No	Pain	NRS

Table 2. Cont.

No	Author (Year)	Sample Size	Gender, Age (Mean Age and/or Range, Ratio)	Pre-Medication	TAP Block Technique	Anesthetics Used for Surgical Infiltrations	Analgesia Used (Intra-Operative and Postoperative)	Use of PCA or PCIA	Outcomes	Outcome Measures
38	Sahu (2021) [92]	60	Gender: (male 35, 58.3%; female 25, 41.7%); Age: US-ESP Block: 41.3 ± 11.8; OSTAP Block: 40.2 ± 11.1.	Midazolam 1 mg; Glycopyrrolate 0.2 mg	1. US-ESP Block, Bilateral 2. OSTAP Block, Bilateral	1. 40 mL of 0.2% Ropivacaine + 4 mg of Dexamethasone. 20 mL each to the left and right. 2. 40 mL of 0.2% Ropivacaine + 4 mg of Dexamethasone. 20 mL on each side (i.e., 20 mL left and right).	Intra-operative: Nalbuphine 0.1 mg/kg. Postoperative: Paracetamol 1 g 4-hourly x 24 h, Tramadol 1 mg/kg (rescue), and when pain persists, Diclofenac 75 mg was used as second option.	No	Pain	VAS
39	Saravanan (2021) [93]	60	Gender: (male = 26, 43.3%; female 34, 56.7%); Age: US-Modified BRILMA Block = 47.7 ± 11.12; Subcostal TAP Block 42.8 ± 11.09.	No	1. US-Modified BRILMA Block, 2. US-TAP Block, subcostal	1. 20 mL 0.2% Ropivacaine 2. 20 mL 0.2% Ropivacaine.	Intra-operative: Fentanyl 2 µg/kg, with 1 mcg/kg as maintenance dose, and Paracetamol 1 g. Postoperative: Morphine 0.1 mg/hour with a bolus of 1 mg, and lockout time of 10 min.	Yes	Pain	VAS
40	Vindal (2021) [94]	100	Gender: (male = 11, 11%; female = 89, 89%); Age: TAP Block 35(15.5); Port Site Infiltration: 35(18.25).	No	1. LAP-TAP Block 2. Control (Port Site Infiltration)	1. 40 mL 0.25% Bupivacaine. 10 mL at each of the four marked sites. 2. 40 mL 0.9% Normal Saline. 10 mL at each of the 4 port sites.	Intra-operative: NA Postoperative: Diclofenac sodium 50 mg (rescue) and 50 mg when needed.	No	Pain	VAS
41	Priyanka (2022) [95]	80	Gender: (male 46, 66.7%); female 45.40; US-TAP Block post: 45.29.	The night before surgery: Ranitidine 150 mg, and Tabs Alprazolam 0.5 mg Prior to surgery: Glycopyrrolate 0.005 mg/kg, Midazolam 0.05 mg/kg, and Fentanyl 2 mcg/kg.	1. US-TAP Block Pre, bilateral 2. US-TAP Block Post, bilateral	1. 40 mL of 0.25% Bupivacaine. 20 mL spread to the left and right. 2. 20 mL of 0.25% Bupivacaine. 20 mL spread to the left and right.	Intra-operative: Fentanyl 2 mcg/kg Postoperative: Tramadol 100 mg	No	Pain	VAS
42	Emile (2022) [96]	110	Gender: (male 11, 10%; female 99, 90%); Age: 40.9 ± 11.7.	No	1. US-TAP Block, bilateral 2. LSTAP Block 3. Control (GA only)	1. 20 mL of 0.25% of Bupivacaine + 2% Lidocaine (i.e., 10 mL left and right) + normal saline. 2. 20 mL of 0.25% of Bupivacaine + 2% Lidocaine + normal saline. (i.e., 10 mL left and right).	Intra-operative: NA Postoperative: Paracetamol 1000 mg and Diclofenac were used for unsatisfactory pain relief.	No	Pain	VAS

Table 2. Cont.

No	Author (Year)	Sample Size	Gender, Age (Mean Age and/or Range, Ratio)	Pre-Medication	TAP Block Technique	Anesthetics Used for Surgical Infiltrations	Analgesia Used (Intra-Operative and Postoperative)	Use of PCA or PCIA	Outcomes	Outcome Measures
43	Fargaly (2022) [97]	50	Gender: (male = 8, 16%; female 42, 84%); Age: US-TAP Block = 33.2 ± 9.1; QL Block = 32.7 ± 8.4.	No	1. US-TAP Block Group, bilateral 2. QLB-Group, bilateral	1. 40 mL of 0.25% Bupivacaine. 20 mL for each side (i.e., right and left) 2. 40 mL of 0.25% Bupivacaine. 20 mL for each side (i.e., right and left).	Intra-operative: Fentanyl 1 µg/kg. Postoperative: Paracetamol 1 g 8-hourly, and Ketorolac30 mg 12-hourly. Morphine sulfate 3 mg bolus increments with the highest amount of 15 mg/4 h or 45 mg a day.	No	Pain	VAS
44	Han (2022) [98]	180	Gender: (male = 124, 68.9%; female = 56, 31.2%); Age: Group S = 45.78 ± 17.13; Group N = 44.52 ± 17.71; US-TAPB Block = 46.28 ± 13.18.	No	1. US-TAPB Block Group 2. Group S 3. Group N	1. 20 mL Ropivacaine 0.4% + 10 mg of Tropisetron diluted with normal saline 0.9% 100 mL. 40 mL of 0.25% Bupivacaine + 1 mL saline. 2. 20 mL + 1 mL (for each of the blocks) Sufentanil 2 mg/kg via PCIA pump, + 10 mg of Tropisetron diluted with normal saline 0.9% 100 mL. 3. Nalbuphine 2 mg/kg via PCIA pump, + 10 mg of Tropisetron diluted with normal saline 0.9% 100 mL.	Intra-operative: Sufentanil 0.4–0.6 mcg/kg. Remifentanil 0.05–0.2 mcg/h.	Yes	Pain	VAS
45	Lee (2022) [99]	53	Gender: (male = 31, 54.5%; female = 22, 44.5%); Age: 1. US-TAPB –Block = 44.3 ± 9.8; 2. Control = 45.7 ± 12.0.	No	1. US-TAP Block (0.375% Ropivacaine), 2. US-TAP Block (Normal saline).	1. 40 mL of 0.375% Ropivacaine. 20 mL per side (i.e., right and left). 2. 40 mL of 0.9% Normal Saline. 20 mL per side (i.e., right and left).	Intra-operative: Remifentanil 0.5 mcg/kg and 0.1 mcg/kg/min as maintenance dose. Postoperative: Fentanyl 0.2 mcg/kg bolus and every hour with a 15 min lockout time.	Yes	Pain	VAS
46	Ozcifci (2022) [100]	90	Gender: (male = 24, 26.7%; female 66, 73.3%); Age: Control: 47.46 ± 11.83; TAP Block, unilateral 48.46 ± 12.05; TAP Block, bilateral 51.90 ± 11.40.	Midazolam 0.02 mg/kg	1. TAP Block, Unilateral (right side). 2. TAP Block, Bilateral 3. Control	1. 20 mL of 0.25% Bupivacaine (right only). 2. 40 mL of 0.25% Bupivacaine. 20 mL for each of side.	Intra-operative: Paracetamol 1 g, Tramadol 2 mg/kg, Diclofenac sodium 75 mg. Postoperative: Paracetamol 1 g, Diclofenac sodium, and Tramadol 0.5 mg/kg hourly to a maximum of dose of 500 mg/day.	Yes	Pain	VNRS

Table 2. Cont.

No	Author (Year)	Sample Size	Gender, Age (Mean Age and/or Range, Ratio)	Pre-Medication	TAP Block Technique	Anesthetics Used for Surgical Infiltrations	Analgesia Used (Intra-Operative and Postoperative)	Use of PCA or PCIA	Outcomes	Outcome Measures
47	Paudel (2022) [101]	60	Gender: (male = 14, 23.3%; female = 46, 76.7%); Age: TAP-Block: 41.63 ± 11.99; Control (local infiltration): 40.23 ± 11.42.	Ranitidine 150 mg	1. US-TAP Block, subcostal, bilateral 2. Control (Local Port Sites Infiltration).	1. 40 mL of 0.25% Bupivacaine. 20 mL to each side (i.e., right and left). 2. 20 mL of 0.25% Bupivacaine at the port sites.	Intra-operative: Fentanyl 2 mcg/kg. Postoperative: NA	No	Pain	VAS
48	Rahimzadeh (2022) [102]	76	Gender: NR; Age: US-TAP (post-surgery) Block = 44.46 ± 8.30; US-TAP (after induction of anaesthesia) = 45.0 ± 10.87.	Fentanyl 2 mcg/kg and Midazolam 0.12 mg/kg	1. US-TAP Block, bilateral (postop group) 2. Pre-emptive Group, block (after induction)	1. 40 mL of 0.25% Ropivacaine. 20 mL to the right and left. 2. 40 mL of 0.25% Ropivacaine. 20 mL to the right and left.	Intra-operative: Fentanyl 2 μg/kg Postoperative: Acetaminophen 20 mg/mL, and Ketorolac 0.6 mg/mL bolus and 2 mL every 15 min.	Yes	Pain	NRS

Total study population: N = 3651; Male = 1090, 29.9%; Female = 1822, 49.9%; Unspecified genders = 739, 20.2%. Measures: VAS = 30, 62.5%; NRS = 12, 25%; VNRS = 3, 6.25%; Unspecified = 1, 2.1%; VAPA = 1, 2.1%; NA = 1, 2.1%.

GA = general anesthesia; VNRS = Verbal Numerical Rating Scale; PCA = patient-controlled analgesia; IV-PCA = intravenous patient-controlled analgesia; PCIA = patient-controlled intravenous analgesia; NAS = not available; NAS = Numeric Analogue Scale; VAS = Visual Analog Scale; NR = not reported; NRS = Numerical Rating Scale; US-TAP = ultrasound-guided transversus abdominis plane block; OSTAP = oblique subcostal transversus abdominis plane; US-OSTAP = ultrasound-guided oblique subcostal transversus abdominis plane; TAP block = transversus abdominis plane block; Subcostal TAP block: subcostal transversus abdominis plane block; US-STA = subcostal ultrasound transversus abdominis; US-Posterior TAP = ultrasound-guided posterior transversus abdominis plane block; US-STA block = ultrasound-guided subcostal transversus abdominis plane block; US-ESP = ultrasound-guided erector spinae plane; US-TAPB = ultrasound-guided transversus abdominis plane block; RSB = rectus sheath block; LAI = local anesthetic infiltration; TAPB = transversus abdominis plane block; IPLA = intraperitoneal local anesthetic injection; Modified BRILMA block = blocking the branches of intercostal nerves at the level of mid-axillary line; LSTAP = laparoscopic subcostal TAP; LAI-Group = received preoperational administration of 0.5% Ropivacaine plus 1 mcg of Dexamethasone at the trocar entrance; TL-Group = received preoperational administration of 0.5% Ropivacaine plus 1 mcg of Dexamethasone at the trocar entrance alongside posterior US-TAP block; TR-Group = US-TAP block combined with rectus sheath block.

15.3.1. Analgesic Efficacy of Ultrasound-Guided Transversus Abdominis Plane Block Versus General Anesthesia Only

As shown in Table 3, Morphine consumption was greater in the control compared to the intervention group. Notably, the mean change in the intervention group from the start to the end of laparoscopic cholecystectomy was 9.6, $p < 0.005$, and the control group had a mean change of 20.5, $p < 0.005$ [59]. Between the first 20 min and 24 h postoperative, the two US-TAP groups using 0.25% and 0.5% Levobupivacaine reported lower postoperative pain scores of 3.3 to 1.6 and 3.2 to 1.3, respectively, compared with those receiving anesthesia alone (8.6 to 4.4) [7]. In addition, analgesic requirements between 20 min and 12 h postoperative were higher in the control group (-4.2 to -0.7) than in patients receiving 0.25% Levobupivacaine (-1.7 to -0.5) and 0.5% Levobupivacaine (-1.9 to -0.5) [7]. Similarly, the control group appeared to have higher pain scores between 0 and 24 h postop (2.35 to 1.3) compared to those who received posterior US-TAP block (1.2 to 0.8) and subcostal US-TAP block (0.85 to 0.15) [6]. Analgesic requirement between 0 and 12 h is also higher in the control group (-1.0 to -0.6) than in the posterior US-TAP block (-0.4 to -1.0) and subcostal US-TAP block (-0.7 to -0.65) [6]. Moreover, pain perception between 10 min and 24 h postoperative was higher in the control group at rest (6.6 to 2.1) than in the US-TAP group (4.2 to 2.1) and during cough (7.5 to 3.0 and 4.7 to 2.9, respectively [61]. The need for analgesics between 10 min and 6 h was also higher in the control group (-4.5 to -1.2) than in US-TAP (-1.8 to -1.8) [61].

As shown in Supplementary Table S1, the most commonly used intra-operative opioid analgesic was Fentanyl ($n = 27$), followed by Remifentanil ($n = 10$). Intra-operative opioids were switched to Tramadol ($n = 14$), Morphine ($n = 12$), Ketorolac ($n = 5$), and Nalbuphine ($n = 1$). However, in some cases, Diclofenac sodium ($n = 6$) and acetaminophen ($n = 1$) were also used.

Table 3. Adverse reactions, side effects, and recorded complications associated with local anesthetics used in laparoscopic cholecystectomy procedures.

No	Author/Year	Side Effects	Adverse Events	Complications	Drugs Used	Dose in mL or mg/kg
1	Ra (2010) [7]					
	US-TAP block (0.25%)	Sleep disturbance (n = 2)			Levobupivacaine 0.25%	30 mL
	US-TAP block 0.5%	Sleep disturbance (n = 0)			Levobupivacaine 0.5%	30 mL
	Control	Sleep disturbance (n = 6)				
2	Petersen (2012) [21]					
	US-TAP block (Ropivacaine)	Nausea scores 0–24 h (n = 0), with no difference in sedation scores.			Ropivacaine 0.5% + 2 mL of normal saline	22 mL
	US-TAP block (saline)	Nausea scores 0–24 h (n = 0), with no difference in sedation scores.			Ropivacaine 0.375%	20 mL
3	Shin (2014) [61]				Ropivacaine 0.375%	40 mL
	US-OSTAP block	Nausea: none (n = 15), mild (n = 0), moderate (n = 0), severe (n = 0), and shoulders pain (n = 2).				
	US-TAP block	Nausea: none (n = 12), mild (n = 2), moderate (n = 1), severe (n = 0), and shoulders pain (n = 0).				
	Control	Nausea: none (n = 11), mild (n = 1), moderate (n = 3), severe (n = 0), and shoulders pain (n = 1).				
4	Huang (2016) [67]					
	Control		Nausea (n = 3, vomiting n = 2, and abnormal sedation n = 2)			
	US-TAP Block, bilateral		Nausea (n = 1, vomiting n = 0, and abnormal sedation n = 0)		Ropivacaine 0.375%	30 mL
	US-TAP block + 2 mL of Dexamethasone		Nausea (n = 0, vomiting n = 0, and abnormal sedation n = 0)		Ropivacaine 0.375%	32 mL
5	Choi (2017) [71]					
	US-TAP block (indwelling catheter inserted)		Nausea (n = 11), vomiting (n = 2), dizziness (n = 2), headache (n = 0), urinary retention (n = 11), pain at the needle insertion site (n = 0), and hematoma (n = 0).		Ropivacaine 0.2%	20 mL
	US-TAP block + PCA		Nausea (n = 15), vomiting (n = 2), dizziness (n = 1), headache (n = 3), urinary retention (n = 3), pain at the needle insertion site (n = 0), and hematoma (n = 1).		Ropivacaine 0.2%	20 mL
	Control (PCA only)		Nausea (n = 9), vomiting (n = 2), dizziness (n = 2), headache (n = 1), urinary retention (n = 0), pain at the needle insertion site (n = 2), and hematoma (n = 1).			
6	Houben (2019) [79]				100 mL of normal saline + 40 mg Oxycodone and 180 mg of Ketorolac	

Table 3. Cont.

No	Author/Year	Side Effects	Adverse Events	Complications	Drugs Used	Dose in mL or mg/kg
	US-TAP block (Levobupivacaine)	1. Fatigue median data (1 h n = 5, 2 h n = 5, 4 h n = 4.5, and 24 h = 4). 2. Nausea median data (1 h n = 1, 2 h n = 0, 4 h n = 0, and 24 h = 0).			Levobupivacaine 0.375% + Epinephrine 5 mcg/mL	40 mL
	US-TAP block (saline)	1. Fatigue median data (1 h n = 5, 2 h n = 5, 4 h n = 3, and 24 h = 4). 2. Nausea median data (1 h n = 0, 2 h n = 0, 4 h n = 0, and 24 h = 0).			40 mL 0.9% normal saline + Epinephrine 5 mcg/mL	40 mL
7	Janjua (2019) [80]					
	US-TAP block, unilateral			Respiratory depression (7.89%); others unclear	Bupivacaine 0.25%	0.4 mL/kg
	Control (port site infiltration)			Respiratory depression (2.56%); others unclear	Bupivacaine 0.25%	0.4 mL/kg
8	Siriwardana (2019) [84]					
	LAP-TAP + port site infiltration (× 4)	Vomiting episodes 0(0–4)			Bupivacaine 0.25%	40 mL + 12 – 20 mL
	Control (port site infiltration × 4)	Vomiting episodes 0(0–2)			Bupivacaine 0.25%	12–20 mL
9	Liang (2020) [88]					
	Group H	Postoperative nausea and vomiting were not significantly different between the 4 groups at 24 h (p = 0.180, p = 0.644).			Ropivacaine 0.75%	20 mL
	Group M				Ropivacaine 0.5%	20 mL
	Group L				Ropivacaine 0.2%	20 mL
	Group C				Normal saline 0.9%	20 mL
10	Ergin (2021) [90]					
	LAI Group			39 (97.5%)	Bupivacaine 0.5%	20 mL
	TAPB Group			40 (100%)	Bupivacaine 0.5% + 20 cc of physiologic saline	40 mL (20 + 20)
	IPLA Group			39 (97.5%)	Bupivacaine 0.5%	20 mL
	Control			40 (100%)		
11	Jung (2021) [91]					
	BD-TAP block, bilateral	Nausea (n = 4), and desaturation (n = 3).			Ropivacaine 0.25%	60 mL
	Control (sham block), bilateral	Nausea (n = 7), and desaturation (n = 2).			Normal saline 0.9%	60 mL
12	Han (2022) [98]					
	US-TAP block		Nausea and vomiting (n = 1), skin itching (n = 0), dizziness (n = 0), respiratory depression (n = 1), and puncture site hematoma (n = 0).		Ropivacaine 0.4% + 10 mg Tropisetron + 100 mL normal saline	142 mL
	Group S				Sufentanil 2 mg/kg via PCA + 10 mg Tropisetron + 100 mL normal saline	100 mL

Table 3. Cont.

No	Author/Year	Side Effects	Adverse Events	Complications	Drugs Used	Dose in mL or mg/kg
	Group N		Nausea and vomiting (n = 8), skin itching (n = 1), dizziness (n = 0), respiratory depression (n = 2), and puncture site hematoma (n = 0).		Nalbuphine 2 mg/kg via PCA + 10 mg Tropisetron + 100 mL normal saline	100 mL
13	Lee (2022) [99]					
	US-TAP block (Ropivacaine)	1 h: nausea (n = 5), vomiting (n = 0); 8 h: nausea (n = 3), vomiting (n = 0); 24 h: nausea (n = 0), vomiting (n = 0).			Ropivacaine 0.375%	40 mL
	US-TAP block (normal saline)	1 h: nausea (n = 12), vomiting (n = 1); 8 h: nausea (n = 8), vomiting (n = 2); 24 h: nausea (n = 3), vomiting (n = 0).			Normal saline 0.9%	40 mL
14	Paudel (2022) [101]					
	US-TAP block	Nausea (n = 0), and vomiting (n = 0).			Bupivacaine 0.25%	40 mL
	Control (port site infiltration)	Nausea (n = 1), and vomiting (n = 2).			Bupivacaine 0.25%	20 mL

TAI Group = local anesthetic infiltration; TAPB Group = transversus abdominis plane block; IPLA Group = intraperitoneal local anesthetic injection; PCA = patient-controlled analgesia; US-TAP = ultrasound-guided transversus abdominis plane.

Opioid consumption was found to be lower in those receiving US-TAP block with 0.25% Bupivacaine 2.1(0.5) and Bupivacaine 0.25% plus Magnesium Sulfate 0.5 g, 2.2(0.5) compared with those receiving general anesthesia alone 2.8(0.6) [65]. Compared with the control group, the first need for rescue analgesics was delayed in the US-TAP and US-TAP (Dexamethasone) groups (403.0, 436.0 versus 152.3, $p < 0.01$). Patients in the US-TAP and US-TAP (perineural Dexamethasone) groups had lower pain scores on the numeric rating scale ($p > 0.01$) and used fewer postoperative analgesics ($p < 0.01$) [67]. The need for analgesics was higher in the control group than in the group US-TAP [68]. The number of patients requiring additional analgesics (Morphine and Ketorolac) was higher in the group of patients receiving US-TAP block with in situ indwelling catheters than in the control group and the group of patients receiving US-TAP block + PCA [71]. There was a significant reduction in pain perception with US-TAP block (4.4 to 1.4) when compared with the control group (6.4 to 2.2) [96]. Again, the mean analgesic requirement between the first 2 and 24 h after surgery was found to be higher in the control group (-42 to -1.0) than in the US-TAP group (-3.0 to -0.5) [96].

Comparing the unilateral and bilateral US-TAP block with the control group, both strategies appear to be effective. Pain perception at rest and during coughing was lower with the unilateral (right) US-TAP (3.10 to 1.23 and 3.37 to 1.8, respectively) and the bilateral US-TAP block (3.33 to 1.23 and 3.47 to 1.57, respectively), compared with the control group (6.03 to 2.10 and 6.33 to 3.07) [100]. Analgesic requirements between 1 and 12 h postoperative both at rest and during cough were higher in the control group (-3.39 to -0.07 and -3.26 to -0.06, respectively) compared with US-TAP block (unilateral) (-1.87 to -0.17 and -1.57 to -0.2, respectively) and US-TAP block (bilateral) (-2.1 to -0.4 and -1.9 to -0.26, respectively) [100].

15.3.2. Analgesic Efficacy of Ultrasound-Guided Transversus Abdominis Plane Block versus Port SITES Infiltration

Between the onset of surgery and 24 h after surgery, the demand for opioids (Morphine) was slightly higher in the US-TAP block group (14.6) than in the port infiltration group (14.4) [20]. This demand pattern continued after 24 h with 11.1 for the US-STAP block group and 9.6 for the port group [20]. However, there seems to be no difference in the need for hydrocodone [20]. The port infiltration group appears to have a higher need for diclofenac (0.65), Paracetamol (21.0), and Fentanyl (3.1) compared with the US-STA block group (diclofenac (0.58), Paracetamol (16.0), and Fentanyl (3.0) [60]. In the US-TAP group and the local infiltration group, the 24 h Morphine requirements (mean) were 34.57 mg and 32.76 mg, respectively ($p = 0.688$). A total of eight patients in the US-TAP group and 16 patients in the local infiltration group required additional fentanyl intra-operatively ($p = 0.028$). In the immediate postoperative period, local infiltration levels were significantly higher at rest and during cough ($p = 0.034$ and $p = 0.007$, respectively) [66]. Patients who received subcostal US-TAP block had a statistically significant reduction in postoperative pain within the first 24 h after surgery compared with port infiltration. In the subcostal TAP block group, opioid consumption was lower over 24 h (125 mg versus 175 mg $p < 0.001$). US-TAP block and local infiltration had significantly different postoperative pain scores (VAS) at 0, 2, 6, 12, and 24 h [101]. The VAS score is significantly higher in the local infiltration group than in the US-TAP block group ($p < 0.001$) [101].

Patients receiving the subcostal block US-TAP had a greater delay in requesting rescue analgesics (3.20 versus. 1.70, $p < 0.001$) [73]. Time to first analgesic (mean) was 292.7 and 510.3 min in the portsite infiltration and subcostal US-TAP block groups, respectively, and mean Tramadol requirements were 141.8 mg and 48.69 mg ($p = 0.001$ for both) [76]. Mean NRS at 2, 3, 6, 12, and 24 h was significantly lower in the subcostal block US-TAP group (0.03, 0.43, 1.35, 0.93, and 1.13) than in the port infiltration group (0.30, 2.05, 3.10, 2.48, and 2.25) [76]. Mean analgesic requirements at 2, 3, 6, and 12 h per group were higher in the port infiltration group (1.95, 0.2, -0.85, and -0.23) than in the US-TAP block group (1.1, 0.7, -0.22, and 0.2) [76]. Similarly, mean pain scores between 0 and 24 h postoperative were higher in the port infiltration group (4.42, 4.64, 5.08, 1.52, and 3.92) than in the unilateral US-TAP block group (2.65, 3.20, 3.47, 1.36, and 2.67) [80]. Likewise, analgesic requirements between 0 and 8 h were higher in the port infiltration group (−0.5, −0.72, −1.16, and 2.4) than in the US-TAP block group (0.02, −0.53, −0.8, and 1.31) [80]. There was a significant difference between the US-TAP block group and the local infiltration group at 10 min, 30 min, 1 h, and 2 h [2 (0–2.5) versus 0.011]; [1.5 (0–3) versus 3 (2–5); $p = 0.001$]; [1.5 (0–2) versus 2 (2–3); $p = 0.001$; and [2 (0–2) versus 2 (1.5–2.5); $p = 0.010$] [81]. Additionally, US-TAP block patients were significantly less likely to require intra-postoperative opioids and rescue analgesia ($n = 5$, $n = 8$, $p< 0.001$) compared to port site infiltration ($n = 38$, and 30, $p < 0.001$) [81]. Finally, the US-TAPB block group had significantly lower resting VAS values than the addition of 2 mg/kg Sufentanil or Nalbuphinevia PCA at 2, 6, 12, 24, and 48 h postop ($p < 0.05$) [98].

It is noteworthy that a similar pattern of changes, in which the US-TAP block group had a lower pain experience and analgesic requirement compared with the port infiltration groups, was observed in a study by Khandelwal, Parag, Singh, Anand, and Govil [82] and by Arık, Akkaya, Ozciftci, Alptekin, and Balas [86]. A similar pattern of changes was observed and the time to rescue analgesia was equally longer in patients receiving subcostal US-TAP block (3.63 h) compared to the port infiltration group (1.73 h, $p = 0.0002$) [87].

Uniquely, Liang, Chen, Zhu, and Zhou [88] used different concentrations of Ropivacaine (0.5% and 0.25%) plus 1 mcg/kg Dexamethasone in addition to preoperative administration of solution at the trocar site before surgery (group LAI), with additional US-TAP block in the TL group, while the TR group received rectus sheath block in addition to US-TAP block; however, the three groups did not differ in pain scores at any time point within the 48 h period.

15.3.3. Analgesic Efficacy of Ultrasound-Guided Transversus Abdominis Plane Block before Induction of Anesthesia and after Surgery

Although there does not appear to be a significant difference between the two groups, mean meperidine consumption (mg) was higher in those receiving US-TAP block (after surgery) (34.21) than in those receiving US-TAP block (induction) (32.11) [102]. Postoperative pain perception in the first 30 min to 24 h was also higher in those who received a US-TAP block (post-surgery) (4.96 to 4.63) compared to US-TAP block (pre-induction) (3.18 to 3.47) [95]. Likewise, analgesic requirements in the first 30 min to 12 h after surgery were higher for the US-TAP block group (post-surgery) (−0.33 to −0.08) compared with the US-TAP block group (pre-induction) (0.29 to −0.06) [95]. On the contrary, time to first analgesic request was shorter for US-TAP blockade group (after surgery) (2.22, $p = 0.089$) than for US-TAP blockade group (induction) (5.80, $p = 0.089$) [102].

15.3.4. Analgesic Efficacy of Ultrasound-Guided Transversus Abdominis Plane Block Using Different Concentrations of Local Anesthetics versus Normal Saline

We found that the US-TAP block group (saline) had higher 24hfentanyl consumption (877.8 mcg) than the US-TAP block group (0.5% bupivacaine + normal saline) (566.7 mcg) or the US-TAP block group (0.5% Bupivacaine + Sufentanil) (555.6 mcg; $p = 0.03$) [64]. Compared with the US-TAP (0.5% bupivacaine + normal saline) and US-TAP (0.5% Bupivacaine + Sufentanil) block groups, the postoperative pain score was higher with the US-TAP (saline) block group ($p = 0.006$); however, the intervention groups did not differ significantly [64]. Time to first fentanyl requirement was significantly less with US-TAP block (saline) (79.44) than with US-TAP block (0.5% Bupivacaine + Sufentanil) (206.38; $p = 0.001$) [64]. Intra-operative consumption of Remifentanil and postoperative VAS scores show that the US-TAP group (Bupivacaine plus 20 mL of normal saline) received a larger volume of local anesthetic solution, albeit at a lower concentration, and required fewer postoperative analgesics than the US-TAP group (Bupivacaine plus 10 mLof normal saline) [72]. The percentage of patients requiring Paracetamol ($p < 0.002$) and Nalbuphine ($p < 0.001$) as rescue analgesics was significantly lower in the US-TAP block (0.25% Bupivacaine) group (17.0, 68% and 2, 8.0%%) than in the US-TAP block (0.9% normal saline) group (25, 100%, and 24, 96%) [74]. In contrast, it has been found that Levobupivacaine 0.375% and 0.9% saline groups consumed similar amounts of opioids 24 h after surgery: 21.2 mg versus 25.2 oral Morphine equivalent; $p = 0.48$ [79]. Mean Morphine consumption after surgery in patients receiving US-TAP block (Esmolol) was 5.83 mg ($p = 0.204$) compared with US-TAP block (saline) (7.5 mg, $p = 0.204$) [89]. The US-TAP block (Esmolol) group had significantly lower early postoperative pain scores ($p = 0.05$) [89]. From arrival at PACU to 12 h postoperative, the mean analgesic requirement appears to be higher for the US-TAP block (saline) (2.5 to 0.1) than for the US-TAP block (Esmolol) (2.16 to −0.04) (Abdelfatah& Amin, 2021). The median Morphine consumption at 0–2 h postoperative was 7.5 mg for the US-TAP block (saline) compared with 5 mg for the US-TAP block (Ropivacaine) [21].

15.3.5. Analgesic Efficacy of Ultrasound-Guided Transversus Abdominis Plane Block Using Different Concentrations of Local Anesthetics

It appears that the higher the concentration of anesthetics used for the US-TAP block, the lower the experience of pain. Of note, Ra et al. [7] used 0.25% and 0.5% Levobupivacaine differently; however, patients who received 0.5% had less pain in the first 20 min to 12 h after surgery. In contrast, the need for a analgesics in this group seems to be higher in the first 20 to 60 min after the procedure [7]. Interestingly, patients who received US-TAP block with 0.25% Levobupivacaine reported a high need for analgesia (−1.0) compared to those receiving 0.5% Levobupivacaine (−0.1) six hours later [7]. Similarly, the mean pain experience at 24 h was higher for those who received US-TAP block with 0.25% Levobupivacaine (1.6) compared to 0.5% Levobupivacaine (1.3) [7]. After 10, 30, and 60 min, patients receiving ultrasound-guided TAP blocks (0.375% Ropivacaine) had significantly lower pain scores than patients receiving US-TAP blocks (0.25% bupivacaine) [69]. The median [interquartile range] of postoperative analgesic requirements and cumulative rescue analgesic requirements were the same for both drugs (0.75% bupivacaine for US-TAP block versus 0.375% Ropivacaine for US-TAP block, $p = 0.366$) [69].

15.3.6. Comparison of Analgesic Efficacy of Ultrasound-Guided Oblique Subcostal Transversus Abdominis Block versus Transversus Abdominis Plane Block

Because US-OSTAP is a relatively new technology that is essentially the same as TAP block procedures, we compared the analgesic efficacy of ultrasound-guided oblique subcostal transversus abdominis block with transversus abdominis plane block. Intra-operatively, there appears to be no difference between the US-TAP and US-OSTAP blocks in terms of Ketorolac consumption; however, the two groups differ in terms of intra-operative fentanyl consumption (US-TAP: 72.4 and US-OSTAP: 78.1) and postoperative Nalbuphine consumption (US-TAP: 7.3 and US-OSTAP: 8.0), with US-TAP block reporting less consumption [61]. In contrast, the US-TAP block group consumed more fentanyl postoperatively (US-TAP: 10.0 and US-OSTAP: 6.7) [61]. Mean postoperative pain scores between 10 min and 24 h at rest/coughing were also higher in the US-TAP group (4.3 to 2.1)/(4.7 to 2.9) than in the US-OSTAP (2.3 to 1.3)/(2.9 to 2.1) [61]. In addition, comparing the effects of the US-OSTAP procedure with only general anesthesia, the VAS pain scores at rest and upon movement were significantly lower in the OSTAP group on arrival at PACU and 2 h postoperative [62]. Total postoperative Tramadol requirements were significantly lower in the OSTAP group at 0–2 h (31.6) and 2–24 h (126.3) than in the control group at 0–2 h (80.3) and 2–24 h (267.1) [62]. In addition, a high proportion of patients who received US-OSTAP block (17, 85%) did not require additional analgesia compared with the US-TAP group (11, 55%) [68].

It should be noted that we compared US-OSTAP (normal saline) with US-OSTAP (Pethidine); however, US-OSTAP (Pethidine) significantly reduced pain scores at 0, 2, 4, 6, 12, and 24 h ($p = 0.001$) [70]. US-OSTAP (Pethidine) patients consumed significantly fewer opioids during surgery than US-OSTAP (normal saline) (150 versus 400 mg, $p = 0.001$), and opioid consumption during the first 24 h was significantly lower (20.4 versus 78 mg, $p = 0.001$) [70]. There were statistically significant differences between the US-OSTAP (bupivacaine) and US-OSTAP (Pethidine) groups when comparing VAS scores of US-

OSTAP (bupivacaine) and US-OSTAP (Pethidine) (0 h) for pain intensity [70]. Therefore, as an alternative to 0.25% bupivacaine, 1% Pethidine might be used to achieve OSTAP blockade during laparoscopic cholecystectomy [70]. Pain experience was higher with US-OSTAP (normal saline) blockade from 0 to 24 h (2.21 to 1.52) than with US-OSTAP (Ropivacaine) blockade (0.71 to 0.38) [83]. Similarly, analgesic requirements were equally higher in the US-OSTAP (normal saline) block group (-0.69 to -1.19) compared with the US-OSTAP (Ropivacaine) block group (-0.33 to 0.18) from 0 to 6 h postoperative [83].

The US-OSTAP block (Ropivacaine) had a low fentanyl consumption of 122 mcg intraoperatively compared to US-OSTAP (normal saline) block (126.19 mcg [83]. Opioid consumption at PACU within the first 8 h after surgery was higher for the US-OSTAP (normal saline) block (9.52 mg) compared with the US-OSTAP (Ropivacaine) block (4.64 mg) [83]. In contrast, the US-OSTAP (Ropivacaine) block appears to have a higher opioid requirement between 8 and 16 h but not after 24 h [83].

15.3.7. Analgesic Efficacy of Ultrasound-Guided Transversus Abdominis Plane Blockade with Equal Anesthetic Concentration and Adjuvant of Dexamethasone, and Dexmedetomidine versus Normal Saline

Postoperatively, it took 485.6 min for the first analgesic to be requested in US-TAP block (Dexmedetomidine), compared with 289.8 min in US-TAP block (normal saline) [75]. Patients in the US-TAP block group (Dexmedetomidine) consumed less cumulative Morphine in the first 24 h than patients in the US-TAP block group (normal saline) [75].

15.3.8. Analgesic Efficacy of Ultrasound-Guided Subcostal Transversus Abdominis Plane versus Quadratus Lumborum Blocks

The time for first analgesic consumption using the US-TAP block was 63.72 min compared with the quadratus lumborum block at 70.00 min [78]. Similarly, Tramadol consumption (mg) was higher in the quadratus lumborum 86.66 mg than in the US-TAP block 83.43 [78]. Using the VAS scale, with the exception of 12 h postoperative, pain perception seems to be higher in the US-TAP block group (1.33 to 0.47) compared to quadratus lumborum (1.03 to 0.42) from 0 to 6 h [78]. However, this seems to differ in 12 and 24 h for the US-TAP block group (0.20 and 0.11) compared to the quadratus lumborum (0.22 to 0.09) [78]. In other words, pain perception using the DVAS scale appeared to be the same at 0 h but was higher in the US-TAP block group at 1 h (1.94) and at 12 h (1.00) [78]. In contrast, this pattern of change was observed in the quadratus lumborum after 6 h (1.50) and after 12 h (0.46) [78].

15.3.9. Analgesic Efficacy of Ultrasound-Guided Transversus Abdominis Versus Quadratus Lumborum Blocks

The analgesic request was found to be higher among those receiving the US-TAP block (18, 72%) as compared to the quadratus lumborum block (14, 56%). Cumulative daily Morphine consumption was significantly higher in the US-TAP block group (6 mg (6–9)) than in the quadratus lumborum block group (3 mg (3–6)), $p = 0.001$ [97]. The median time to first analgesic request was longer in the quadratus lumborum block group (17 h (12, 24)) than in the US-TAP block group (8 h (6, 24)), $p \leq 0.001$ [97].

b. Comparison of different approaches to laparoscopic-assisted transversus abdominal blockade

15.3.10. Comparison of Analgesic Efficacy Analgesic Efficacy of Laparoscopic-Assisted Transversus Abdominal Block with Bupivacaine versus Normal Saline

In the LAP-TAP group (Bupivacaine + periportal saline injection), numerical pain assessment scores were significantly decreased after 1, 3, and 6 h of rest ($p = 0.025$, $p = 0.03$, and $p = 0.007$, respectively) as compared to normal saline [63].

15.3.11. Analgesic Efficacy of Laparoscopic-Assisted Transversus Abdominal Block versus Port Sites Infiltration

Compared to port site infiltration, there seems to be no change in LAP-TAP block for pain at rest between the first 3 and 6 h postoperative [94]. However, it appears that the port infiltration group had more pain 24 h postoperative (3.0) and at discharge (2.0) [94]. In addition, a significant mean change was observed between the two groups in pain upon cough 6 h postop (LAP-TAP: 4.0, port site infiltration: 5.0) and on discharge (LAP-TAP: 1.5, port site infiltration: 3.0) [94]. On the contrary, the LAP-TAP block participants experienced higher pain scores ($p = 0.043$) and opioid requirements ($p = 0.021$) at 6 h than port infiltration group participants [84].

15.3.12. Analgesic Efficacy of Laparoscopic-Assisted Infiltration Using Different Doses of Local Anesthetic versus Normal Saline

The results of this review show that patients who received 0.9% normal saline for infiltration during laparoscopy reported a high need for rescue analgesia both in the ward (21, 70%) and at PACU (13, 43.3%) [88]. Compared with the other two groups, a higher proportion of those who received Ropivacaine at low concentrations (0.25%) required rescue anesthesia in the ward (5 (16.7%) [88]. The values of the control group VAS were significantly higher than those of the groups TAI, TAPB, and IPLA after 1, 2, 4, 6, 12, and 24 h [90]. In addition, the VAS values of the IPLA group were significantly higher than those of the LAI and TAPB groups at 1, 2, 4, 6, 12, and 24 h [90]. VAS values at 1, 2, 4, 6, and 24 h were not significantly different between TAI and the TAPB group. A significant difference was observed between the TAI and TAPB groups in terms of VAS values at 12 h [90].

c. Other known techniques

When bilateral double transversus abdominis plane blockade (BD-TAP) was compared with sham control, higher pain sensation was observed postoperatively in the control group at rest (2 h), during coughing (2, 6, and 48 h), and during walking (2, 6, and 48 h), with no change between the two groups at 24 h [91]. Ultrasound-guided modified BRILMA block (US-BRILMA) was compared with US-TAP block (subcostal), and it was found that postoperative Morphine consumption was higher in the US-BRILMA group (5.67 mg) than in the US-TAP block group (5.17 mg) [93]. The time to request rescue analgesia was higher in the US-BRILMA group (845) than in the US-TAP group (759.33) [93]. The efficacy of erector spinae block and oblique subcostal transversus abdominis block was compared, and the mean pain of the two groups between 2 and 24 h differed, with the OSTAP block group reporting more pain experience (2.27 to 0.70) [92]). The US-TAPB block group had significantly lower resting VAS values than the two groups receiving PCIA with Sufentanil and Nalbuphineat 2, 6, 12, 24, and 48 h postop ($p < 0.05$) (Han et al., 2022). Postoperatively, dynamic VAS was significantly lower in the US-TAPB block group ($p < 0.05$) than in the two groups receiving PCIA with Sufentanil and Nalbuphine [98].

16. Long-Term Effects

As shown in Table 3, all studies examined participants between 0 and 48 h or on the first postoperative day, with only one study examining pain intensity one week postop. Therefore, we cannot infer from this study that TAP block anesthesia has a long-term effect.

Objective #4. Clinical Significance of TAP Block

As shown in Table 4, the minimal clinically significant differences between the US-TAP block and port infiltration groups all had a large effect size index; however, the US-TAP block group had a higher effect.

Table 4. Clinical significance of TAP.

No	Author (Year)	Drugs Used	Mean$_{post}$	Mean$_{pre}$	SDpre	Effect Size Index
1	Ortiz (2012) [20]	Morphine 24 h				
		US-TAP block	16.1	1.5	1.8	8.1
		Port infiltration	15.4	0.9	2.0	7.3

17. Discussion

To our knowledge, this is the first review to comprehensively compare the analgesic efficacy of different procedures for laparoscopic cholecystectomy.

The seven classes of drugs used before anesthesia (pre-medication) include benzodiazepines (e.g., Midazolam), analgesics (e.g., Paracetamol), prokinetics (e.g., Metoclopramide), anticholinergics (Glycopyrrolate), 5-HT3 antagonists (Ondansetron), H2 receptor blockers (e.g., ranitidine), and alkalinizing agents (ringer lactate solution) [20,60,68,71,74,76]. Common local anesthetics used for various block procedures in laparoscopic cholecystectomy include Bupivacaine (0.25–0.375%), Ropivacaine (0.2–0.75%), and Levobupivacaine (0.25–0.375%). In all, 20 mL and 10 mL of local anesthetics could be the optimal dose for US-TAP or US-OSTAP blockade procedures and port infiltration.

Evidence from this study has shown that US-TAP blockade in addition to general anesthesia is more effective than general anesthesia alone for postoperative pain management [59]. Use of the US-TAP block is associated with a reduced need for analgesics within the first 24 h postoperative [7]. In addition, using US-TAP block before induction of anesthesia and after the surgery might be associated with less need for analgesics within the first 24 h after laparoscopic cholecystectomy, although the two groups do not differ significantly [95]. The lower the concentration of local anesthetics used for laparoscopic infiltration, the higher the need for rescue analgesics [7]. Similarly, the higher the concentration of the solution used for US-TAP block, the lower the need for intra-operative or postoperative analgesia [7,72,98].

Apparently, the addition of 20 mL of normal saline to 0.5% bupivacaine for the US-TAP block might be associated with a lower need for analgesics than in patients who received 10 mL of normal saline to 0.5% bupivacaine [72]. US-TAP blockade with 0.375% Ropivacaine plus 2 mL Dexamethasone is more effective in relieving pain than US-TAP blockade with the same concentration of Ropivacaine or general anesthesia alone [67]. However, the addition of a lesser amount of Dexamethasone 1 mcg to 0.5% Ropivacaine does not result in any significant change [88]. Again, the same concentration of 0.2% Ropivacaine with an additional 4 mg/kg Dexamethasone was used for different TAP block procedures, and the US-ESP group had less postoperative pain and required fewer opioids than the OSTAP block group [92]. The addition of 0.5 mg/kg Esmolol to the local anesthetic for TAP block infiltration is more effective for pain management than the addition of 0.9% normal saline [89]. Again, administration of a local anesthetic percutaneously or subcutaneously or between obliquus internus and transversus abdominis or in the sub-diaphragmatic and pericholecystic areas is more effective than normal saline. In another development, the addition of 0.4% Ropivacaine to 100 mL of 0.9% saline and 10 mg/kg Tropisetron for US-TAP blockade could provide better pain relief than the addition of 2 mg/kg Sufentanil or Nalbuphine via PCA [98]. Patients receiving 0.5 mcg/kg Dexmedetomidine over 0.375% Ropivacaine consumed fewer opioids and took longer to request initial analgesia than patients receiving 2 mL of 0.9% saline over 0.375% Ropivacaine [75]. Magnesium Sulfate (0.5 g) was added on top of 0.25% Bupivacaine and achieved a reduction pain and in intra-operative opioid consumption [65]. The addition of 5 mcg Epinephrine to 0.375% Levobupivacaine is associated with lower postoperative and total opioid consumption [79]. Ketorolac (180 mg) was administered in combination with Oxycodone (40 mg) in addition to 100 mL of 0.9% saline, compared with patients receiving 20 mL of 0.2% Ropivacaine and those receiving additional patient-controlled analgesia; however, patients without local anesthetic had a greater need for analgesia than the others [71]. It was found that the addition of 2 mL of Sufentanil to 0.5% Bupivacaine prolonged the time to the first analgesia request in 24 h compared with patients who received 2 mL of normal saline or normal saline alone in addition to Bupivacaine [64].

US-TAP blockade with 2 mLof Sufentanil on 0.5% Bupivacaine might be associated with a lower opioids requirement than the use of 2 mL of 0.9% saline on 0.5% Bupivacaine or normal saline alone [64]. Uniquely, US-TAP blockade with 1% of Pethidine (40 mL) in addition to general anesthesia was found to be more effective for pain than US-TAP blockade with normal saline [70]. In particular, it is associated with lower intra-operative Fentanyl consumption and lower postoperative Morphine requirements [70].

Postoperative opioid consumption differs for the different types of blocks, with US-TAP consuming more Fentanyl and US-OSTAP consuming more Nalbuphine [61]. Although US-OSTAP was a relatively new technology, the results seemed consistent with US-TAP. Notably, when comparing the analgesic efficacy of the US-OSTAP and US-TAP block procedures, there appears to be no intra-operative difference between the two procedures in terms of Ketorolac (NSAID) consumption; however, US-OSTAP consumed more Fentanyl (opioids) than US-TAP block [61]. In contrast, more Fentanyl (opioids) was consumed postoperatively during the US-TAP block than during the US-OSTAP block [61]. However, Nalbuphine (opioids) consumption was higher in US-OSTAP block than in US-TAP block [61].

US-OSTAP blockade with Ropivacaine is more effective against pain and requires fewer analgesics than normal saline during and after surgery and at PACU [83]. In particular, US-OSTAP blockade appears to be associated with less pain and less need for opioids 2 h postop and at PACU compared with US-TAP [83]. US-TAP Subcostal block is associated with less pain experience and opioid consumption compared with quadratus lumborum [78]. Between 0 and 6 h postop, the US-TAP subcostal block appeared to be associated with higher pain perception; in contrast, the quadratus lumborum was perceived as more painful between 12 and 24 h [97]. To view it differently, quadratus lumborum reportedly had lower pain perception, lower cumulative daily Morphine consumption, and longer median time to first analgesic request compared with US-TAP block [97]. Therefore, further quantification is needed to clarify the pattern of analgesic consumption during different TAP blockade procedures.

Laparoscopically assisted TAP blockade with Bupivacaine plus Periportal injection of normal saline is associated with pain reduction between 1 and 6 h postoperative compared with those who received saline TAP blockade with a periportal injection of Bupivacaine [63]. The use of normal saline for LAP-TAP correlates with a higher need for rescue analgesia both in the ward and at PACU [88].

The port infiltration group seems to have a higher need for analgesics than the US-STA or US-TAP groups [94]. Notably, in the US-TAP block group, there seems to be a delay in requesting the first analgesics compared to the port infiltration group [94]. Within 3–6 h postoperative and at discharge, there appeared to be no significant difference between LAP-TAP and the port infiltration group; however, at 24 h, the port infiltration group had a greater demand for analgesia [94]. In contrast, the LAP-TAP group had a greater need for opioids and greater pain perception 6 h postoperative [94].

Subcostal US-TAP blockade is associated with lower postoperative opioid consumption compared with US-BRILMA [93]. Likewise, the time to request rescue analgesia was higher with the US-BRILMA blockade than with the US-TAP subcostal blockade [93]. In addition, US-ESP blockade was found to result in less pain between 2 and 24 h postoperative compared with OSTAP blockade [77]. Moreover, the bilateral double blockade of the transversus abdominis plane with Ropivacaine was associated with less pain perception at 2 h at rest and at 2, 6, and 48 h during walking and coughing, compared with the sham control group with normal saline [91].

The optimal dose means that symptoms and side effects can be most effectively controlled with the lowest dose of a drug [103]. From this study, we can infer that the optimal dose of local anesthetic for the blocks US-TAP or US-OSTAP could be 20 mL of

Ropivacaine, Bupivacaine, or Levobupivacaine and 0.4 mL/kg for port site infiltration (Table 4). This is because we recorded a low number of side effects, adverse events, and complications (Table 4). However, caution should be exercised in using these data because of insufficient evidence. Overall, the effects of the interventions in this study were short-term effects, and we could not find evidence of long-term effects because in most cases, the studies assessed outcomes between 0 and 24 h, and very few studied subjects 48 h or a week postoperative.

Corroborating the extant literature, our study confirmed the reduction in analgesic consumption 24 h after laparoscopic surgery with TAP blockade or general anesthesia with TAP blockade compared with general anesthesia or no TAP blockade or placebo treatment, with analgesic consumption also reduced after 24 h [45]. Consistent with the results of our study, Kalu et al. [104] submitted that postoperative opioid consumption was influenced by the use of the US-TAP block procedure both preoperatively and postoperatively. Notably, there was no significant difference between groups in opioid consumption, but the US-TAP blockade reduced postoperative pain in both groups. From this review, the higher the concentration of local anesthetic used for local infiltration, the greater the effect on pain. Notably, this study found that 30 mL of 0.5% Levobupivacaine was more effective than 0.2% at 6 h postoperative; El-Dawlatly et al. [59] also used 30 mL of 0.5% Bupivacaine for US-TAP procedures and achieved a reduction in opioid consumption for 24 h postoperative. Similarly, 0.375% Ropivacaine was equally more effective against pain compared with 0.25% between 10 and 60 min after surgery when administered by the same route [69]. The route of local anesthetic administration has been controversial; however, in previous studies, different routes of administration of Ropivacaine were found to be more effective than Bupivacaine [105,106]. Although Bupivacaine and Ropivacaine have been compared at various concentrations in the context of different surgical procedures, there appears to be a paucity of evidence comparing these local anesthetics in US-TAP blockade for laparoscopic cholecystectomy. Therefore, future studies should compare the analgesic efficacy of Ropivacaine and Bupivacaine in different routes of administration for laparoscopic cholecystectomy.

The modified BRILMA block has been used and was found to reduce intra-operative Fentanyl consumption and postoperative Morphine consumption in supra-umbilical open surgeries such as cholecystectomy and gastrectomy [107]. OSTAP block was found to reduce postoperative pain scores more than intravenous multimodal analgesics, and TAP for laparoscopic cholecystectomy [68]. In a similar study, Basaran et al. [62] showed significant improvement in respiratory function and postoperative pain with OSTAP blockade. As our study shows, the OSTAP block reduced postoperative Tramadol consumption significantly more than the ESP block; however, the ESP block did not reduce postoperative Tramadol consumption as significantly as the OSTAP block.

Opioid consumption varies by plane block procedure. While there are no intra-operative differences between US-TAP and US-OSTAP for Ketorolac, the US-OSTAP group consumed more Fentanyl, while the US-TAP group consumed more Nalbuphine postoperatively using 0.375% of Ropivacaine 40 mL [61]. However, there is contradictory evidence in the literature. It is worth noting that the US-TAP block reduced intra-operative consumption of Remifentanil or Sufentanil when 30 mL of Bupivacaine or Levobupivacaine was used [7,59]. Ortiz et al. [20] used 30 mL of 0.5% Ropivacaine and achieved lower intra-operative consumption of Morphine and Fentanyl compared to the port site infiltration. In addition, analgesic consumption and the need for rescue analgesia were reduced [7,59]. To look at it another way, 20 mL of Ropivacaine was previously found to reduce pain when coughing but not at rest [21]. US-TAP blocks following general anesthesia were significantly associated with lower Morphine consumption in the 24 h following surgery compared with patients receiving general anesthesia alone [59]. Therefore, future studies should be designed to clarify the analgesic efficacy of different block procedures using similar dosages.

The results of this review have shown that the use of adjuvant in addition to local anesthetics for TAP block procedures could be effective for pain management in laparoscopic cholecystectomy. To improve recovery after surgery and reduce postoperative opioid consumption, opioid-sparing techniques are increasingly used in anesthesia. Evidently, it was found that local anesthetics may be improved, and additional analgesics need to be administered less frequently when Dexmedetomidine is added to local anesthetics during central neuraxial blocks and peripheral nerve blocks [108]. Additionally, a study has shown that postoperative Fentanyl requirements were significantly lower in patients in the Esmolol group [109]. Perineural Dexamethasone combined with posterior TAP block was found to have a prolonged analgesic effect [110]. The pharmacokinetics of Ropivacaine were studied after the addition of Epinephrine for abdominal trunk blocks; however, this was found to attenuate the systemic absorption of Ropivacaine [111]. Previous studies have shown that multimodal analgesia with TAP blockade in combination with Nalbuphine PCIA is likely to be more beneficial for hemodynamic stability than Sufentanil or Nalbuphine PCIA, which is in line with this study outcome [112]. In abdominal TAP procedures, Magnesium Sulfate in addition to Bupivacaine reduced opioid requirements, duration of anesthesia, and pain intensity without adverse effects [113]. For OSTAP blockade, Pethidine was used in comparison with Bupivacaine and normal saline, and it proved to be as effective as Bupivacaine. The result is consistent with previous studies on the efficacy of US-OSTAP blocks in laparoscopic cholecystectomy [47,60].

Study results by McDonnell et al. [114] and [115] suggest that local anesthetics in TAP are cleared only after 36 to 48 h, possibly because TAP has fewer blood vessels compared to other body regions. Because there are no blood vessels in TAP, there is less risk of systemic toxicity from local anesthetics, which can occur when blood vessels are punctured, a common complication of peripheral nerve blocks. An effective method for relieving abdominal pain is to block the abdominal wall nerves (intercostal nerves, T7-T12, and ilioinguinal and iliohypogastric nerves, L1) [7]. There are two nerves that cross the intercostal plane between the obliquus internus muscle and the transversus abdominis muscle [7]. TAP blocking eliminates the pain caused by abdominal distension due to pneumoperitoneum during four accesses to laparoscopic cholecystectomy, even though the gallbladder is a supra-umbilical organ [69]. Unlike conventional blind techniques, ultrasound allows direct visualization of the target plane, virtually eliminating the limitations of anatomic and marker access. In patients with limited cardiac status, TAP blockade has also been used as an effective analgesic during abdominal surgery [116,117].

A few studies have contributed to the understanding of the modulation of postoperative pain by Esmolol, although its role in modulating pain still remains unclear [89]. Analgesic effects of beta-adrenergic antagonists are mediated by G proteins that are activated in isolated cell membranes [108]. Clonidine, which also acts on G proteins, produces central analgesia by activating these proteins [108]. Clinical studies have shown that the use of Magnesium Sulfate as an adjunct to local anesthetics is effective for pain in regional procedures [7,21,59]. However, the mechanism by which it acts remains unclear. It has been postulated that it may potentiate analgesic effects through local or systemic actions [65]. For magnesium to exert analgesic effects, it must block calcium influx into nerve fibers and block the NMDA (*n*-methyl D-aspartate) receptors [118–120]. These effects may interfere with the release of neurotransmitters at synaptic junctions or enhance the effects of local anesthetics [121]. There are many sites in the body where this NMDA receptor is found, including nerve endings, and it plays a well-defined role in modulating pain and various other functions [122–124]; therefore, blocking NMDA receptors could prevent peripheral nociceptive stimuli from causing central sensitization [125]. Specifically, as magnesium prevents NMDA receptor activation, calcium and sodium influx into the cell and potassium outflow into space activate peripheral nociceptive stimulation, resulting in central sensitization and enhancement [65].

The mechanism by which Dexamethasone might affect pain management also remains unclear; however, the lack of local blood vessels makes the TAP blockade lasts a long time because of the slow breakdown of local analgesia [114,126]. Aside from that, the literature has shown that different approaches to TAP blockade affect nerves differently [38,127]. In the past, Dexamethasone prolonged intercostal nerve blockade in sheep when added to Bupivacaine microspheres [128]. In addition, blockade of the sciatic nerves was induced in rats with Dexamethasone microspheres added to Bupivacaine [129]. Increasing systemic absorption and intraneural clearance of local anesthetics may be decreased because the vasoconstrictive effects of Epinephrine antagonize their inherent vasodilator effects and they may be redistributed intraneurally [130]. With shorter-acting agents, Epinephrine significantly prolongs both infiltration anesthesia and peripheral nerve blockade; it may also increase blockade somewhat, but with Bupivacaine, it prolongs epidural or peripheral blockade only slightly [131]. Research has shown that the use of different analgesics for multiple targets can result in satisfactory postoperative pain management [98]. There are several previous studies indicating a reduction in postoperative pain scores and opioid consumption after classic mid-axillary blocks US-TAP; a sensory blockade occurs between dermatomes T6 and T10 when TAP subcostal is reached [132,133]. As a result, OSTAP is used in the upper abdomen to relieve pain [134].

18. Limitations

The present systematic review has some limitations. Although all included studies were searched from different countries, we are subject to publication bias because this systematic review includes studies published in English only. Because of the lack of sufficient data, we could not draw conclusions about the clinical significance of the various TAP block procedures. We were also unable to provide information on the long-term effects of the TAP blockade procedures because of a lack of evidence. There were numerous RCTs whose data were not suitable for meta-analysis, either because of a pictorial representation of the data, different methods of measuring outcomes, or inappropriate statistical analysis (e.g., reporting median and mean values with a range) or the lack of baseline data. Furthermore, the ASA grade and BMI in the baseline data of patients could have an impact on the tolerance of local anesthetics. Again, the broader inclusion criteria and overall objective may be a limiting factor to consider when planning further studies. In view of these problems, it is advisable to not generalize conclusions from this study to broader clinical settings. However, further studies are needed to clarify the analgesic efficacy of different TAP block procedures at similar doses. The optimal long-term effect of local anesthetics in TAP blockade procedures and the toxicity of local anesthetics should be further investigated.

19. Conclusions

Four different types of anesthetics (Bupivacaine, Ropivacaine, Levobupivacaine, and Lidocaine) have been reported to be used in concentrations ranging from 0.2% to 0.375% for LC procedures. Ten different types of drugs (normal saline, Dexamethasone, Dexmedetomidine, Magnesium Sulfate, Oxycodone, Ketorolac, Epinephrine, Esmolol, Tropisetron, and Sufentanil) were reportedly used as supportive agents in addition to local anesthetics for LC. Although concentrations of LA may vary, 20 mL is probably the optimal dose for TAP block procedures and 0.4 mg/kg for port infiltration. However, further quantification is needed to clarify the optimal dose for different anesthetic concentrations. US-TAP blockades performed in addition to general anesthesia were more effective for pain than port infiltration or general anesthesia alone. Postoperative pain perception and opioid consumption were higher in those who received a US-TAP block after surgery than in those who received a block before induction; however, it took a shorter time for those who received a US-TAP block after surgery to require the first analgesics. US-TAP block with normal saline reportedly had higher opioid consumption in 24 h compared with those with Bupivacaine over normal saline or Bupivacaine over Sufentanil. It appears that the higher the concentration of the anesthetic used for US-TAP blockade, the lower the pain sensation, and that an adjuvant to LA could enhance its analgesic effect. Evidently, those who received Ropivacaine at low concentrations required rescue anesthesia in the ward. There seems to be no significant difference between the US-TAP and US-OSTAP. Time to first analgesic intake/request was higher in the groups with US-TAP block compared with quadratus lumborum. However, pain perception between 12 and 24 h was lower in the US-TAP group than in the quadratus lumborum group. This should be clarified in further studies. Compared with the port infiltrations, the LAP-TAP block group reportedly had less pain at rest in the first 3–6 h after surgery. The minimal clinically significant differences for both TAP block procedures and port infiltration appeared to have a large effect size index, but this should be taken with caution because of insufficient evidence. Subcostal US-TAP blockade may be correlated with lower postoperative opioid consumption and reduced need for rescue analgesics compared with US-BRILMA. US-ESP proved to be more effective than US-OSTAP block for postoperative pain within 24 h. Finally, multimodal analgesia could be another strategy for pain management. Analgesia with the TAP blockade significantly reduces opioid consumption and also provides effective analgesia.

Supplementary Materials: The following supporting information can be downloaded at: https://www.mdpi.com/article/10.3390/jcm11236896/s1, Table S1: Within Group Effects of the Interventions.

Author Contributions: Conceptualization, A.F.A., F.H.A., Y.S.A. and D.S.; methodology, A.F.A., F.H.A., Y.S.A. and D.S.; software, A.F.A. and D.S.; validation, A.F.A., F.H.A. and Y.S.A.; formal analysis, D.S.; investigation, A.F.A., F.H.A., Y.S.A. and D.S.; resources, A.F.A. and D.S.; data curation, F.H.A. and Y.S.A.; writing—original draft preparation, F.H.A., Y.S.A. and D.S.; writing—review and editing, A.F.A.; visualization, A.F.A., F.H.A., Y.S.A. and D.S.; supervision, A.F.A. All authors have read and agreed to the published version of the manuscript.

Funding: The authors extend their appreciation to the Deanship of Scientific Research at Jouf University for funding this work through research grant no. DSR2020-04-2628.

Institutional Review Board Statement: The study did not require ethical approval.

Informed Consent Statement: Not applicable.

Data Availability Statement: The data that support the findings of this study are available from the corresponding author upon reasonable request.

Conflicts of Interest: The authors declare no conflict of interest.

References

1. Mitra, S.; Khandelwal, P.; Roberts, K.; Kumar, S.; Vadivelu, N. Pain relief in laparoscopic cholecystectomy—A review of the current options. *Pain Pract.* **2012**, *12*, 485–496.
2. Bisgaard, T.; Warltier, D.C. Analgesic treatment after laparoscopic cholecystectomy: A critical assessment of the evidence. *Anesthesiology* **2006**, *104*, 835–846. [CrossRef]
3. Johns, N.; O'Neill, S.; Ventham, N.; Barron, F.; Brady, R.; Daniel, T. Clinical effectiveness of transversus abdominis plane (TAP) block in abdominal surgery: A systematic review and meta-analysis. *Color. Dis.* **2012**, *14*, e635–e642.
4. Tekeli, A.E.; Eker, E.; Bartin, M.K.; Öner, M.Ö. The efficacy of transversus abdominis plane block for postoperative analgesia in laparoscopic cholecystectomy cases: A retrospective evaluation of 515 patients. *J. Int. Med. Res.* **2020**, *48*, 1–9. [CrossRef]
5. Abrahams, M.S.; Horn, J.-L.; Noles, L.M.; Aziz, M.F. Evidence-based medicine: Ultrasound guidance for truncal blocks. *Reg. Anesthesia Pain Med.* **2010**, *35*, S36–S42. [CrossRef]
6. Bhatia, N.; Arora, S.; Jyotsna, W.; Kaur, G. Comparison of posterior and subcostal approaches to ultrasound-guided transverse abdominis plane block for postoperative analgesia in laparoscopic cholecystectomy. *J. Clin. Anesth.* **2014**, *26*, 294–299. [CrossRef]
7. Ra, Y.S.; Kim, C.H.; Lee, G.Y.; Han, J.I. The analgesic effect of the ultrasound-guided transverse abdominis plane block after laparoscopic cholecystectomy. *Korean J. Anesthesiol.* **2010**, *58*, 362–368. [CrossRef]
8. Wassef, M.; Lee, D.Y.; Levine, J.; Ross, R.E.; Guend, H.; Vandepitte, C.; Hadzic, A.; Teixeira, J. Feasibility and analgesic efficacy of the transversus abdominis plane block after single-port laparoscopy in patients having bariatric surgery. *J. Pain Res.* **2013**, *6*, 837–841. [CrossRef]
9. Statzer, N.; Cummings, K.C. Transversus abdominis plane blocks. *Adv. Anesth.* **2018**, *36*, 163–180.
10. Rafi, A.N. Abdominal field block: A new approach via the lumbar triangle. *Anaesthesia* **2001**, *56*, 1024–1026. [CrossRef]

11. Rozen, W.; Tran, T.; Ashton, M.; Barrington, M.; Ivanusic, J.; Taylor, G. Refining the course of the thoracolumbar nerves: A new understanding of the innervation of the anterior abdominal wall. *Clin. Anat.* **2008**, *21*, 325–333. [CrossRef]
12. Szental, J.; Webb, A.; Weeraratne, C.; Campbell, A.; Sivakumar, H.; Leong, S. Postoperative pain after laparoscopic cholecystectomy is not reduced by intraoperative analgesia guided by analgesia nociception index (ANI®) monitoring: A randomized clinical trial. *Br. J. Anaesth.* **2015**, *114*, 640–645.
13. Brogi, E.; Kazan, R.; Cyr, S.; Giunta, F.; Hemmerling, T.M. Transversus abdominal plane block for postoperative analgesia: A systematic review and meta-analysis of randomized-controlled trials. *Can. J. Anaesth.* **2016**, *63*, 1184–1196. [CrossRef]
14. Champaneria, R.; Shah, L.; Geoghegan, J.; Gupta, J.K.; Daniels, J.P. Analgesic effectiveness of transversus abdominis plane blocks after hysterectomy: A meta-analysis. *Eur. J. Obstet. Gynecol. Reprod. Biol.* **2012**, *166*, 1–9. [CrossRef]
15. Elkassabany, N.; Ahmed, M.; Malkowicz, S.B.; Heitjan, D.F.; Isserman, J.A.; Ochroch, E.A. Comparison between the analgesic efficacy of transversus abdominis plane (TAP) block and placebo in open retropubic radical prostatectomy: A prospective, randomized, double-blinded study. *J. Clin. Anesth.* **2013**, *25*, 459–465. [CrossRef]
16. Abdallah, F.W.; Laffey, J.G.; Halpern, S.H.; Brull, R. Duration of analgesic effectiveness after the posterior and lateral transversus abdominis plane block techniques for transverse lower abdominal incisions: A meta-analysis. *Br. J. Anaesth.* **2013**, *111*, 721–735. [CrossRef]
17. Maeda, A.; Shibata, S.C.; Kamibayashi, T.; Fujino, Y. Continuous subcostal oblique transversus abdominis plane block provides more effective analgesia than single-shot block after gynaecological laparotomy. *Eur. J. Anaesthesiol.* **2015**, *32*, 514–515. [CrossRef]
18. Niraj, G.; Kelkar, A.; Hart, E.; Kaushik, V.; Fleet, D.; Jameson, J. Four quadrant transversus abdominis plane block and continuous transversus abdominis plane analgesia: A 3-year prospective audit in 124 patients. *J. Clin. Anesth.* **2015**, *27*, 579–584. [CrossRef]
19. Hutchins, J.L.; Kesha, R.; Blanco, F.; Dunn, T.; Hochhalter, R. Ultrasound-guided subcostal transversus abdominis plane blocks with liposomal bupivacaine vs. non-liposomal bupivacaine for postoperative pain control after laparoscopic hand-assisted donor nephrectomy: A prospective randomised observer-blinded study. *Anaesthesia* **2016**, *71*, 930–937. [CrossRef]
20. Ortiz, J.; Suliburk, J.; Wu, K.; Bailard, N.S.; Mason, C.; Minard, C.G.; Palvadi, R.R. Bilateral Transversus Abdominis Plane Block Does Not Decrease Postoperative Pain After Laparoscopic Cholecystectomy When Compared with Local Anesthetic Infiltration of Trocar Insertion Sites. *Reg. Anesth. Pain Med.* **2012**, *37*, 188–192. [CrossRef]
21. Petersen, P.L.; Stjernholm, P.; Kristiansen, V.B.; Torup, H.; Hansen, E.G.; Mitchell, A.U.; Moeller, A.; Rosenberg, J.; Dahl, J.B.; Mathiesen, O. The Beneficial Effect of Transversus Abdominis Plane Block After Laparoscopic Cholecystectomy in Day-Case Surgery. *Anesth. Analg.* **2012**, *115*, 527–533. [CrossRef]
22. Kaye, A.; Urman, R.; Rappaport, Y.; Siddaiah, H.; Cornett, E.; Belani, K.; Salinas, O.; Fox, C. Multimodal analgesia as an essential part of enhanced recovery protocols in the ambulatory settings. *J. Anaesthesiol. Clin. Pharmacol.* **2019**, *35*, 40–45. [CrossRef]
23. Koyyalamudi, V.; Sen, S.; Patil, S.; Creel, J.B.; Cornett, E.M.; Fox, C.J.; Kaye, A.D. Adjuvant Agents in Regional Anesthesia in the Ambulatory Setting. *Curr. Pain Headache Rep.* **2017**, *21*, 6. [CrossRef]
24. Bisgaard, T.; Klarskov, B.; Rosenberg, J.; Kehlet, H. Characteristics and prediction of early pain after laparoscopic cholecystectomy. *Pain* **2001**, *90*, 261–269.
25. Desai, N.; El-Boghdadly, K.; Albrecht, E. Epidural vs. transversus abdominis plane block for abdominal surgery–a systematic review, meta-analysis and trial sequential analysis. *Anaesthesia* **2021**, *76*, 101–117.
26. Grape, S.; Kirkham, K.R.; Akiki, L.; Albrecht, E. Transversus abdominis plane block versus local anesthetic wound infiltration for optimal analgesia after laparoscopic cholecystectomy: A systematic review and meta-analysis with trial sequential analysis. *J. Clin. Anesth.* **2021**, *75*, 110450.
27. Panda, A.; Saxena, S.; Pathak, M.; Rath, S. Laparoscopic assisted versus ultrasound guided transversus abdominis plane block in laparoscopic surgeries: A systematic review and meta-analysis. *Trends Anaesth. Crit. Care* **2022**, *44*, 20–26. [CrossRef]
28. Peng, K.; Ji, F.-H.; Liu, H.-Y.; Wu, S.-R. Ultrasound-Guided Transversus Abdominis Plane Block for Analgesia in Laparoscopic Cholecystectomy: A Systematic Review and Meta-Analysis. *Med. Princ. Pract.* **2016**, *25*, 237–246.
29. Howle, R.; Ng, S.-C.; Wong, H.-Y.; Onwochei, D.; Desai, N. Comparison of analgesic modalities for patients undergoing midline laparotomy: A systematic review and network meta-analysis. *Can. J. Anaesth.* **2021**, *69*, 140–176.
30. Liheng, L.; Siyuan, C.; Zhen, C.; Changxue, W. Erector Spinae Plane Block versus Transversus Abdominis Plane Block for Postoperative Analgesia in Abdominal Surgery: A Systematic Review and Meta-Analysis. *J. Investig. Surg.* **2022**, *35*, 1711–1722.
31. Liu, X.; Song, T.; Chen, X.; Zhang, J.; Shan, C.; Chang, L.; Xu, H. Quadratus lumborum block versus transversus abdominis plane block for postoperative analgesia in patients undergoing abdominal surgeries: A systematic review and meta-analysis of randomized controlled trials. *BMC Anesthesiol.* **2020**, *20*, 1–10.
32. Qin, C.; Liu, Y.; Xiong, J.; Wang, X.; Dong, Q.; Su, T.; Liu, J. The analgesic efficacy compared ultrasound-guided continuous transverse abdominis plane block with epidural analgesia following abdominal surgery: A systematic review and meta-analysis of randomized controlled trials. *BMC Anesthesiol.* **2020**, *20*, 1–9.
33. Yu, N.; Long, X.; Lujan-Hernandez, J.R.; Succar, J.; Xin, X.; Wang, X. Transversus abdominis-plane block versus local anesthetic wound infiltration in lower abdominal surgery: A systematic review and meta-analysis of randomized controlled trials. *BMC Anesthesiol.* **2014**, *14*, 121. [CrossRef]

34. Zhang, D.; Zhou, C.; Wei, D.; Ge, L.; Li, Q. Dexamethasone added to local anesthetics in ultrasound-guided transversus abdominis plain (TAP) block for analgesia after abdominal surgery: A systematic review and meta-analysis of randomized controlled trials. *PLoS ONE* **2019**, *14*, 1–15. [CrossRef]
35. Hain, E.; Maggiori, L.; à la Denise, P.; Panis, Y. Transversus abdominis plane (TAP) block in laparoscopic colorectal surgery improves postoperative pain management: A meta-analysis. *Colorectal. Dis.* **2018**, *20*, 279–287.
36. Peltrini, R.; Cantoni, V.; Green, R.; Greco, P.A.; Calabria, M.; Bucci, L.; Corcione, F. Efficacy of transversus abdominis plane (TAP) block in colorectal surgery: A systematic review and meta-analysis. *Tech. Coloproctol.* **2020**, *24*, 787–802.
37. Guo, Q.; Li, R.; Wang, L.; Zhang, D.; Ma, Y. Transversus abdominis plane block versus local anaesthetic wound infiltration for postoperative analgesia: A systematic review and meta-analysis. *Int. J. Clin. Exp. Med.* **2015**, *8*, 17343.
38. Abdallah, F.W.; Halpern, S.H.; Margarido, C.B. Transversus abdominis plane block for postoperative analgesia after Caesarean delivery performed under spinal anaesthesia? A systematic review and meta-analysis. *Br. J. Anaesth.* **2012**, *109*, 679–687.
39. Aamir, M.A.; Sahebally, S.M.; Heneghan, H. Transversus Abdominis Plane Block in Laparoscopic Bariatric Surgery—A Systematic Review and Meta-Analysis of Randomized Controlled Trials. *Obes. Surg.* **2021**, *31*, 133–142.
40. Chaw, S.H.; Lo, Y.L.; Goh, S.-L.; Cheong, C.C.; Tan, W.K.; Loh, P.S.; Wong, L.F.; Shariffuddin, I.I. Transversus Abdominis Plane Block Versus Intraperitoneal Local Anesthetics in Bariatric Surgery: A Systematic Review and Network Meta-analysis. *Obes. Surg.* **2021**, *31*, 4305–4315.
41. Abdou, S.A.; Daar, D.A.; Wilson, S.C.; Thanik, V. Transversus Abdominis Plane Blocks in Microsurgical Breast Reconstruction: A Systematic Review and Meta-analysis. *J. Reconstr. Microsurg.* **2020**, *36*, 353–361.
42. Hamid, H.K.; Emile, S.H.; Saber, A.A.; Ruiz-Tovar, J.; Minas, V.; Cataldo, T.E. Laparoscopic-Guided Transversus Abdominis Plane Block for Postoperative Pain Management in Minimally Invasive Surgery: Systematic Review and Meta-Analysis. *J. Am. Coll. Surg.* **2020**, *231*, 376–386.e315.
43. Koo, C.-H.; Hwang, J.-Y.; Shin, H.-J.; Ryu, J.-H. The Effects of Erector Spinae Plane Block in Terms of Postoperative Analgesia in Patients Undergoing Laparoscopic Cholecystectomy: A Meta-Analysis of Randomized Controlled Trials. *J. Clin. Med.* **2020**, *9*, 2928.
44. Ni, X.; Zhao, X.; Li, M.; Li, Q.; Liu, Z. The effect of transversus abdominis plane block for pain after laparoscopic cholecystectomy: A meta-analysis of randomized controlled trials. *Int. J. Clin. Exp. Med.* **2016**, *9*, 9974–9982.
45. Zhao, X.; Tong, Y.; Ren, H.; Ding, X.-B.; Wang, X.; Zong, J.-Y.; Jin, S.-Q.; Li, Q. Transversus abdominis plane block for postoperative analgesia after laparoscopic surgery: A systematic review and meta-analysis. *Int. J. Clin. Exp. Med.* **2014**, *7*, 2966–2975.
46. Ma, N.; Duncan, J.K.; Scarfe, A.J.; Schuhmann, S.; Cameron, A.L. Clinical safety and effectiveness of transversus abdominis plane (TAP) block in post-operative analgesia: A systematic review and meta-analysis. *J. Anesth.* **2017**, *31*, 432–452.
47. Ripollés, J.; Mezquita, S.M.; Abad, A.; Calvo, J. Analgesic efficacy of the ultrasound-guided blockade of the transversus abdominis plane–A systematic review. *Braz. J. Anesthesiol. Engl. Ed.* **2015**, *65*, 255–280.
48. Wang, W.; Wang, L.; Gao, Y. A Meta-Analysis of Randomized Controlled Trials Concerning the Efficacy of Transversus Abdominis Plane Block for Pain Control After Laparoscopic Cholecystectomy. *Front. Surg.* **2021**, *8*, 700318.
49. Wang, Y.; Wang, X.; Zhang, K. Effects of transversus abdominis plane block versus quadratus lumborum block on postoperative analgesia: A meta-analysis of randomized controlled trials. *BMC Anesthesiol.* **2020**, *20*, 1–9.
50. Keir, A.; Rhodes, L.; Kayal, A.; Khan, O.A. Does a transversus abdominal plane (TAP) local anaesthetic block improve pain control in patients undergoing laparoscopic cholecystectomy? A best evidence topic. *Int. J. Surg.* **2013**, *11*, 792–794.
51. Parums, D.V. Editorial: Review Articles, Systematic Reviews, Meta-Analysis, and the Updated Preferred Reporting Items for Systematic Reviews and Meta-Analyses (PRISMA) 2020 Guidelines. *Med. Sci. Monit.* **2021**, *27*, e934475. [CrossRef]
52. de Morton, N.A. The PEDro scale is a valid measure of the methodological quality of clinical trials: A demographic study. *Aust. J. Physiother.* **2009**, *55*, 129–133.
53. Batchelor, F.; Hill, K.; Mackintosh, S.; Said, C. What works in falls prevention after stroke? A systematic review and meta-analysis. *Stroke* **2010**, *41*, 1715–1722.
54. Macedo, L.G.; Elkins, M.R.; Maher, C.G.; Moseley, A.M.; Herbert, R.D.; Sherrington, C. There was evidence of convergent and construct validity of Physiotherapy Evidence Database quality scale for physiotherapy trials. *J. Clin. Epidemiol.* **2010**, *63*, 920–925.
55. Silverman, S.R.; Schertz, L.A.; Yuen, H.K.; Lowman, J.D.; Bickel, C.S. Systematic review of the methodological quality and outcome measures utilized in exercise interventions for adults with spinal cord injury. *Spinal Cord* **2012**, *50*, 718–727.
56. Higgins, J.P.; Thomas, J.; Chandler, J.; Cumpston, M.; Li, T.; Page, M.J.; Welch, V.A. *Cochrane Handbook for Systematic Reviews of Interventions*; John Wiley & Sons: Hoboken, NJ, USA, 2019.
57. Watt, J.A.; Veroniki, A.A.; Tricco, A.C.; Straus, S.E. Using a distribution-based approach and systematic review methods to derive minimum clinically important differences. *BMC Med. Res. Methodol.* **2021**, *21*, 1–7.
58. Sullivan, G.M.; Feinn, R. Using effect size—Or why the P value is not enough. *J. Grad. Med. Educ.* **2012**, *4*, 279–282.
59. El-Dawlatly, A.A.; Turkistani, A.; Kettner, S.C.; Machata, A.-M.; Delvi, M.B.; Thallaj, A.; Kapral, S.; Marhofer, P. Ultrasound-guided transversus abdominis plane block: Description of a new technique and comparison with conventional systemic analgesia during laparoscopic cholecystectomy. *Br. J. Anaesth.* **2009**, *102*, 763–767.
60. Tolchard, S.; Davies, R.; Martindale, S. Efficacy of the subcostal transversus abdominis plane block in laparoscopic cholecystectomy: Comparison with conventional port-site infiltration. *J. Anaesthesiol. Clin. Pharmacol.* **2012**, *28*, 339.

61. Shin, H.-J.; Oh, A.-Y.; Baik, J.-S.; Kim, J.-H.; Han, S.-H.; Hwang, J.-W. Ultrasound-guided oblique subcostal transversus abdominis plane block for analgesia after laparoscopic cholecystectomy: A randomized, controlled, observer-blinded study. *Minerva Anestesiol.* **2014**, *80*, 185–193.
62. Basaran, B.; Basaran, A.; Kozanhan, B.; Kasdogan, E.; Eryilmaz, M.A.; Ozmen, S. Analgesia and respiratory function after laparoscopic cholecystectomy in patients receiving ultrasound-guided bilateral oblique subcostal transversus abdominis plane block: A randomized double-blind study. *Med. Sci. Monit. Int. Med. J. Exp. Clin. Res.* **2015**, *21*, 1304–1312.
63. Elamin, G.; Waters, P.S.; Hamid, H.; O'Keeffe, H.M.; Waldron, R.M.; Duggan, M.; Khan, W.; Barry, M.K.; Khan, I.Z. Efficacy of a Laparoscopically Delivered Transversus Abdominis Plane Block Technique during Elective Laparoscopic Cholecystectomy: A Prospective, Double-Blind Randomized Trial. *J. Am. Coll. Surg.* **2015**, *221*, 335–344.
64. Saliminia, A.; Azimaraghi, O.; Babayipour, S.; Ardavan, K.; Movafegh, A. Efficacy of transverse abdominis plane block in reduction of postoperation pain in laparoscopic cholecystectomy. *Acta Anaesthesiol. Taiwanica* **2015**, *53*, 119–122.
65. Al-Refaey, K.; Usama, E.; Al-Hefnawey, E. Adding magnesium sulfate to bupivacaine in transversus abdominis plane block for laparoscopic cholecystectomy: A single blinded randomized controlled trial. *Saudi J. Anaesth.* **2016**, *10*, 187.
66. Bava, E.P.; Ramachandran, R.; Rewari, V.; Chandralekha; Bansal, V.K.; Trikha, A. Analgesic efficacy of ultrasound guided transversus abdominis plane block versus local anesthetic infiltration in adult patients undergoing single incision laparoscopic cholecystectomy: A randomized controlled trial. *Anesth. Essays Res.* **2016**, *10*, 561.
67. Huang, S.-H.; Lu, J.; Gan, H.-Y.; Li, Y.; Peng, Y.-G.; Wang, S.-K. Perineural dexamethasone does not enhance the analgesic efficacy of ultrasound-guided subcostal transversus abdominis plane block during laparoscopic cholecystectomy. *Hepatobiliary Pancreat. Dis. Int.* **2016**, *15*, 540–545.
68. Oksar, M.; Koyuncu, O.; Turhanoglu, S.; Temiz, M.; Oran, M.C. Transversus abdominis plane block as a component of multimodal analgesia for laparoscopic cholecystectomy. *J. Clin. Anesth.* **2016**, *34*, 72–78.
69. Sinha, S.; Palta, S.; Saroa, R.; Prasad, A. Comparison of ultrasound-guided transversus abdominis plane block with bupivacaine and ropivacaine as adjuncts for postoperative analgesia in laparoscopic cholecystectomies. *Indian J. Anaesth.* **2016**, *60*, 264.
70. Breazu, C.M.; Ciobanu, L.; Bartos, A.; Bodea, R.; Mircea, P.A.; Ionescu, D. Pethidine efficacy in achieving the ultrasound-guided oblique subcostal transversus abdominis plane block in laparoscopic cholecystectomy: A prospective study. *Bosn. J. Basic Med. Sci.* **2017**, *17*, 67.
71. Choi, Y.-M.; Byeon, G.-J.; Park, S.-J.; Ok, Y.-M.; Shin, S.-W.; Yang, K. Postoperative analgesic efficacy of single-shot and continuous transversus abdominis plane block after laparoscopic cholecystectomy: A randomized controlled clinical trial. *J. Clin. Anesthesia* **2017**, *39*, 146–151.
72. Şahin, A.S.; Ay, N.; Şahbaz, N.A.; Akay, M.K.; Demiraran, Y.; Derbent, A. Analgesic effects of ultrasound-guided transverse abdominis plane block using different volumes and concentrations of local analgesics after laparoscopic cholecystectomy. *J. Int. Med. Res.* **2017**, *45*, 211–219.
73. Baral, B.; Poudel, P.R. Comparison of Analgesic Efficacy of Ultrasound Guided Subcostal Transversus Abdominis Plane Block with Port Site Infiltration Following Laparoscopic Cholecystectomy. *J. Nepal Health Res. Counc.* **2018**, *16*, 457–461.
74. Bhalekar, P.; Gosavi, R.; Mutha, S.; Mahajan, V.; Phalgune, D. Efficacy of ultrasound-guided subcostal transversus abdominis plane block for analgesia after laparoscopic cholecystectomy. *Indian Anaesth. Forum.* **2018**, *19*, 73.
75. Sarvesh, B.; Shivaramu, B.T.; Sharma, K.; Agarwal, A. Addition of dexmedetomidine to ropivacaine in subcostal transversus abdominis plane block potentiates postoperative analgesia among laparoscopic cholecystectomy patients: A prospective randomized controlled trial. *Anesth. Essays Res.* **2018**, *12*, 809–813.
76. Suseela, I.; Anandan, K.; Aravind, A.; Kaniyil, S. Comparison of ultrasound-guided bilateral subcostal transversus abdominis plane block and port-site infiltration with bupivacaine in laparoscopic cholecystectomy. *Indian J. Anaesth.* **2018**, *62*, 497.
77. Altıparmak, B.; Toker, M.K.; Uysal, A.I.; Kuşçu, Y.; Demirbilek, S.G. Ultrasound-guided erector spinae plane block versus oblique subcostal transversus abdominis plane block for postoperative analgesia of adult patients undergoing laparoscopic cholecystectomy: Randomized, controlled trial. *J. Clin. Anesthesia* **2019**, *57*, 31–36.
78. Baytar, Ç.; Yılmaz, C.; Karasu, D.; Topal, S. Comparison of Ultrasound-Guided Subcostal Transversus Abdominis Plane Block and Quadratus Lumborum Block in Laparoscopic Cholecystectomy: A Prospective, Randomized, Controlled Clinical Study. *Pain Res. Manag.* **2019**, *2019*, 1–6.
79. Houben, A.M.; Moreau, A.-S.J.; Detry, O.M.; Kaba, A.; Joris, J.L. Bilateral subcostal transversus abdominis plane block does not improve the postoperative analgesia provided by multimodal analgesia after laparoscopic cholecystectomy: A randomised placebo-controlled trial. *Eur. J. Anaesthesiol.* **2019**, *36*, 772–777.
80. Janjua, S.; Aslam, K.Z.; Sarfraz, S.; Qarni, A.; Niazi, W.; Sarfraz, M.B. Comparison of modified unilateral ultrasound guided subcostal transversus abdominis plane block with conventional port-site and intraperitoneal infiltration of bupivacaine for postoperative pain relief in laparoscopic cholecystectomy. *PAFMJ* **2019**, *69*, 800–807.
81. Karnik, P.P.; Dave, N.M.; Shah, H.B.; Kulkarni, K. Comparison of ultrasound-guided transversus abdominis plane (TAP) block versus local infiltration during paediatric laparoscopic surgeries. *Indian J. Anaesth.* **2019**, *63*, 356–360.
82. Khandelwal, H.; Parag, K.; Singh, A.; Anand, N.; Govil, N. Comparison of subcostal transversus abdominis block with intraperitoneal instillation of levobupivacaine for pain relief after laparoscopic cholecystectomy: A prospective study. *Anesth. Essays Res.* **2019**, *13*, 144.

83. Ribeiro, K.N.S.; Misquith, J.C.; Eapen, A.; A Naik, S. Ultrasound Guided Oblique Subcostal Transverse Abdominis Plane Block using Local Anaesthetic Versus Saline for Laparoscopic Cholecystectomies: A Randomised Controlled Trial. *J. Clin. Diagn. Res.* **2019**, *13*, 7–10.
84. Siriwardana, R.C.; Kumarage, S.K.; Gunathilake, B.M.; Thilakarathne, S.B.; Wijesinghe, J.S. Local infiltration versus laparoscopic-guided transverse abdominis plane block in laparoscopic cholecystectomy: Double-blinded randomized control trial. *Surg. Endosc.* **2019**, *33*, 179–183.
85. Wu, L.; Wu, L.; Sun, H.; Dong, C.; Yu, J. Effect of Ultrasound-Guided Peripheral Nerve Blocks of the Abdominal Wall on Pain Relief After Laparoscopic Cholecystectomy [Corrigendum]. *J. Pain Res.* **2019**, *13*, 2169–2170.
86. Arık, E.; Akkaya, T.; Ozciftci, S.; Alptekin, A.; Balas, Ş. Unilateral transversus abdominis plane block and port-site infiltration. *Der Anaesthesist* **2020**, *69*, 270–276.
87. Kharbuja, K.; Singh, J.; Ranjit, S.; Pradhan, B.B.; Shrestha, A.; Tandukar, A.; Shalike, N. Efficacy of The Subcostal Transversus Abdominis Plane Block in Laparoscopic Cholecystectomy: A Comparison with Conventional Port- Site Infiltration. *J. KIST Med. Coll.* **2020**, *2*, 42–47.
88. Liang, M.; Chen, Y.; Zhu, W.; Zhou, D. Efficacy and safety of different doses of ropivacaine for laparoscopy-assisted infiltration analgesia in patients undergoing laparoscopic cholecystectomy: A prospective randomized control trial. *Medicine* **2020**, *99*, e22540.
89. Abdelfatah, F.A.; Amin, S.R. Does esmolol infusion have an adjuvant effect on transversus abdominis plane block for pain control in laparoscopic cholecystectomy? A randomized controlled double-blind trial. *Egypt. J. Anaesth.* **2021**, *37*, 418–424.
90. Ergin, A.; Aydin, M.T.; Çiyiltepe, H.; Karip, A.B.; Fersahoğlu, M.M.; Özcabi, Y.; Ar, A.Y. Effectiveness of local anesthetic application methods in postoperative pain control in laparoscopic cholecystectomies: A randomised controlled trial. *Int. J. Surg.* **2021**, *95*, 106134.
91. Jung, J.; Jung, W.; Ko, E.Y.; Chung, Y.-H.; Koo, B.-S.; Chung, J.C.; Kim, S.-H. Impact of Bilateral Subcostal Plus Lateral Transversus Abdominis Plane Block on Quality of Recovery After Laparoscopic Cholecystectomy: A Randomized Placebo-Controlled Trial. *Anesthesia Analg.* **2021**, *133*, 1624–1632.
92. Sahu, L.; Behera, S.K.; Satapathy, G.C.; Saxena, S.; Priyadarshini, S.; Sahoo, R.K. Comparison of Analgesic Efficacy of Erector Spinae and Oblique Subcostal Transverse Abdominis Plane Block in Laparoscopic Cholecystectomy. *J. Clin. Diagn. Res.* **2021**, *15*, UC09–UC13.
93. Saravanan, R.; Venkatraman, R.; Karthika, U. Comparison of Ultrasound-Guided Modified BRILMA Block with Subcostal Transversus Abdominis Plane Block for Postoperative Analgesia in Laparoscopic Cholecystectomy—A Randomized Controlled Trial. *Local Reg. Anesth.* **2021**, *14*, 109.
94. Vindal, A.; Sarda, H.; Lal, P. Laparoscopically guided transversus abdominis plane block offers better pain relief after laparoscopic cholecystectomy: Results of a triple blind randomized controlled trial. *Surg. Endosc.* **2021**, *35*, 1713–1721.
95. Priyanka, B.G.; Krishnamurthy, P.K.D.; Rohit, S. Comparative Study of Pre-Operative Ultrasound Guided Transversus Abdominis Plane Block Versus Post-Operative Ultrasound Guided Transversus Abdominis Plane Block on Perioperative Hemodynamic Status and Post Operative Analgesic Requirement in Patients Undergoing Laparoscopic Abdominal Surgeries. *Eur. J. Mol. Clin. Med.* **2022**, *9*, 2781–2789. Available online: https://ejmcm.com/article_17726.html (accessed on 17 August 2022).
96. Emile, S.H.; Elfeki, H.; Elbahrawy, K.; Sakr, A.; Shalaby, M. Ultrasound-guided versus laparoscopic-guided subcostal transversus abdominis plane (TAP) block versus No TAP block in laparoscopic cholecystectomy: A randomized double-blind controlled trial. *Int. J. Surg.* **2022**, *101*, 106639.
97. Fargaly, O.S.; Boules, M.L.; Hamed, M.A.; Abbas, M.A.A.; Shawky, M.A. Lateral Quadratus Lumborum Block versus Transversus Abdominis Plane Block in Laparoscopic Surgery: A Randomized Controlled Study. *Anesthesiol. Res. Pract.* **2022**, *2022*, 1–6.
98. Han, K.; Zhang, Y.; Bai, R.; An, R.; Zhang, S.; Xue, M.; Shen, X. Application of Ultrasound-Guided Transversus Abdominis Plane Block Combined with Nalbuphine Patient-Controlled Intravenous Analgesia in Postoperative Analgesia After Laparotomy: A Randomized Controlled Trial. *Pain Ther.* **2022**, *11*, 627–641.
99. Lee, S.Y.; Ryu, C.G.; Koo, Y.H.; Cho, H.; Jung, H.; Park, Y.H.; Kang, H.; Lee, S.E.; Shin, H.Y. The effect of ultrasound-guided transversus abdominis plane block on pulmonary function in patients undergoing laparoscopic cholecystectomy: A prospective randomized study. *Surg. Endosc.* **2022**, *18*, 1–9.
100. Ozciftci, S.; Sahiner, Y.; Sahiner, I.T.; Akkaya, T. Is Right Unilateral Transversus Abdominis Plane (TAP) Block Successful in Postoperative Analgesia in Laparoscopic Cholecystectomy? *Int. J. Clin. Pract.* **2022**, *2022*, 2668215.
101. Paudel, B.; Paudel, S.; Rai, P.; Dahal, S.; Pokhrel, A. Comparison of Ultrasound Guided Bilateral Subcostal Transversus Abdominis Plane Block versus Local Infiltration of Port Site with Bupivacaine in Patients Undergoing Laparoscopic Cholecystectomy under General Anesthesia. *Birat J. Health Sci.* **2021**, *6*, 1642–1646.
102. Rahimzadeh, P.; Faiz, S.H.R.; Latifi-Naibin, K.; Alimian, M. A Comparison of effect of preemptive versus postoperative use of ultrasound-guided bilateral transversus abdominis plane (TAP) block on pain relief after laparoscopic cholecystectomy. *Sci. Rep.* **2022**, *12*, 1–7.
103. Mukherjee, A.; Pal, A.; Agrawal, J.; Mehrotra, A.; Dawar, N. Intrathecal nalbuphine as an adjuvant to subarachnoid block: What is the most effective dose? *Anesth. Essays Res.* **2011**, *5*, 171.
104. Kalu, R.; Boateng, P.; Carrier, L.; Garzon, J.; Tang, A.; Reickert, C.; Stefanou, A. Effect of preoperative versus postoperative use of transversus abdominis plane block with plain 0.25% bupivacaine on postoperative opioid use: A retrospective study. *BMC Anesthesiol.* **2021**, *21*, 1–6.

105. Marret, E.; Gentili, M.; Bonnet, M.P.; Bonnet, F. Intra-articular ropivacaine 0.75% and bupivacaine 0.50% for analgesia after arthroscopic knee surgery: A randomized prospective study. *Arthrosc. J. Arthrosc. Relat. Surg.* **2005**, *21*, 313–316.
106. Sinardi, D.; Marino, A.; Chillemi, S.; Siliotti, R.; Mondello, E. Sciatic nerve block with lateral popliteal approach for hallux vagus correction. Comparison between 0.5% bupivacaine and 0.75% ropivacaine. *Minerva Anestesiol.* **2004**, *70*, 625–629.
107. Martín, M.F.; Álvarez, S.L.; Herrero, M.P. Bloqueo interfascial serrato-intercostal como estrategia ahorradora de opioides en cirugía supraumbilical abierta. *Revista Española de Anestesiología y Reanimación* **2018**, *65*, 456–460.
108. Esmaoglu, A.; Yegenoglu, F.; Akin, A.; Turk, C.Y. Dexmedetomidine Added to Levobupivacaine Prolongs Axillary Brachial Plexus Block. *Anesth. Analg.* **2010**, *111*, 1548–1551.
109. Lahiri, S.; Das, S.; Basu, S.R. Effect of intraoperative esmolol infusion on postoperative analgesia in laparoscopic cholecystectomy patients: A randomised controlled trial. *J. Evol. Med. Dent. Sci.* **2015**, *4*, 14143–14152.
110. Akkaya, A.; Yıldız, İ.; Tekelioğlu, Ü.Y.; Demirhan, A.; Bayır, H.; Özlü, T.; Bilgi, M. Dexamethasone added to levobupivacaine in ultrasound-guided tranversus abdominis plain block increased the duration of postoperative analgesia after caesarean section: A randomized, double blind, controlled trial. *Eur. Rev. Med. Pharmacol. Sci.* **2014**, *18*, 717–722.
111. Kitayama, M.; Wada, M.; Hashimoto, H.; Kudo, T.; Takada, N.; Hirota, K. Effects of adding epinephrine on the early systemic absorption kinetics of local anesthetics in abdominal truncal blocks. *J. Anesth.* **2014**, *28*, 631–634.
112. Bacal, V.; Rana, U.; McIsaac, D.I.; Chen, I. Transversus Abdominis Plane Block for Post Hysterectomy Pain: A Systematic Review and Meta-Analysis. *J. Minim. Invasive Gynecol.* **2019**, *26*, 40–52.
113. Abd-Elsalam, K.A.; Fares, K.M.; Mohamed, M.A.; Mohamed, M.F.; El-Rahman, A.M.A.; Tohamy, M.M. Efficacy of Magnesium Sulfate Added to Local Anesthetic in a Transversus Abdominis Plane Block for Analgesia Following Total Abdominal Hysterectomy: A Randomized Trial. *Pain Physician.* **2017**, *20*, 641.
114. McDonnell, J.G.; Curley, G.; Carney, J.; Benton, A.; Costello, J.; Maharaj, C.H.; Laffey, J.G. The Analgesic Efficacy of Transversus Abdominis Plane Block After Cesarean Delivery: A Randomized Controlled Trial. *Anesth. Analg.* **2008**, *106*, 186–191. [CrossRef]
115. O'Donnell, B.D. The transversus abdominis plane (TAP) block in open retropubic prostatectomy. *Reg. Anesth. Pain Med.* **2006**, *31*, 91.
116. Hebbard, P.; Fujiwara, Y.; Shibata, Y.; Royse, C. Ultrasound-guided transversus abdominis plane (TAP) block. *Anaesth. Intensiv. Care* **2007**, *35*, 616–618.
117. Niraj, G.; Searle, A.; Mathews, M.; Misra, V.; Baban, M.; Kiani, S.; Wong, M. Analgesic efficacy of ultrasound-guided transversus abdominis plane block in patients undergoing open appendicectomy. *Br. J. Anaesth.* **2009**, *103*, 601–605.
118. Dean, C.; Douglas, J. Magnesium and the obstetric anaesthetist. *Int. J. Obstet. Anesth.* **2013**, *22*, 52–63.
119. Gutiérrez-Román, C.I.; Carrillo-Torres, O.; Pérez-Meléndez, E.S. Uses of magnesium sulfate in anesthesiology. *Revista Médica del Hospital General de México* **2022**, *85*, 25–33.
120. Herroeder, S.; Schoenherr, M.E.; De Hert, S.G.; Hollmann, M.W.; Warner, D.S. Magnesium—Essentials for anesthesiologists. *J. Am. Soc. Anesthesiol.* **2011**, *114*, 971–993.
121. Goyal, P.; Jaiswal, R.; Hooda, S.; Goyal, R.; Lal, J. Role of magnesium sulphate for brachial plexus analgesia. *Int. J. Anesth.* **2008**, *21*, 1.
122. Barbosa, F.T.; Barbosa, L.T.; Jucá, M.J.; da Cunha, R.M. Applications of Magnesium Sulfate in Obstetrics and Anesthesia. *Braz. J. Anesthesiol.* **2010**, *60*, 104–110.
123. Bottiger, B.A.; Esper, S.A.; Stafford-Smith, M. Pain Management Strategies for Thoracotomy and Thoracic Pain Syndromes. In *Seminars in Cardiothoracic and Vascular Anesthesia*; SAGE Publications: Los Angeles, CA, USA, 2014; Volume 18, pp. 45–56.
124. Buvanendran, A.; Kroin, J.S. Useful adjuvants for postoperative pain management. *Best Pract. Res. Clin. Anaesthesiol.* **2007**, *21*, 31–49.
125. Dabbagh, A.; Elyasi, H.; Razavi, S.S.; Fathi, M.; Rajaei, S. Intravenous magnesium sulfate for post-operative pain in patients undergoing lower limb orthopedic surgery. *Acta Anaesthesiol. Scand.* **2009**, *53*, 1088–1091.
126. Murphy, G.S.; Szokol, J.W.; Greenberg, S.B.; Avram, M.J.; Vender, J.S.; Nisman, M.; Vaughn, J. Preoperative dexamethasone enhances quality of recovery after laparoscopic cholecystectomy: Effect on in-hospital and postdischarge recovery outcomes. *J. Am. Soc. Anesthesiol.* **2011**, *114*, 882–890.
127. Milan, Z.; Tabor, D.; McConnell, P.; Pickering, J.; Kocarev, M.; du Feu, F.; Barton, S. Three different approaches to transversus abdominis plane block: A cadaveric study. *Med. Glas.* **2011**, *8*, 181–184.
128. Drager, C.; Benziger, D.; Gao, F.; Berde, C.B. Prolonged Intercostal Nerve Blockade in Sheep Using Controlled-release of Bupivacaine and Dexamethasone from Polymer Microspheres. *Anesthesiology* **1998**, *89*, 969–974.
129. Castillo, J.; Curley, J.; Hotz, J.; Uezono, M.; Tigner, J.; Chasin, M.; Wilder, R.; Langer, R.; Berde, C. Glucocorticoids Prolong Rat Sciatic Nerve Blockade In Vivo from Bupivacaine Microspheres. *Anesthesiology* **1996**, *85*, 1157–1166.
130. Sinnott, C.J.; Cogswell, L.P.; Johnson, A.; Strichartz, G.R. On the mechanism by which epinephrine potentiates lidocaine's peripheral nerve block. *J. Am. Soc. Anesthesiol.* **2003**, *98*, 181–188.
131. Eisenach, J.C.; Grice, S.C.; Dewan, D.M. Epinephrine Enhances Analgesia Produced by Epidural Bupivacaine during Labor. *Anesth. Analg.* **1987**, *66*, 447–451.
132. Chatrath, V.; Khetarpal, R.; Kumari, H.; Kaur, H.; Sharma, A. Intermittent transcutaneous electrical nerve stimulation versus transversus abdominis plane block for postoperative analgesia after infraumbilical surgeries. *Anesth. Essays Res.* **2018**, *12*, 349.

133. Chou, R.; Gordon, D.B.; de Leon-Casasola, O.A.; Rosenberg, J.M.; Bickler, S.; Brennan, T.; Carter, T.; Cassidy, C.L.; Chittenden, E.H.; Degenhardt, E.; et al. Management of Postoperative Pain: A Clinical Practice Guideline from the American Pain Society, the American Society of Regional Anesthesia and Pain Medicine, and the American Society of Anesthesiologists' Committee on Regional Anesthesia, Executive Committee, and Administrative Council. *J. Pain* **2016**, *17*, 131–157.
134. Hebbard, P.D.; Barrington, M.J.; Vasey, C. Ultrasound-guided continuous oblique subcostal transversus abdominis plane blockade: Description of anatomy and clinical technique. *Reg. Anesth. Pain Med.* **2010**, *35*, 436–441.

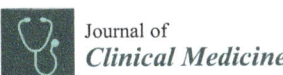

Review

Effect of Intravenous Ketamine on Hypocranial Pressure Symptoms in Patients with Spinal Anesthetic Cesarean Sections: A Systematic Review and Meta-Analysis

Xiaoshen Liang [1], Xin Yang [1], Shuang Liang [1], Yu Zhang [1], Zhuofeng Ding [1], Qulian Guo [1,2] and Changsheng Huang [1,2,*]

1. Department of Anesthesiology, Xiangya Hospital Central South University, Changsha 410008, China; 198112351@csu.edu.cn (X.L.); doctorxinyang@hotmail.com (X.Y.); liangshuang@csu.edu.cn (S.L.); zhangy20210618@163.com (Y.Z.); dzfzhuofeng@163.com (Z.D.); qulianguo@hotmail.com (Q.G.)
2. National Clinical Research Center for Geriatric Disorders, Xiangya Central South University, Changsha 410008, China
* Correspondence: changsheng.huang@csu.edu.cn; Tel./Fax: +86-731-84327413

Abstract: Background: Pregnant women are more likely to suffer post-puncture symptoms such as headaches and nausea due to the outflow of cerebrospinal fluid after spinal anesthesia. Because ketamine has the effect of raising intracranial pressure, it may be able to improve the symptoms of perioperative hypocranial pressure and effectively prevent the occurrence of hypocranial pressure-related side effects. Method: Keywords such as ketamine, cesarean section, and spinal anesthesia were searched in databases including Medline, Embase, Web of Science, and Cochrane from 1976 to 2021. Thirteen randomized controlled trials were selected for the meta-analysis. Results: A total of 12 randomized trials involving 2099 participants fulfilled the inclusion criteria. There was no significant association between ketamine and the risk of headaches compared to the placebo (RR = 1.12; 95% CI: 0.53, 2.35; $p = 0.77$; $I^2 = 62\%$). There was no significant association between ketamine and nausea compared to the placebo (RR = 0.66; 95% CI: 0.40, 1.09; $p = 0.10$; $I^2 = 57\%$). No significant associations between ketamine or the placebo and vomiting were found (RR = 0.94; 95% CI: 0.53, 1.67; $p = 0.83$; $I^2 = 72\%$). Conclusion: Intravenous ketamine does not improve the symptoms caused by low intracranial pressure after spinal anesthesia in patients undergoing cesarean section.

Keywords: cesarean section; ketamine; spinal anesthesia; intracranial hypotension; post-dural puncture headache

1. Introduction

The proportion of cesarean sections in deliveries is increasing due to the gradual maturation of birth assistance techniques and social factors [1,2]. Cesarean delivery can help pregnant women who are not allowed to deliver normally due to problems such as pelvic stenosis, uterine opening insufficiency, and placenta previa, as well as avoiding the occurrence of pelvic floor injury, urinary incontinence, vaginal relaxation and other complications caused by natural labor [3,4]. However, weight gain during pregnancy leads to subcutaneous fat thickening and unclear exposure between vertebrae, which inevitably increases the risk of spinal anesthesia and post-puncture complications [5]. Hypocranial pressure caused by cerebrospinal fluid outflow is one of the common complications after spinal anesthesia, mainly manifested as headache after dural puncture [6], especially in terms of obstetric anesthesia [7]. In addition, low intracranial pressure can cause nausea and vomiting [8]. Ketamine is known as a non-competitive, high-affinity N-methyl-D-aspartic acid (NMDA) receptor antagonist. Unlike sedative drugs such as propofol and etomidate, it also has a good analgesic effect, which has led to its common use in postoperative analgesia in patients undergoing surgery [9]. Another characteristic of ketamine is that it can increase the intracranial pressure [10,11], and by this compensatory effect, it can relieve headaches caused by low intracranial pressure [12]. However, evidence from other studies is inconsistent regarding whether ketamine reduces the incidence of headaches in patients undergoing cesarean delivery. Therefore, as evidence accumulated, we integrated relevant randomized controlled trials (RCTs) and performed a systematic review and meta-analysis to assess whether ketamine reduced the incidence of headaches in patients undergoing cesarean section under spinal anesthesia. Herein, we hypothesize that ketamine may be an effective agent for the prevention of hypocranial pressure syndrome. We hope to provide evidence for the value of ketamine in the prevention of headaches caused by low cranial pressure.

2. Materials and Methods

2.1. Search Strategy and Selection Criteria

This study was designed according to the Preferred Reporting Items for Systematic Reviews and Meta-Analyses (PRISMA) guidelines. We searched the Medline, Embase, Web of Science, and Cochrane databases from 1976 to 2021 (search strategies are detailed in Appendix A), resulting in the inclusion of 2099 patients. The search policy was designed and executed by two authors (Xing, Yang, and Shuang, Liang).

The inclusion criteria were as follows: (a) randomized controlled trial; (b) American Society of Anesthesiologists (ASA) I–II; (c) patient undergoing cesarean section with spinal anesthesia; (d) participant treated intravenously with ketamine; (e) article written in English. The exclusion criteria were as follows: (a) unpublished clinical trial; (b) full text unavailable; (c) control group received a drug other than normal saline.

2.2. Data Extraction and Quality Assessment

The data included in each study were independently extracted by two researchers and summarized in an Excel spreadsheet (Xiaoshen Liang and Yu Zhang). We extracted the following information from these studies: the first author's name, year of publication, number of patients, age, BMI (height and weight values were provided in some studies), ketamine dose, needle size, relevant outcomes (the incidence of perioperative headaches, nausea, and vomiting), and reported results. This analysis assessed the outcomes, including the incidence of perioperative headaches, nausea, and vomiting, which are clinical manifestations of low cranial pressure (Table 1). Two other investigators (Xing, Yang, and Shuang, Liang) independently evaluated the included studies according to the Cochrane Handbook for Systematic Reviews of Interventions 5.0. The specific contents of the assessment's "risk of bias" table included the following: adequate sequence generation, allocation of concealment, blinding, incomplete outcome data, free of selective reporting, and free of other bias.

2.3. Statistical Analysis

We evaluated the dichotomous data using risk ratios with 95% confidence intervals. Heterogeneity is reported using I^2 statistics; $I^2 > 50\%$ indicates significant heterogeneity. When there was significant heterogeneity between the two included studies ($p < 0.05$ or $I^2 > 50\%$), the size of the combined effect was calculated using the random-effects model; otherwise, the fixed-effects model was used. If significant heterogeneity existed, we omitted a study and instead looked for potential sources of heterogeneity. We also performed heterogeneity analysis by subgroup analysis. A leave-one-out test, consisting of calculating the pooled risk ratio by sequentially excluding one study, was performed to identify studies with a strong influence on the results. The publication bias was assessed by using funnel plots. Review Manager Version 5.3 (The Cochrane Collaboration, Software Update, Oxford, UK) was used to perform the meta-analyses. p-Values <0.05 were considered statistically significant.

Table 1. Characteristics of the included studies.

First Author	Year	Number (K; C)	Age, Years (K; C)	BMI	Height, cm (K; C)	Weight, kg (K; C)	Surgery Time, min (K; C)	Ketamine Dose (mg/kg)	Needle Size (G)	Relevant Outcomes	Reported Results (K; C)
Sen, S. et al. [13].	2005	30; 30	26.3 ± 5.3; 27.1 ± 4.6	/	162 ± 6.1; 160.0 ± 5.2	78.1 ± 7.8; 73.2 ± 9.4	41.9 ± 9.2; 48.3 ± 6.4	0.15	25	Headache, nausea	1. Headache 2; 5 2. Nausea 2; 3
Menkiti, I. D. et al. [14].	2012	28; 28	30.3 ± 4.0; 29.8 ± 3.1	/	1.64 ± 0.03; 1.61 ± 0.12	73.7 ± 6.2; 72.2 ± 5.0	56.3 ± 8.6; 55.6 ± 8.6	0.15	26	Headaches, nausea, and vomiting	1. Headaches 1; 1 2. Nausea 0; 2 3. Vomiting 2; 1
Rahmanian, M. et al. [15].	2015	80; 80	27.4 ± 4.8; 27.6 ± 4.4	/	/	78.5 ± 11.9; 77.7 ± 10.8	40.2 ± 3.8; 39.8 ± 3.2	0.25	25	Headaches, nausea, and vomiting	1. Headaches 21; 27 2. Nausea 26; 25 3. Vomiting 15; 28
Edipoglu, I. S. et al. [16].	2017	60; 60	28.68 ± 5.82; 28.43 ± 4.82	33.54 ± 4.61; 33.85 ± 4.94	/	/	27.30 ± 7.36; 27.93 ± 5.34	0.15	26	Headaches, nausea, and vomiting	1. Headaches 0; 2 2. Nausea 2; 11 3. Vomiting 2; 11
Xu, Y. et al. [17].	2017	162; 163	31 ± 4; 32 ± 4	27 ± 3; 28 ± 3	/	/	43.8 ± 14.4; 44.0 ± 12.6	0.25	25	Headaches and vomiting	1. Headaches 8; 1 2. Vomiting 7; 2
Zangouei, A. et al. [12].	2019	32; 32	/	/	/	/	/	0.15	27	Headaches	1. Headaches 10; 14
Yao, J. et al. [18].	2020	153; 155	30 ± 4; 30 ± 3	29 ± 3; 28 ± 3	/	/	/	0.25	/	Headaches	1. Headache 15; 3
Kose, E. A. et al. [19].	2013	(30 + 30); 30	[28.2 (18–43) + 26.8 (20–45)]; 27.3 (18–43)	(26.9 ± 5.9 + 26.3 ± 6.1]; 27.8 ± 6.8	/	/	68 ± 6; 71 ± 5; 65 ± 7	0.25 and 0.5	25	Nausea and vomiting	1. Nausea 10; 13 2. Vomiting 5; 6
Hassanein, A. et al. [20].	2015	45; 45	29.4 ± 7.2; 30 ± 6	/	163 ± 4; 162 ± 6.5	72 ± 9; 69 ± 13	/	0.4	25	Nausea and vomiting	1. Nausea 6; 13 2. Vomiting 4; 9
Lema, G. F. et al. [21].	2017	41; 41	26 (6); 26 (7)	/	160 (10); 160 (11)	60 (9); 60 (14)	50 (20); 45 (20)	0.2	22–25	Nausea and vomiting	1. Nausea 5; 6 2. Vomiting 5; 6
Ma, J. H. et al. [22].	2019	327; 327	/	27.5 ± 3.1; 29.4 ± 26.6	/	/	/	0.5	25	Vomiting	1. Vomiting 62; 30
Sarshivi, F. et al. [23].	2020	45; 45	30.8 (±4.5); 29.8 (±4.5)	29.4 ± 3.3; 29.1 ± 8.8	159.12 ± 4.52; 158.14 ± 4.22	68.19 ±5.48; 67.37 ± 8.12	51 (±18); 54 (±15)	0.3	25	Nausea and vomiting	1. Nausea 18; 12 2. Vomiting 14; 8

Table notes: K, ketamine group; C, control group; BMI, body mass index.

3. Results

3.1. Eligible Studies and the Characteristics

By searching the databases mentioned above, 208 studies were retrieved for the systematic review. Eighty-seven duplicate studies were excluded. After screening the titles and abstracts, only thirty studies were considered eligible for full reading. Twelve studies met all the selection criteria [12–23] as determined through browsing the titles, abstracts, and full texts (Figure 1). The included articles were published between 2005 and 2020, with sample sizes ranging from 28 to 163. All of the patients were delivered by cesarean section under spinal anesthesia and injected with ketamine intravenously at 0.15–0.5 mg/kg. The baseline characteristics of all the studies were statistically similar. The characteristics of the included randomized controlled trials are summarized below (Table 1).

Of all the included studies, three documented the incidence of postoperative headaches at different time points; the remaining studies did not explain the specific time points of occurrence. Therefore, the number with the highest incidence in these studies was chosen as the overall incidence figure based on the authors' description of the recording method. One study used two doses of ketamine compared to a placebo group, so we combined the two into one group when extracting data. In all the included articles, we could only calculate the respective totals of postoperative headaches, nausea, and vomiting in each study, as most articles did not include headaches, nausea, or vomiting as primary outcomes. Only one study [12] documented, in detail, the incidence of headaches occurring immediately postoperatively, 4 h postoperatively, 12 h postoperatively, and 24 h postoperatively. And in this study, a significant difference was found in the incidence of headaches between the ketamine and control groups in the immediate postoperative period and 4 h postoperatively, while no significant difference was found in the 12-h and 24-h postoperative periods. However, in another study [18], who recorded the incidence of headaches at 5 min postoperatively, 15 min postoperatively, and at the time of leaving the operating room, the incidence of headaches was higher in the ketamine group than in the control group.

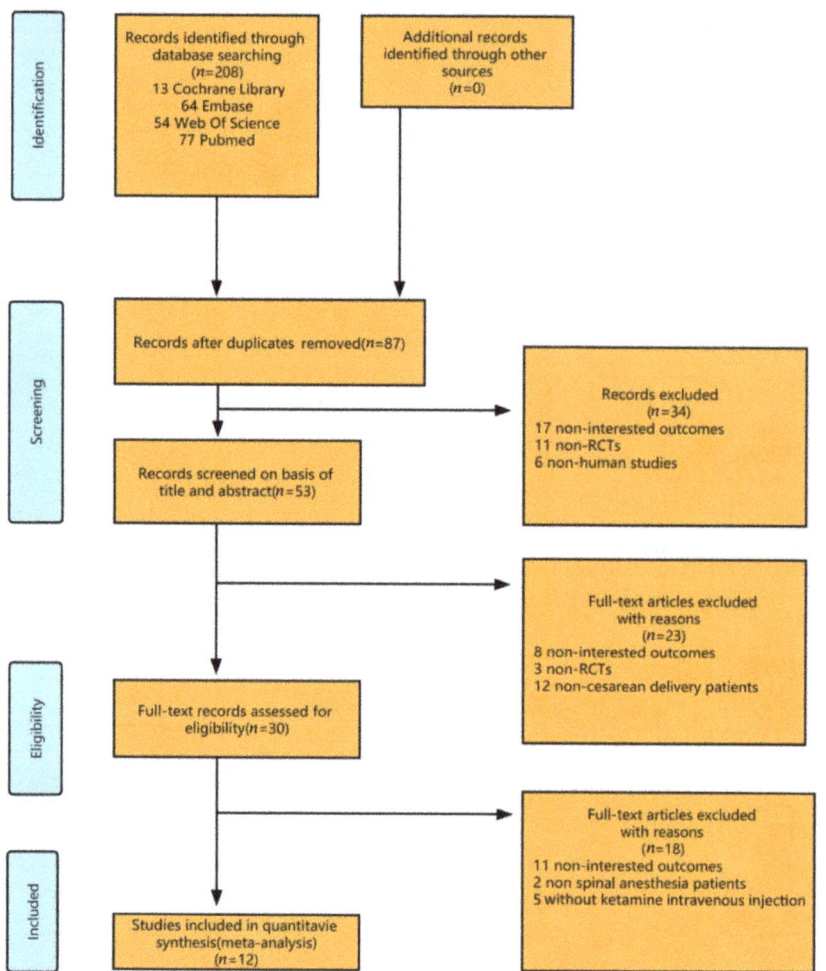

Figure 1. Flow diagram of the study selection.

3.2. Quality Assessment of the Selected Studies

The Cochrane Quality Assessment Form indicated that the majority of the studies were regarded as "low risk" or "unclear risk". The risk after consolidation is shown in Figure 2.

3.3. Effect of Interventions
3.3.1. Headaches

The incidence of postoperative headaches was assessed in this meta-analysis. Considering the significant heterogeneity ($I^2 > 50\%$), we used the random-effects model to calculate the pooled effect size. There was no significant improvement in the ketamine group compared to the placebo (RR = 1.12; 95% CI: 0.53, 2.35; p = 0.77; I^2 = 62%) (Figure 3).

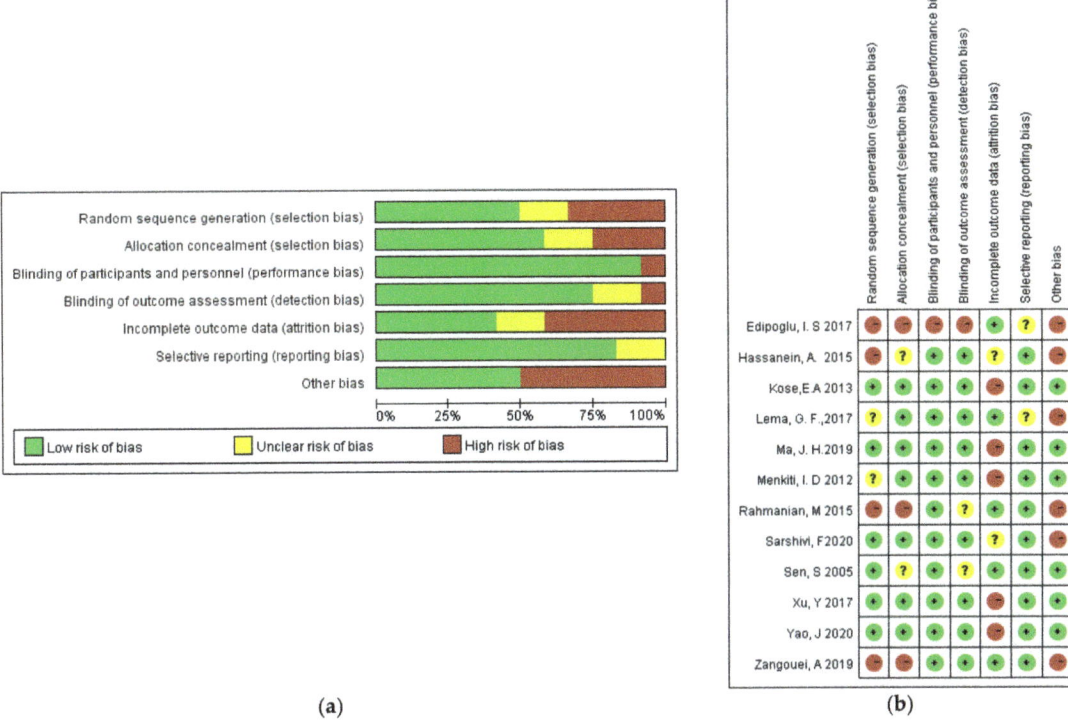

Figure 2. Risk of bias: (**a**) a summary table of the review authors' judgements for each risk of bias item for each study; (**b**) a plot of the distribution of the review authors' judgements across studies for each risk of bias item [12–23]. "+" Low risk of bias; "?" unclear risk of bias; "−" high risk of bias.

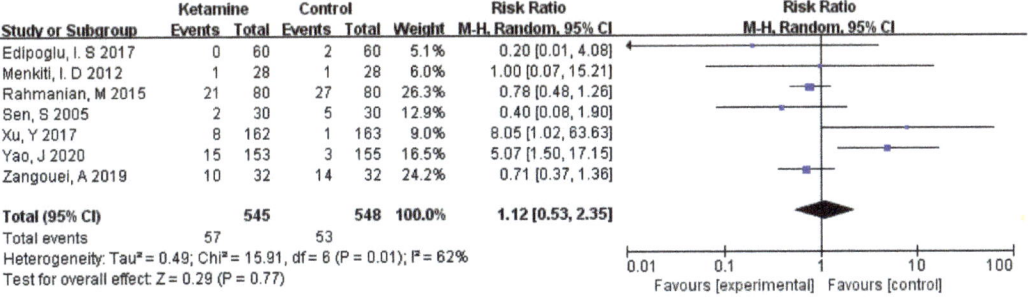

Figure 3. Forest plot of headaches [12–18].

3.3.2. Nausea

The incidence of postoperative nausea was assessed in this meta-analysis. We used the random-effects model to calculate the pooled effect size. The nausea was not significantly different between the two groups (RR = 0.66; 95% CI: 0.40, 1.09; p = 0.10; I^2 = 57%) (Figure 4).

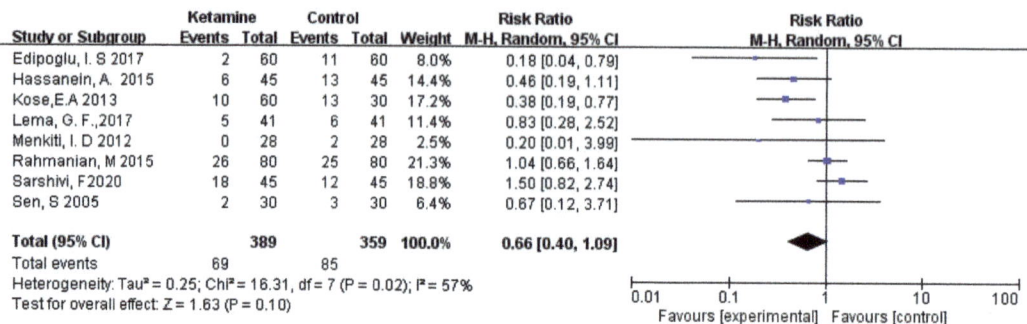

Figure 4. Forest plot of nausea [13–16,19–21,23].

3.3.3. Vomiting

The incidence of postoperative vomiting was assessed in this meta-analysis. We used the random-effects model to calculate the pooled effect size. Vomiting was not significantly different between the two groups (RR = 0.94; 95% CI: 0.53, 1.67; p = 0.83; I^2 = 72%) (Figure 5).

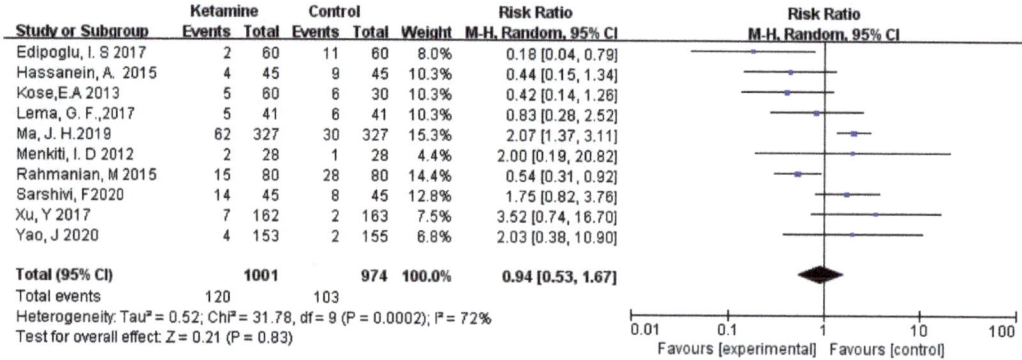

Figure 5. Forest plot of vomiting [14–23].

3.4. Subgroup Analysis

Considering that different durations of ketamine administration may be one of the important factors affecting the outcome indicators, we conducted a subgroup analysis of the included studies, which were divided into two subgroups: pre-delivery administration and post-delivery administration. However, the results of the three outcome measures did not change, and there was still no significant difference between the ketamine and control groups (Figure 6a–c).

3.5. Sensitivity Analysis and Publication Bias

In sensitivity analyses, we calculated the combined effect size by the consecutive exclusion of one study, but the indicators remained non-significantly different between the two groups, indicating that our primary estimates of headaches, nausea, and vomiting were robust. No obvious publication bias was found through the visual inspection of the funnel plots (Figure 7a–c).

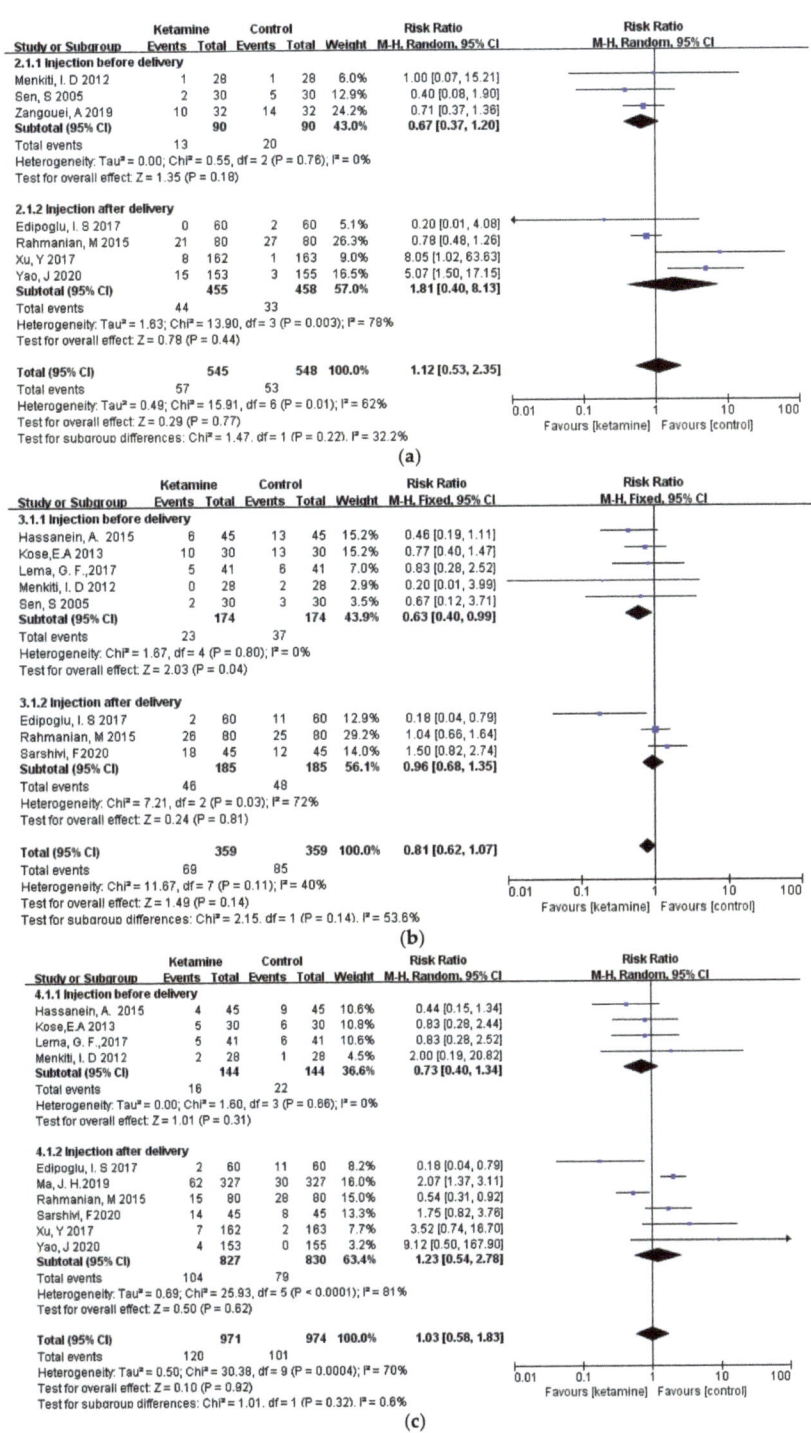

Figure 6. Forest plot of subgroups [12–23]: (**a**) headaches; (**b**) nausea; (**c**) vomiting.

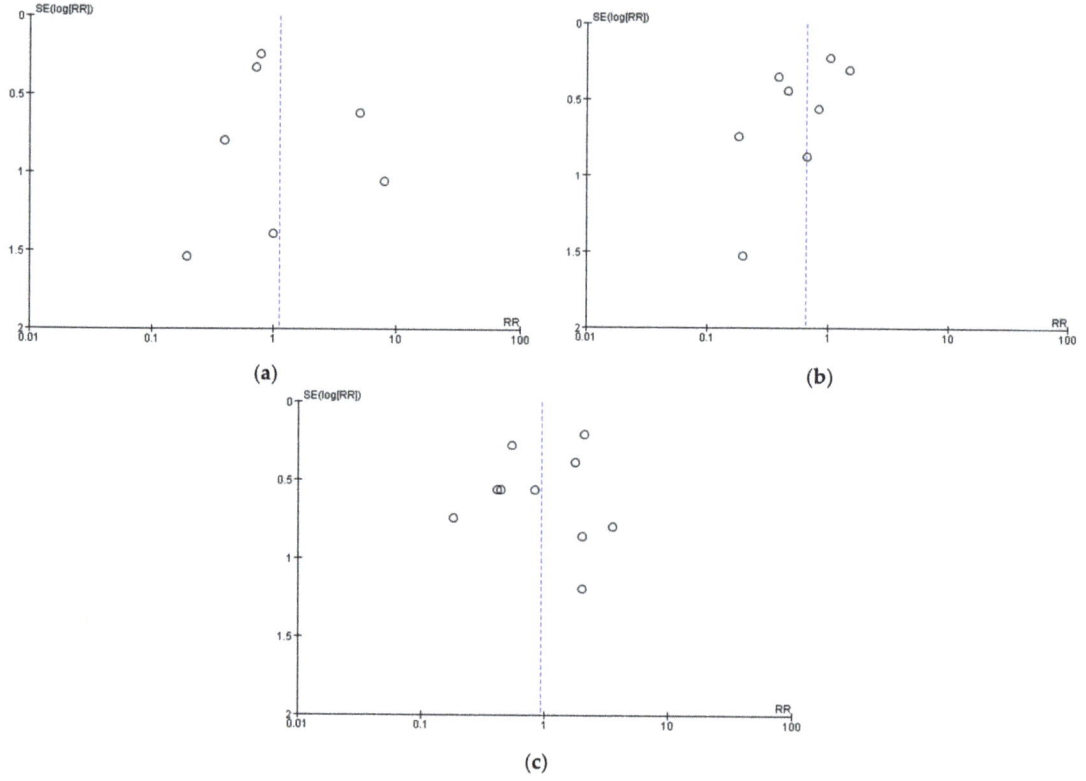

Figure 7. Funnel plot of comparison: (**a**) headaches; (**b**) nausea; (**c**) vomiting.

4. Discussion

A cesarean section is one of the most common operations in the operating room, and spinal anesthesia can provide sufficient surgical anesthesia [24]. Among the many complications of spinal anesthesia, post-dural puncture headaches are one of the more common, usually due to cerebrospinal fluid flowing out of the patient's dural puncture site [25,26]. Moreover, due to significant weight gain during pregnancy, most pregnant women have thickened subcutaneous fat, making the administration of spinal anesthesia more difficult, which also leads to an increased risk of cerebrospinal fluid outflow leading to hypocranial pressure [27,28]. Headaches are a characteristic symptom of low intracranial pressure [29], most importantly, postural headaches, accompanied by nausea and vomiting [30]. Therefore, we regard the incidence of headaches, nausea, and vomiting as an indicator for assessing the treatment of hypocranial pressure. Studies have shown that hypocranial pressure syndrome affects the prognosis and recovery of pregnant women [31]. Although different treatment modalities are available depending on the severity, including lying down, massive fluid administration, analgesic medications, and epidural blood patches [32,33], the effective prevention of PDPH is important.

Ketamine is a traditional intravenous anesthetic that not only has sympathetic excitatory effects [34], but also increases cerebral blood flow by dilating cerebral blood vessels, triggering an increase in intracranial pressure [35]. The mechanism by which ketamine increases intracranial pressure has been discerned, and it is noteworthy that ketamine can cause an increase in intracranial pressure by increasing the partial pressure of carbon dioxide and thus dilating the cerebral vasculature while preserving natural respiration [36]. Therefore, the intracranial pressure-raising effect of ketamine was allowed during spontaneous breathing in the cesarean section patients included in our study. Furthermore, although other studies have suggested that ketamine may cause a decrease in intracranial pressure [37,38] or have no significant effect on intracranial pressure [36,39,40], the prevailing view remains that ketamine has an increased effect on intracranial pressure. However, it is unclear whether this increase in intracranial pressure is sustained and whether it has associated adverse effects in the perioperative period.

In this meta-analysis, we demonstrate that intravenous ketamine does not improve headaches, nausea, and vomiting due to low cranial pressure in patients undergoing spinal anesthesia for cesarean delivery. Considering that the different time points of intravenous ketamine administration may be a key variable in this assessment, we performed a subgroup analysis with fetal delivery as the dividing line, but no difference between the ketamine and control groups was demonstrated. We concluded that the different time points of administration had no effect on the therapeutic effect of ketamine.

The main limitation of this study is that, for most of the included studies, we do not know whether the patients experienced cerebrospinal fluid leakage—this would affect our ability to accurately determine whether these patients had low cranial pressure. Thus, we could not distinguish whether the patients' headaches, nausea, and vomiting were caused by low cranial pressure or the psychiatric-related side effects of ketamine [41,42]. Therefore, based on the available evidence, we believe that ketamine (range 0.15 mg/kg to 0.5 mg/kg) is not effective in preventing hypocranial-pressure-related symptoms in patients undergoing cesarean section under spinal anesthesia. However, esketamine, with its stronger analgesic effect and fewer psychiatric side effects, has gradually replaced ketamine in clinical anesthesia [43]. This drug may be an effective agent for the prevention of hypocranial pressure.

Author Contributions: Conceptualization, X.L.; methodology, X.L.; software, X.L. and S.L.; validation, X.L., X.Y. and Y.Z.; formal analysis, X.L.; investigation, Z.D.; resources, X.L. and X.Y; data curation, X.L.; writing—original draft preparation, X.L.; writing—review and editing, X.L., X.Y. and S.L.; supervision, C.H. and Q.G.; project administration, C.H. All authors have read and agreed to the published version of the manuscript.

Funding: This research received no external funding.

Institutional Review Board Statement: Not applicable.

Informed Consent Statement: Not applicable.

Data Availability Statement: No new data were created in this study. Data sharing is not applicable to this article.

Conflicts of Interest: The authors declare no conflict of interest.

Appendix A

1. Search strategy for CENTRAL, the Cochrane Library

    #1 Mesh descriptor: [Cesarean Section] explode all trees
    #2 Mesh descriptor: [Ketamine] explode all trees
    #3 (Spinal anesthesia): ti, ab, kw OR (Epidural): ti, ab, kw
    #4 (#1 AND #2 AND #3)

2. Search strategy for web of science (OvidSP)

    #1 TS= (Ketamine OR CI-581 OR CI581 OR CI581 OR Ketalar OR Ketaset OR Ketanest OR Calipsol OR Kalipsol OR Kalipsol OR Ketamine Hydrochloride)
    #2 TS= (Cesarean section OR cesarean Sections OR Delivery, Abdominal OR Abdominal Deliveries OR Deliveries, Abdominal OR Caesarean Section OR Caesarean Sections OR Abdominal Delivery OR C-Section OR C Section OR Postcesarean Section)
    #3 TS= (Anesthesia, Epidural OR Anesthesia, Peridural OR Anesthesia, Peridural OR Peridural Anesthesia OR Peridural Anesthesia's OR Anesthesia, Extradural OR Anesthesia, Extradural OR Extradural Anesthesia OR Extradural Anesthesia's OR Epidural Anesthesia OR Anesthesias, Epidural OR Epidural Anesthesias)

#4 TS= (Anesthesia, Spinal OR Anesthesia, Spinal OR Spinal Anesthesia OR Spinal Anesthesias)
#5 '#4 OR #3'
#6 '#5 AND #2 AND #1'

3. Search strategy for Embase (OvidSP)

#1 ('controlled study': ab, ti OR random*: ab, ti OR 'trial*: ab, ti)
#2 ('ketamine'/exp)
#3 (keta*: ab, ti)
#4 (#2 AND #3)
#5 ('cesarean section'/exp)
#6 ('cesarean section*': ab, it OR deliver*: ab, it OR 'abdominal deliver*': ab, ti OR 'c section*': ab, ti OR 'postcesarean section': ab, ti OR cesarean: ab, ti)
#7 (#5 AND #6)
#8 (#1 AND #4 AND #7)

4. Search strategy for MEDLINE (OvidSP)

#1 ("ketamine"[Mesh Terms] OR "keta*"[Mesh Terms])
#2 ("cesarean section*"[Title/Abstract] OR "deliver*"[Title/Abstract] OR "abdominal deliver*"[Title/Abstract] OR "c section*"[Title/Abstract] OR "postcesarean section" [Title/Abstract] OR "cesarean section"[Mesh Terms])
#3 ("Randomized Controlled Trial"[Publication Type] OR "Controlled Clinical Trial" [Publication Type] OR "Clinical Trials as Topic"[Mesh Terms: noexp] OR "randomized" [Title/Abstract] OR "placebo" [Title/Abstract] OR "randomly"[Title/Abstract] OR "trial" [Title/Abstract]) NOT ("Animals"[Mesh Terms] NOT "Humans"[Mesh Terms])
#4 (#1 AND #2 AND #3)

References

1. Belizán, J.M.; Minckas, N.; McClure, E.M.; Saleem, S.; Moore, J.L.; Goudar, S.S.; Esamai, F.; Patel, A.; Chomba, E.; Garces, A.L.; et al. An approach to identify a minimum and rational proportion of caesarean sections in resource-poor settings: A global network study. *Lancet Glob. Health* **2018**, *6*, e894–e901. [CrossRef]
2. Stjernholm, Y.; Petersson, K.; Eneroth, E. Changed indications for cesarean sections. *Acta Obstet. Gynecol. Scand.* **2010**, *89*, 49–53. [CrossRef] [PubMed]
3. Gregory, K.D.; Curtin, S.C.; Taffel, S.M.; Notzon, F.C. Changes in indications for cesarean delivery: United States, 1985 and 1994. *Am. J. Public Health* **1998**, *88*, 1384–1387. [CrossRef]
4. Mylonas, I.; Friese, K. Indications for and Risks of Elective Cesarean Section. *Dtsch. Arztebl. Int.* **2015**, *112*, 489–495. [CrossRef] [PubMed]
5. Butwick, A.; Carvalho, B.; Danial, C.; Riley, E. Retrospective analysis of anesthetic interventions for obese patients undergoing elective cesarean delivery. *J. Clin. Anesth.* **2010**, *22*, 519–526. [CrossRef]
6. Ferede, Y.A.; Nigatu, Y.A.; Agegnehu, A.F.; Mustofa, S.Y. Incidence and associated factors of post dural puncture headache after cesarean section delivery under spinal anesthesia in University of Gondar Comprehensive Specialized Hospital, 2019, cross sectional study. *Int. J. Surg. Open* **2021**, *33*, 100348. [CrossRef]
7. Gaiser, R.R. Postdural Puncture Headache: An Evidence-Based Approach. *Anesthesiol. Clin.* **2017**, *35*, 157–167. [CrossRef] [PubMed]
8. D'Antona, L.; Merchan MA, J.; Vassiliou, A.; Watkins, L.D.; Davagnanam, I.; Toma, A.K.; Matharu, M.S. Clinical Presentation, Investigation Findings, and Treatment Outcomes of Spontaneous Intracranial Hypotension Syndrome: A Systematic Review and Meta-analysis. *JAMA Neurol.* **2021**, *78*, 329–337. [CrossRef] [PubMed]
9. Porter, S.B. Perioperative ketamine for acute analgesia and beyond. *Rom. J. Anaesth. Intensiv. Care* **2019**, *26*, 67–73.
10. Gardner, A.; Olson, B.; Lichtiger, M.J.A. Cerebrospinal-fluid pressure during dissociative anesthesia with ketamine. *Anesthesiology* **1971**, *35*, 226–228. [CrossRef]
11. Wyte, S.; Shapiro, H.M.; Turner, P.; Harris, A.B. Ketamine-induced intracranial hypertension. *Anesthesiology* **1972**, *36*, 174–176. [CrossRef] [PubMed]
12. Zangouei, A.; Zahraei, S.A.H.; Sabertanha, A.; Nademi, A.; Golafshan, Z.; Zangoue, M. Effect of low-dose intravenous ketamine on prevention of headache after spinal anesthesia in patients undergoing elective cesarean section: A double-blind clinical trial study. *Anesthesiol. Pain Med.* **2019**, *9*, e97249. [CrossRef]
13. Sen, S.; Ozmert, G.; Aydin, O.N.; Baran, N.; Calskan, E. The persisting analgesic effect of low-dose intravenous ketamine after spinal anaesthesia for caesarean section. *Eur. J. Anaesthesiol.* **2005**, *22*, 518–523. [CrossRef] [PubMed]

14. Menkiti, I.D.; Desalu, I.; Kushimo, O.T. Low-dose intravenous ketamine improves postoperative analgesia after caesarean delivery with spinal bupivacaine in African parturients. *Int. J. Obstet. Anesth.* **2012**, *21*, 217–221. [CrossRef] [PubMed]
15. Rahmanian, M.; Leysi, M.; Hemmati, A.A.; Mirmohammadkhani, M. The effect of low-dose intravenous ketamine on postoperative pain following cesarean section with spinal anesthesia: A randomized clinical trial. *Oman Med. J.* **2015**, *30*, 11–16. [CrossRef]
16. Edipoglu, I.S.; Celik, F.S.; Omaygenc, D.O. Perioperative low-dose ketamine diminishes post-operative caesarean pain, nausea & vomiting after spinal anaesthesia. *J. Istanb. Fac. Med.-Istanb. Tip Fak. Derg.* **2017**, *80*, 7–12.
17. Xu, Y.; Li, Y.; Huang, X.; Chen, D.; She, B.; Ma, D. Single bolus low-dose of ketamine does not prevent postpartum depression: A randomized, double-blind, placebo-controlled, prospective clinical trial. *Arch. Gynecol. Obstet.* **2017**, *295*, 1167–1174. [CrossRef]
18. Yao, J.; Song, T.; Zhang, Y.; Guo, N.; Zhao, P. Intraoperative ketamine for reduction in postpartum depressive symptoms after cesarean delivery: A double-blind, randomized clinical trial. *Brain Behav.* **2020**, *10*, e01715. [CrossRef]
19. Kose, E.A.; Honca, M.; Dal, D.; Akinci, S.B.; Aypar, U. Prophylactic ketamine to prevent shivering in parturients undergoing Cesarean delivery during spinal anesthesia. *J. Clin. Anesth.* **2013**, *25*, 275–280. [CrossRef]
20. Hassanein, A.; Mahmoud, E. Effect of low dose ketamine versus dexamethasone on intraoperative nausea and vomiting during cesarean section under spinal anesthesia. *Egypt. J. Anaesth.* **2015**, *31*, 59–63. [CrossRef]
21. Lema, G.F.; Gebremedhn, E.G.; Gebregzi, A.H.; Desta, Y.T.; Kassa, A.A. Efficacy of intravenous tramadol and low-dose ketamine in the prevention of post-spinal anesthesia shivering following cesarean section: A double-blinded, randomized control trial. *Int. J. Womens Health* **2017**, *9*, 681–688. [CrossRef] [PubMed]
22. Ma, J.H.; Wang, S.-Y.; Yu, H.-Y.; Li, D.-Y.; Luo, S.-C.; Zheng, S.-S.; Wan, L.-F.; Duan, K.-M. Prophylactic use of ketamine reduces postpartum depression in Chinese women undergoing cesarean section. *Psychiatry Res.* **2019**, *279*, 252–258. [CrossRef] [PubMed]
23. Sarshivi, F.; Ghaderi, E.; Sarshivi, A.; Shami, S.; Nasseri, K. Intravenous ketamine for the prevention of post anesthetic shivering in spinal anesthesia: A randomized double-blind placebo-controlled trial. *Acta Med. Iran.* **2020**, *58*, 479–485. [CrossRef]
24. Sachs, A.; Smiley, R. Post-dural puncture headache: The worst common complication in obstetric anesthesia. *Semin. Perinatol.* **2014**, *38*, 386–394. [CrossRef]
25. Grände, P.O. Mechanisms behind postspinal headache and brain stem compression following lumbar dural puncture—A physiological approach. *Acta Anaesthesiol. Scand.* **2005**, *49*, 619–626. [CrossRef] [PubMed]
26. Davignon, K.R.; Dennehy, K.C. Update on postdural puncture headache. *Int. Anesthesiol. Clin.* **2002**, *40*, 89–102. [CrossRef]
27. Antoine, C.; Young, B.K. Cesarean section one hundred years 1920–2020: The Good, the Bad and the Ugly. *J. Perinat. Med.* **2020**, *49*, 5–16. [CrossRef]
28. Kuntz, K.; Kokmen, E.; Stevens, J.C.; Miller, P.; Offord, K.P.; Ho, M.M. Post-lumbar puncture headaches: Experience in 501 consecutive procedures. *Neurology* **1992**, *42*, 1884. [CrossRef]
29. Brownridge, P. The management of headache following accidental dural puncture in obstetric patients. *Anaesth. Intensiv. Care* **1983**, *11*, 4–15. [CrossRef]
30. Haider, A.; Sulhan, S.; Watson, I.T.; Leonard, D.; Arrey, E.N.; Khan, U.; Nguyen, P.; Layton, K.F. Spontaneous Intracranial Hypotension Presenting as a "Pseudo-Chiari 1". *Cureus* **2017**, *9*, e1034. [CrossRef]
31. Angle, P.; Thompson, D.; Szalai, J.P.; Tang, S.L.T. Expectant management of postdural puncture headache increases hospital length of stay and emergency room visits. *Can. J. Anaesth.* **2005**, *52*, 397–402. [CrossRef] [PubMed]
32. International Headache Society. Headache classification subcommittee of the international headache society. *Cephalgia* **2004**, *24*, 9–160.
33. Ahmed, S.; Jayawarna, C.; Jude, E. Post lumbar puncture headache: Diagnosis and management. *Postgrad. Med. J.* **2006**, *82*, 713–716. [CrossRef] [PubMed]
34. Dakwar, E.; Levin, F.; Foltin, R.W.; Nunes, E.V.; Hart, C.L. The Effects of Subanesthetic Ketamine Infusions on Motivation to Quit and Cue-Induced Craving in Cocaine-Dependent Research Volunteers. *Biol. Psychiatry* **2014**, *76*, 40–46. [CrossRef] [PubMed]
35. Sari, A.; Okuda, Y.; Takeshita, H. The effect of ketamine on cerebrospinal fluid pressure. *Anesth. Analg.* **1972**, *51*, 560–565. [CrossRef]
36. Himmelseher, S.; Durieux, M.E. Revising a dogma: Ketamine for patients with neurological injury? *Anesth. Analg.* **2005**, *101*, 524–534. [CrossRef]
37. Zeiler, F.; Teitelbaum, J.; West, M.; Gillman, L.M. The ketamine effect on intracranial pressure in nontraumatic neurological illness. *J. Crit. Care* **2014**, *29*, 1096–1106. [CrossRef]
38. Godoy, D.; Badenes, R.; Pelosi, P.; Robba, C. Ketamine in acute phase of severe traumatic brain injury "an old drug for new uses?". *Crit. Care* **2021**, *25*, 19. [CrossRef]
39. Albanese, J.; Arnaud, S.; Rey, M.; Thomachot, L.; Alliez, B.; Martin, C. Ketamine decreases intracranial pressure and electroencephalographic activity in traumatic brain injury patients during propofol sedation. *Anesthesiology* **1997**, *87*, 1328–1334. [CrossRef]
40. Cohen, L.; Athaide, V.; Wickham, M.E.; Doyle-Waters, M.M.; Rose, N.G.; Hohl, C.M. The effect of ketamine on intracranial and cerebral perfusion pressure and health outcomes: A systematic review. *Ann. Emerg. Med.* **2015**, *65*, 43–51.e2. [CrossRef]
41. Morgan, C.J.; Mofeez, A.; Brandner, B.; Bromley, L.; Curran, H.V. Acute effects of ketamine on memory systems and psychotic symptoms in healthy volunteers. *Neuropsychopharmacology* **2004**, *29*, 208–218. [CrossRef] [PubMed]

42. Wan, L.B.; Levitch, C.F.; Perez, A.M.; Brallier, J.W.; Iosifescu, D.V.; Chang, L.C.; Foulkes, A.; Mathew, S.J.; Charney, D.S.; Murrough, J.W. Ketamine safety and tolerability in clinical trials for treatment-resistant depression. *J. Clin. Psychiatry* **2015**, *76*, 247–252. [CrossRef] [PubMed]
43. Wang, J.; Huang, J.; Yang, S.; Cui, C.; Ye, L.; Wang, S.-Y.; Yang, G.-P.; Pei, Q. Pharmacokinetics and Safety of Esketamine in Chinese Patients Undergoing Painless Gastroscopy in Comparison with Ketamine: A Randomized, Open-Label Clinical Study. *Drug. Des. Dev. Ther.* **2019**, *13*, 4135–4144. [CrossRef] [PubMed]

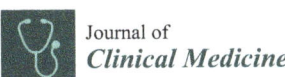

Article

No Gender Differences in Pain Perception and Medication after Lumbar Spine Sequestrectomy—A Reanalysis of a Randomized Controlled Clinical Trial

Christa K. Raak [1,2,*], Thomas Ostermann [3], Anna-Li Schönenberg-Tu [2], Oliver Fricke [1,4], David D. Martin [1], Sibylle Robens [3] and Wolfram Scharbrodt [1,2]

1. Institute of Integrative Medicine, Witten/Herdecke University, 58313 Herdecke, Germany; o.fricke@gemeinschaftskrankenhaus.de (O.F.); david.martin@uni-wh.de (D.D.M.); w.scharbrodt@gemeinschaftskrankenhaus.de (W.S.)
2. Integrative Neuromedicine, Community Hospital Herdecke, Witten/Herdecke University, 58313 Herdecke, Germany; anna_tu@gmx.de
3. Department of Psychology and Psychotherapy, Witten/Herdecke University, 58448 Witten, Germany; thomas.ostermann@uni-wh.de (T.O.); sibylle.robens@uni-wh.de (S.R.)
4. Department of Child and Adolescent Psychiatry, Psychotherapy and Child Neurology, Witten/Herdecke University, 58313 Herdecke, Germany
* Correspondence: christa.raak@uni-wh.de

Abstract: Background: Gender issues have received increasing attention in clinical research of the past years, and biological sex has been introduced as a moderating variable in experimental pain perception. However, in clinical studies of acute pain and gender, there are conflicting results. In particular, there are limited data on the impact of gender differences after spinal sequestrectomy. The aim of this work is to examine gender differences in postoperative pain and pain medication consumption in an inpatient clinical setting. Methods: Data of a completed double-blind RCT was subdivided by gender and reanalyzed by means of an analysis of variance in repeated measures. Outcomes included pain severity measured on a VAS, affective (SES-A) and sensory pain perception (SES-S) and morphine equivalent doses (MED) of analgesics after spinal sequestrectomy. Results: In total, 42 female (47.73%) and 46 male (52.27%) patients were analyzed. No differences in pain severity (VAS: Gender × Time F = 0.35; (df = 2, 86); $p = 0.708$), affective and sensory pain perception (SES-A: Gender × Time F = 0.08; (df = 2, 86); $p = 0.919$; SES-S: Gender × Time F = 0.06; (df = 2, 86); $p = 0.939$) or post-operative opioid use between men and women (MEDs: Gender × Time F = 1.44; (df = 2, 86); $p = 0.227$) could be observed. Conclusions: This reanalysis of an RCT with respect to gender differences is to our knowledge the first attempt to investigate the role of gender in pain perception and medication after lumbar spine sequestrectomy. In contrast to other studies, we were not able to show significant differences between male and female patients in all pain-related outcomes. Apart from well-established pain management, psychological reasons such as gender-specific response biases or the observer effect might explain our results. Trial registration: The study was registered as a regulatory phase IV study at the German Clinical Trials Register (DRKS), an open-access online register for clinical trials conducted in Germany (Reg-No: DRKS00007913).

Keywords: gender differences; clinical trial; lumbar sequestrectomy; postoperative pain

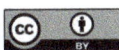

1. Introduction

According to recent statistics, the incidence of disc herniation is 5 to 20 cases per 1000 adults per year [1]. It is most common in people in their third to fifth decade of life, with a male-to-female ratio of 2:1. The approximate prevalence is about 1–3 percent of patients for symptomatic herniated discs of the lumbar spine [2]. In such cases, lumbar spine surgery is one of the most common procedures in the Western world. According to several studies and systematic reviews, there has been a rising trend in the total number of surgical interventions by 71% since 2007 in Germany [3].

Gender-specific perception of pain has been discussed frequently and has gained increasing attention in pain research in recent years [4]. Differences between women and men in pain appear to be related to both sex and gender. In abbreviated terms, the word "sex" refers to differences in human anatomy, physiology or organ systems, and the word "gender" refers to psychosocial interactions [5]. Most pain conditions have a higher prevalence in women, and women report more severe pain, longer pain duration and more frequent pain [6]. Studies have shown that female patients have higher pain intensity and require higher doses of opioids compared to male patients in the immediate postoperative period to achieve a similar level of analgesia [7]. In a brief review, Pieretti et al. examined literature on sex differences in experimental and clinical pain, focusing on biological mechanisms that have been suggested to be responsible for the observed sex differences. They found that biological factors such as sex hormones are considered to be one of the main mechanisms explaining differences in pain sensitivity in males and females [8].

Although gender differences in pain perception is a current research topic, little is known about its role in the field of degenerative diseases of the lumbar spine. Given these challenges, Maclean et al. [9] recently conducted a scoping review to map and synthesize the adult surgical literature regarding gender differences in pre- and postoperative patient-reported clinical assessment scores for patients diagnosed with lumbar degenerative disease. Postoperatively, female patients showed worse absolute pain, disability and quality of life, but showed equal or greater interval change compared with men [9]. Several clinical studies observed higher analgesic consumption after lumbar surgery in women than in men [10–12]. Most authors, however, conclude that further studies are needed to investigate gender differences in the effects of spine surgery.

Hence, we aimed at reanalyzing a recently conducted randomized, controlled clinical trial of patients undergoing elective, monosegmental, lumbar sequestrectomy [13] with respect to gender differences in pain perception, severity and pain medication use.

2. Materials and Methods

The original study was a regulatory, randomized controlled trial of phase IV, comparing additional treatment with potentized *Hypericum perforatum* to standard pain medication alone. The study was approved by the local ethics committee and the Federal Institute for Drugs and Medical Devices (BfArM, Bonn, Germany, EudraCT–No.: 2013-001383-31) [14].

2.1. Patients

A total of 114 study participants were recruited from November 2015 to August 2018 from patients receiving a monosegmental spinal sequestrectomy due to a lumbar disc herniation at the Department of Neurosurgery at the Community Hospital Herdecke. Of those, twelve patients were excluded and thus, a total of 88 patients were eligible for statistical analysis. Of those, two did not meeting inclusion criteria, ten declined to participate, twelve did not receive allocated intervention and two patients were excluded for other reasons. Thus, a total of 88 patients were included for statistical analysis. Figure 1 provides a flow chart of the patients included in the study.

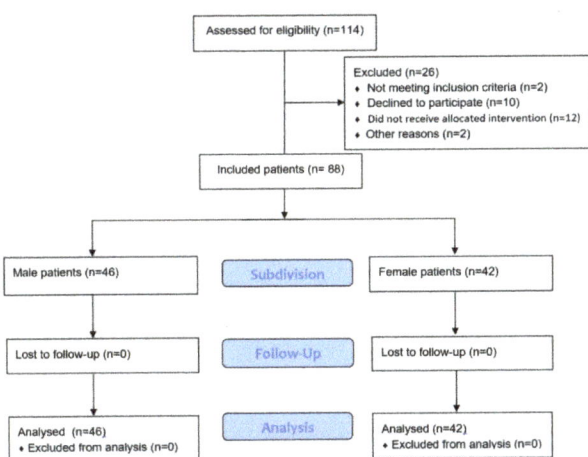

Figure 1. Flow chart of the patients included in the study.

2.2. Pain Medication and Outcomes

Patients were followed several times per day for their pain perception and medication use during their hospital stay. Standard pain medication included Ibuprofen and Metamizole, and in less frequent cases, Oxycodone, Tilidine or Tapentadol. If necessary, patients in few cases also received Morphine, Piritramide or Tramadol. Their number and dosages (mg) were extracted from the medical record folder and converted to morphine-equivalent doses (MEDs) in accordance with other trials on analgesic intake [13].

Pain perception was measured on a 100-mm visual analog scale (VAS) four times each day and then averaged for further evaluation. In addition, the German Version of the Pain Perception Scale introduced by Geissner was used to access the dimensions of "Affective Pain" (SES-A) and "Sensory Pain" (SES-S). The SES was scored at baseline and during postoperative study visits on days one, three and five [15].

2.3. Statistical Analysis

Baseline summary data of the total study population subdivided by gender were calculated using descriptive analyses and univariate statistics. To test for gender differences in pain management and perception, outcomes were modeled as a function of gender, duration of surgery and pain intensity at baseline within an ANOVA, including days after surgery as repeated measures (SAS-procedure PROC MIXED). A two-tailed error probability of $\alpha = 5\%$ was used to test for gender differences. Results were reported using mean values and standard deviations for sample description and 95% confidence intervals for inferential statistics.

3. Results

In total, 42 female (47.73%) and 46 male (52.27%) patients were analyzed.

No significant differences were observed between the groups at baseline: female patients were aged between 25 and 82 years with a mean of 52.74 ± 12.85 years while male patients were aged between 18 and 79 years and on average 1.25 years younger (50.5 ± 14.42 years). Duration of surgery for all patients was about one hour (64.70 ± 24.73 min) without being significantly different between female (60.83 ± 23.35 min) and male (68.24 ± 25.66 min) patients. Body mass index also did not differ between females (26.93 ± 5.01) and males (28.02 ± 4.30). With respect to the indication of operation, an equal majority of the patients ($n = 34$, 38.6%) were diagnosed with a herniated disc at lumbar segments L5–S1 and L4–L5, followed by L3–L4 in 14 cases (15.9%), L2–L3 in 5 cases (5.7%) and in one case, L1–L2 (1.1%). As shown in Table 1, there was no significant difference in the distribution of affected lumbar segments between male and female patients. Also, the affected side did not significantly differ between male and female patients ($p = 0.741$): in 15 female (35.7%) and 18 male patients (39.1%) the right side was affected, while the left side was affected in 27 female patients (64.3%) and 28 male patients (60.9%). In two cases (one female, one male) the location according to the classification given in [16] was exclusively intraforaminal, while in one male patient, the location was intra-extraforaminal. Table 1 summarizes the sociodemographic data, anatomical location and surgical duration.

Table 1. Sociodemographics subdivided by gender.

	Total $n = 88$	Female $n = 42$	Male $n = 46$	p-Value
Age (years)				
n	88	42	46	
M ± SD	51.57 ± 13.66	52.74 ± 12.85	50.5 ± 14.42	0.446
Median	53	53.5	53	
Minimum	18	25	18	
Maximum	82	82	79	
Surgery duration				
n	88	42	46	
M ± SD	64.70 ± 24.73	60.83 ± 23.35	68.24 ± 25.66	0.162
Median	60	57.5	65	
Minimum	26	26	33	
Maximum	158	158	133	
BMI				
n	86	42	44	
M ± SD	27.48 ± 4.67	26.93 ± 5.01	28.02 ± 4.30	0.283
Median	27.05	25.31	28.54	
Minimum	19.13	19.13	19.15	
Maximum	40.09	40.09	38.58	
Level of disc herniation				
n	88	42	46	
L1–L2	1 (1.1%)	1 (2.4%)	0 (0.0%)	
L2–L3	5 (5.7%)	2 (4.8%)	3 (6.5%)	
L3–L4	14 (15.9%)	7 (16.7%)	7 (15.2%)	0.828
L4–L5	34 (38.6%)	17 (40.5%)	17 (37.0%)	
L5–S1	34 (38.6%)	15 (35.7%)	19 (41.3%)	
Side				
n	88	42	46	
right	33 (37.5%)	15 (35.7%)	18 (39.1%)	0.741
left	55 (62.5%)	27 (64.3%)	28 (60.9%)	
Location				
n	88	42	46	
exclusively intraforaminal	2 (2.3%)	1 (2.4%)	1 (2.2%)	
intra-extraforaminal	1 (1.1%)	0 (0.0%)	1 (2.2%)	0.629
intraspinal	85 (96.6%)	41 (97.6%)	44 (95.6%)	

3.1. Pain Severity

Figure 2 shows the development of the pain severity as measured with a VAS over the entire inpatient period. Regardless of gender, a clear decrease in pain perception by about 60% from 6.21 ± 2.59 at hospital admission to 2.46 ± 2.52 at day 5 was observed without being significantly different between gender in the complete course of time (ANOVA: Gender × Time $F = 0.35$; (df = 2, 86); $p = 0.708$) and for each of the single time points (p between 0.412 and 0.983).

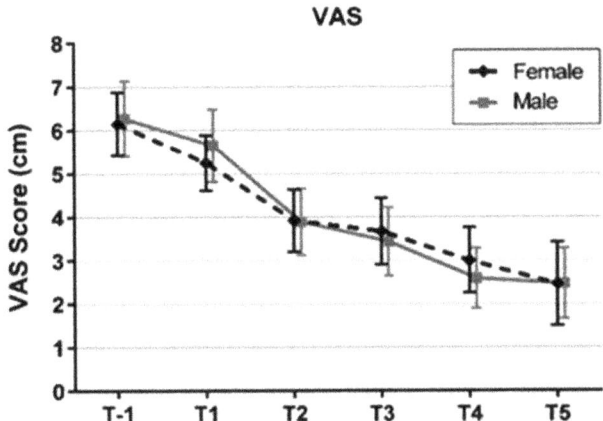

Figure 2. Means and 95% confidence intervals of pain severity from hospital admission (T-1) to day 5 (T5) by gender (VAS: visual analogue scale).

3.2. Affective and Sensory Pain Perception

Data on affective (SES-A) and sensory pain perception (SES-S) are provided in Tables 2 and 3.

Table 2. Affective pain perception (SES-A) from hospital admission (T-1) to day 5 after operation (T5). p-values of t-test comparisons between men and women.

SES-A		Total $n = 88$	Female $n = 42$	Male $n = 46$	t-Test p-Value
T-1	n	88	42	46	
	M ± SD	35.60 ± 11.50	36.71 ± 12.32	34.59 ± 10.74	0.389
	Median	36.00	40.00	35.50	
T1	n	88	42	46	
	M ± SD	24.30 ± 10.43	24.14 ± 10.24	24.43 ± 10.71	0.897
	Median	20.00	20.00	20.50	
T3	n	87	42	45	
	M ± SD	20.55 ± 8.61	20.14 ± 9.38	20.93 ± 7.92	0.671
	Median	17.00	16.50	18.00	
T5	n	37	19	18	
	M ± SD	22.81 ± 10.75	22.53 ± 11.15	23.11 ± 10.62	0.871
	Median	18.00	17.00	18.50	

Table 3. Sensory pain perception (SES-S) from hospital admission (T-1) to day 5 after operation (T5). p-values of t-test comparisons between men and women.

SES-S		Total $n = 88$	Female $n = 42$	Male $n = 46$	t-Test p-Value
T-1	n	87	41	46	
	M ± SD	21.10 ± 7.55	21.29 ± 7.35	20.93 ± 7.80	0.827
	Median	20.00	20.00	19.50	
T1	n	86	41	45	
	M ± SD	16.51 ± 6.70	16.63 ± 6.59	16.40 ± 6.88	0.873
	Median	14.50	14.00	15.00	
T3	n	86	42	44	
	M ± SD	14.06 ± 5.23	14.00 ± 5.06	14.11 ± 5.44	0.920
	Median	12.00	12.00	12.00	
T5	n	37	19	18	
	M ± SD	15.32 ± 6.21	15.32 ± 5.53	15.33 ± 7.02	0.993
	Median	13.00	14.00	13.00	

In both groups there was a significant reduction in sensory pain perception, which resulted in almost identical values for affective pain perception (22.53 ± 11.15 in female patients and 23.11 ± 10.62 in male patients) and sensory pain perception (15.32 ± 5.53 in female patients and 15.33 ± 7.02 in male patients) on day five. Again, the linear mixed model did not reveal any significant differences in the course of time between the groups (ANOVA SES-A: Gender × Time F = 0.08; (df = 2, 86); p = 0.919; SES-S: Gender × Time F = 0.06; (df = 2, 86); p = 0.939).

3.3. Pain Medication

Pain medication measured in MEDs increased from 129.94 ± 155.46 mg MED at admission to 149.97 ± 151.95 mg MED on day one and a maximum of 171.02 ± 148.16 mg MED on day 2 for all patients. Subdivided by gender pain medication showed an almost identical course in women and men, however, MEDs in men except for day three were always below the MEDs of the female patients (Figure 3) but without being significant (ANOVA: Gender × Time F = 1.44; (df = 2, 86); p = 0.227).

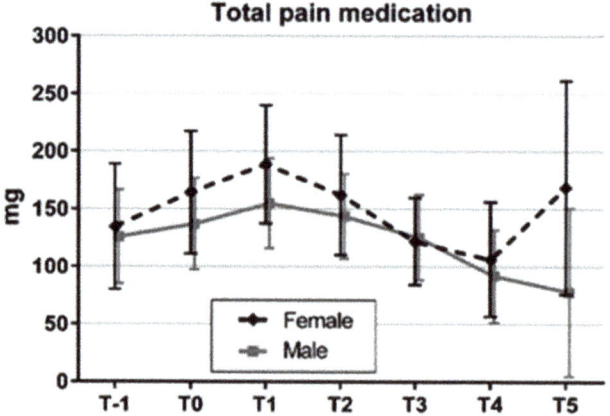

Figure 3. Means and 95% confidence intervals of total pain medication from hospital admission (T-1) to day 5 (T5) by gender.

This is also reflected in the statistical analysis of the total amount of medication in the inpatient period subdivided by gender. Although there is a lower amount of medication in men, the difference is not significant (p = 0.47; Table 4).

Table 4. Total amount of medication in mg MED from day 1 to day 5 after operation by gender.

	Total n = 88	Female n = 42	Male n = 46	t-Test
Sum of day 1 to day 5 Medication	Mean (SD) 569.57 (543.78)	Mean (SD) 614.09 (596.95)	Mean (SD) 528.92 (498.42)	p-value 0.47

4. Discussion

This reanalysis of an RCT with respect to gender differences is to our knowledge the first attempt to investigate the role of gender in pain perception and medication after lumbar spine sequestrectomy. Clinical and anatomical data of our study i.e., data on the level of disc herniation, side and location is in accordance with published data provided in [16–18]. No significant differences were observed between the groups at baseline in terms of age, pain medication, duration of operation and body mass index, which, in terms of preoperative opioid use, is in accordance with [19]. We were able to show that there were no differences between male and female patients for all pain-related outcomes.

Remarkably, pain medication consumption showed an almost identical course in women and men, however, MEDs in men except for day three were always below the MEDs of the female patients but without being significant, in agreement with the results of [20]. The same is seen in the total amount of medication consumption: a lower amount of medication in men, but the difference is not significant, which contrasts with the results of [21] but is in line with the results of [22].

As mentioned in the introduction, most studies examining pain and gender differences find worse outcomes for women. Studies have shown this effect in both pre- and postoperative acute pain settings [8,23], which was also shown by a number of studies from the field of gender differences in surgical management of lumbar degenerative disease [9,24]. In another study of Strömquist et al. (2016) on preoperative data from 15,631 patients who underwent lumbar disc herniation surgery between 2000 and 2010, women were reported to have worse clinical status than men [11]. The study, however, found no evidence-based data to support this difference, and the reason for this finding remained unclear. Part of the explanation for the differences between men and women could be physical constitution, which leads to different biomechanical properties [25].

Sex hormones are often listed as influencing factors for gender differences, in addition to endogenous opioid activation, neurochemical mechanisms or differences in neuroimmunology and genetic factors matter [26,27]. Possible biopsychosocial and psychosocial factor mechanisms underlying sex differences in pain need to be discussed.

The prevalence of chronic low back pain is higher in women than men and increases linearly from the third decade of life to age 60 [28]. Therefore, women are more likely to experience clinical pain symptoms, and they show increased pain sensitivity in experimental pain studies [29].

Finally, these findings may simply reflect gender-specific response biases. Men underreport pain and/or women overreport pain. Humans of different genders also differ in pain management strategies. Male patients tend to prefer problem-solving and instrumental strategies, whereas female patients are more likely to seek social support and tend to focus more on emotional aspects of the pain situation [29,30]. In addition, depression and anxiety are also often associated with physical pain, with a higher prevalence in women [31].

A systematic literature review found that a so-called observer effect often influences studies: female study participants tended to decrease pain when the investigator was of the opposite sex, while men tended to rate pain lower when the investigator was female [32]. In our study, the outcomes were directly documented in the documentation sheets from the patients themselves, so this effect will not have played a role.

5. Limitations

The sample size of the study was based on an efficacy trial investigating the treatment with homeopathic *Hypericum perforatum* as an add-on to standard postoperative pain management. Thus, the trial was not intended to detect small differences such as those in the present reanalysis with regard to gender. However, statistical results with *p*-values clearly above the threshold of significance do not suggest that the low sample size plays an important role.

All patients had been randomly assigned to receive either a placebo or *Hypericum perforatum*; blinding of the patients was carried out properly, and no gender differences in the original study outcomes were observed. Thus, a contamination of the present results due to positive expectancy regarding the therapy, which might have influenced pain perception, can also be ruled out. Moreover, in the original trial, the additional treatment with *Hypericum perforatum* did not show a significant effect with respect to pain perception or opioid consumption. Thus, an influence of the additional treatment with *Hypericum perforatum* can also be excluded [13].

6. Conclusions

The results of this reanalysis are contradictory to most other studies in the field of neurosurgery, as no significant gender differences in pain perception and analgesic consumption after lumbar spinal surgery could be presented. It is possible that biopsychosocial mechanisms and the role of psychological factors that may influence sex differences in pain do not occur during a short postoperative inpatient stay. This should be considered in future research. Moreover, a summary of existing findings, e.g., in terms of a systematic review or meta-analysis, would therefore be desirable.

Author Contributions: Conceptualization, C.K.R., T.O. and W.S.; Data curation, S.R.; Formal analysis, T.O. and S.R.; Investigation, A.-L.S.-T. and W.S.; Methodology, T.O. and S.R.; Project administration, C.K.R.; Supervision, T.O., O.F., D.D.M. and W.S.; Validation, C.K.R. and T.O.; Visualization, S.R.; Writing—original draft, C.K.R. and T.O.; Writing—review and editing, C.K.R., T.O., A.-L.S.-T., O.F., D.D.M., S.R. and W.S. All authors have read and agreed to the published version of the manuscript.

Funding: This research received no external funding.

Institutional Review Board Statement: The ethical approval Authorization N° 49/2013 was obtained on 18 June 2013 from the Institutional Ethics Committee of Witten/Herdecke University. Before data collection, written consent was obtained from all patients. No patient was below the age of 16 at the time of the study.

Informed Consent Statement: Informed consent was obtained from all patients involved in the study.

Data Availability Statement: The datasets used and/or analyzed during the current study are available from the corresponding author upon reasonable request.

Conflicts of Interest: The authors declare no conflict of interest.

References

1. Dydyk, A.M.; Ngnitewe Massa, R.; Mesfin, F.B. *StatPearls: Disc Herniation*; StatPearls Publishing: Treasure Island, FL, USA, 2022.
2. Fjeld, O.R.; Grøvle, L.; Helgeland, J.; Småstuen, M.C.; Solberg, T.K.; Zwart, J.-A.; Grotle, M. Complications, reoperations, readmissions, and length of hospital stay in 34 639 surgical cases of lumbar disc herniation. *Bone Jt. J.* **2019**, *101-B*, 470–477. [CrossRef] [PubMed]
3. Volbracht, E.; Fürchtenicht, A.; Grote-Westrick, M. Back Surgery: Place of residence determines if patients are admitted to hospital, receive conservative treatment, or undergo an operation. *Spotlight Healthc.* **2017**, *7*, 1–8.
4. Fillingim, R.B.; King, C.D.; Ribeiro-Dasilva, M.C.; Rahim-Williams, B.; Riley, J.L., III. Sex, Gender, and Pain: A Review of Recent Clinical and Experimental Findings. *J. Pain* **2009**, *10*, 447–485. [CrossRef] [PubMed]
5. Templeton, K.J. Sex and Gender Issues in Pain Management. *J. Bone Jt. Surg.* **2020**, *102*, 32–35. [CrossRef]
6. Lövgren, A.; Häggman-Henrikson, B.; Fjellman-Wiklund, A.; Begic, A.; Landgren, H.; Lundén, V.; Svensson, P.; Österlund, C. The impact of gender of the examiner on orofacial pain perception and pain reporting among healthy volunteers. *Clin. Oral Investig.* **2021**, *26*, 3033–3040. [CrossRef]
7. Khan, F.A.; Hussain, A.M.; Ahmed, A.; Chawla, T.; Azam, S.I. Effect of gender on pain perception and analgesic consumption in laparoscopic cholecystectomy: An observational study. *J. Anaesthesiol. Clin. Pharmacol.* **2013**, *29*, 337–341. [CrossRef]
8. Pieretti, S.; Di Giannuario, A.; Di Giovannandrea, R.; Marzoli, F.; Piccaro, G.; Minosi, P.; Aloisi, A.M. Gender differences in pain and its relief. *Ann. Dell'istituto Super. Di Sanita* **2016**, *52*, 184–189. [CrossRef]
9. MacLean, M.A.; Touchette, C.J.; Han, J.H.; Christie, S.D.; Pickett, G.E. Gender differences in the surgical management of lumbar degenerative disease: A scoping review. *J. Neurosurg. Spine* **2020**, *32*, 799–816. [CrossRef]
10. Adogwa, O.; Davison, M.A.; Vuong, V.; Desai, S.A.; Lilly, D.T.; Moreno, J.; Cheng, J.; Bagley, C. Sex Differences in Opioid Use in Patients With Symptomatic Lumbar Stenosis or Spondylolisthesis Undergoing Lumbar Decompression and Fusion. *Spine* **2019**, *44*, E800–E807. [CrossRef]
11. Strömqvist, F.; Strömqvist, B.; Jönsson, B.; Karlsson, M.K. Gender differences in patients scheduled for lumbar disc herniation surgery: A National Register Study including 15,631 operations. *Eur. Spine J.* **2015**, *25*, 162–167. [CrossRef]
12. Strömqvist, F.; Strömqvist, B.; Jönsson, B.; Karlsson, M.K. Gender differences in the surgical treatment of lumbar disc herniation in elderly. *Eur. Spine J.* **2016**, *25*, 3528–3535. [CrossRef] [PubMed]
13. Raak, C.K.; Scharbrodt, W.; Berger, B.; Büssing, A.; Schönenberg-Tu, A.; Martin, D.D.; Robens, S.; Ostermann, T. Hypericum perforatum to Improve Postoperative Pain Outcome After Monosegmental Spinal Sequestrectomy (HYPOS): Results of a Randomized, Double-Blind, Placebo-Controlled Trial. *J. Integr. Complement. Med.* **2022**, *Advance online publication*. [CrossRef] [PubMed]

14. Raak, C.; Scharbrodt, W.; Berger, B.; Büssing, A.; Geißen, R.; Ostermann, T. Hypericum perforatum to improve post-operative Pain Outcome after monosegmental Spinal microdiscectomy (HYPOS): A study protocol for a randomised, double-blind, placebo-controlled trial. *Trials* **2018**, *19*, 253. [CrossRef] [PubMed]
15. Geissner, E. The Pain Perception Scale—A differentiated and change-sensitive scale for assessing chronic and acute pain. *Die Rehabil.* **1995**, *34*, XXXV–XLIII.
16. Lofrese, G.; Mongardi, L.; Cultrera, F.; Trapella, G.; De Bonis, P. Surgical treatment of intraforaminal/extraforaminal lumbar disc herniations: Many approaches for few surgical routes. *Acta Neurochir.* **2017**, *159*, 1273–1281. [CrossRef]
17. Sedighi, M.; Haghnegahdar, A. Lumbar Disk Herniation Surgery: Outcome and Predictors. *Glob. Spine J.* **2014**, *4*, 233–243. [CrossRef]
18. Dammers, R.; Koehler, P.J. Lumbar disc herniation: Level increases with age. *Surg. Neurol.* **2002**, *58*, 209–212. [CrossRef]
19. Lee, C.-W.; Lo, Y.T.; Devi, S.; Seo, Y.; Simon, A.; Zborovancik, K.; Alsheikh, M.Y.; Lamba, N.; Smith, T.R.; Mekary, R.A.; et al. Gender Differences in Preoperative Opioid Use in Spine Surgery Patients: A Systematic Review and Meta-analysis. *Pain Med.* **2020**, *21*, 3292–3300. [CrossRef]
20. Siccoli, A.; Staartjes, V.E.; De Wispelaere, M.P.; Schröder, M.L. Gender differences in degenerative spine surgery: Do female patients really fare worse? *Eur. Spine J.* **2018**, *27*, 2427–2435. [CrossRef]
21. Patel, D.V.; Yoo, J.S.; Karmarkar, S.S.; Lamoutte, E.H.; Singh, K. Sex Differences on Postoperative Pain and Disability Following Minimally Invasive Lumbar Discectomy. *Clin. Spine Surg. A Spine Publ.* **2019**, *32*, E444–E448. [CrossRef]
22. Zheng, H.; Schnabel, A.; Yahiaoui-Doktor, M.; Meissner, W.; Van Aken, H.; Zahn, P.; Pogatzki-Zahn, E. Age and preoperative pain are major confounders for sex differences in postoperative pain outcome: A prospective database analysis. *PLoS ONE* **2017**, *12*, e0178659. [CrossRef] [PubMed]
23. Triebel, J.; Snellman, G.; Sandén, B.; Strömqvist, F.; Robinson, Y. Women do not fare worse than men after lumbar fusion surgery: Two-year follow-up results from 4780 prospectively collected patients in the Swedish National Spine Register with lumbar degenerative disc disease and chronic low back pain. *Spine J.* **2017**, *17*, 656–662. [CrossRef] [PubMed]
24. Tschugg, A.; Lener, S.; Wildauer, M.; Hartmann, S.; Neururer, S.; Thomé, C.; Löscher, W.N. Gender differences after lumbar sequestrectomy: A prospective clinical trial using quantitative sensory testing. *Eur. Spine J.* **2016**, *26*, 857–864. [CrossRef]
25. Olsen, M.B.; Jacobsen, L.M.; Schistad, E.I.; Pedersen, L.M.; Rygh, L.J.; Røe, C.; Gjerstad, J. Pain Intensity the First Year after Lumbar Disc Herniation Is Associated with the A118G Polymorphism in the Opioid Receptor Mu 1 Gene: Evidence of a Sex and Genotype Interaction. *J. Neurosci.* **2012**, *32*, 9831–9834. [CrossRef] [PubMed]
26. Kwon, A.H.; Flood, P. Genetics and Gender in Acute Pain and Perioperative Opioid Analgesia. *Anesthesiol. Clin.* **2020**, *38*, 341–355. [CrossRef]
27. Meucci, R.D.; Fassa, A.G.; Faria, N.M.X. Prevalence of chronic low back pain: Systematic review. *Rev. Saude Publica* **2015**, *49*, 1. [CrossRef]
28. Bartley, E.J.; Fillingim, R. Sex differences in pain: A brief review of clinical and experimental findings. *Br. J. Anaesth.* **2013**, *111*, 52–58. [CrossRef]
29. Keogh, E.; Herdenfeldt, M. Gender, coping and the perception of pain. *Pain* **2002**, *97*, 195–201. [CrossRef]
30. Keogh, E.; Eccleston, C. Sex differences in adolescent chronic pain and pain-related coping. *Pain* **2006**, *123*, 275–284. [CrossRef]
31. Donner, N.C.; Lowry, C.A. Sex differences in anxiety and emotional behavior. *Pflügers Archiv.-Eur. J. Physiol.* **2013**, *465*, 601–626. [CrossRef]
32. Racine, M.; Tousignant-Laflamme, Y.; Kloda, L.A.; Dion, D.; Dupuis, G.; Choinière, M. A systematic literature review of 10 years of research on sex/gender and experimental pain perception—Part 1: Are there really differences between women and men? *Pain* **2012**, *153*, 602–618. [CrossRef] [PubMed]

Article

The Lack of Analgesic Efficacy of Nefopam after Video-Assisted Thoracoscopic Surgery for Lung Cancer: A Randomized, Single-Blinded, Controlled Trial

Hyean Yeo [1], Ji Won Choi [2,*], Seungwon Lee [2], Woo Seog Sim [2], Soo Jung Park [2], Heejoon Jeong [2], Mikyung Yang [2], Hyun Joo Ahn [2], Jie Ae Kim [2] and Eun Ji Lee [3]

[1] Department of Anesthesiology and Pain Medicine, CHA Ilsan Medical Center, CHA University, Goyang 10414, Korea
[2] Department of Anesthesiology and Pain Medicine, Samsung Medical Center, Sungkyunkwan University School of Medicine, Seoul 06351, Korea
[3] Department of Anesthesiology and Pain Medicine, Seongnam Citizens Medical Center, Seongnam 13290, Korea
* Correspondence: jiwon0715.choi@samsung.com; Tel.: +82-2-3410-0730

Abstract: Nefopam is a centrally acting non-opioid analgesic, and its efficacy in multimodal analgesia has been reported. This study aimed to assess the analgesic efficacy of intraoperative nefopam on postoperative pain after video-assisted thoracoscopic surgery (VATS) for lung cancer. Participants were randomly assigned to either the nefopam or the control group. The nefopam group received 20 mg of nefopam after induction and 15 min before the end of surgery. The control group received saline. The primary outcome was cumulative opioid consumption during the 6 h postoperatively. Pain intensities, the time to first request for rescue analgesia, adverse events during the 72 h postoperatively, and the incidence of chronic pain 3 months after surgery were evaluated. Ninety-nine patients were included in the analysis. Total opioid consumption during the 6 h postoperatively was comparable between the groups (nefopam group [$n = 50$] vs. control group [$n = 49$], 19.8 [13.5–25.3] mg vs. 20.3 [13.9–27.0] mg; median difference: -1.55, 95% CI: -6.64 to 3.69; $p = 0.356$). Pain intensity during the 72 h postoperatively and the incidence of chronic pain 3 months after surgery did not differ between the groups. Intraoperative nefopam did not decrease acute postoperative opioid consumption or pain intensity, nor did it reduce the incidence of chronic pain after VATS.

Keywords: nefopam; video-assisted thoracoscopic surgery; acute postoperative pain; opioid consumption; chronic post-surgical pain; lung cancer

1. Introduction

Severe postoperative pain after thoracic surgery interferes with deep breathing and coughing and reduces pulmonary function, which increases the incidence of postoperative pulmonary complications [1,2]. Furthermore, severe pain in acute postoperative periods seems to be strongly associated with the development of chronic post thoracotomy pain syndrome (CPTPS) [3–5]. The CPTPS, defined as pain which persists or recurs longer than 3 months after thoracotomy [6], has been reported in its incidence up to 80% of patients at 3 months and 61% 1 year after surgery [1]. The patients with CPTPS suffer from neuropathic or sympathetically mediated pain as well as nociceptive pain, and it can interfere with patients' daily activities and further reduce their quality of life [3,4,6]. Therefore, several efforts have been made to manage or prevent acute and chronic post-thoracotomy pain. Thoracic epidural analgesia was widely used as the gold standard for pain control. However, it has relatively common complications, such as hypotension and urinary retention, and has low cost effectiveness [7,8]. Opioids are also an important component of pain management; however, the indiscriminate use of opioids can result in adverse events, such as decreased consciousness, delayed mobilization and constipation. Currently, multimodal analgesia is recommended to optimize analgesia and minimize opioid-related side effects [1,9,10].

Nefopam is a centrally acting, non-opioid, non-steroidal analgesic drug, and its efficacy in multimodal analgesia has been reported in some previous studies [11,12]. The mechanism of nefopam is not fully understood; however, the inhibition of serotonin, norepinephrine, and dopamine re-uptake is known to play a main role in its analgesic effect. It also reduces the activity of post-synaptic glutamate receptors, such as N-methyl-D-aspartate (NMDA) receptors, by modulating calcium and sodium channels [12–14]. Therefore, we expected that nefopam could decrease postoperative opioids consumption and, based on its mechanisms, contribute to reducing the incidence of CPTPS.

Although the analgesic efficacy of nefopam was reported in several surgeries, including abdominal and orthopedic surgeries [15–18], it has not been assessed in patients undergoing video-assisted thoracoscopic surgery (VATS). Therefore, this prospective study aimed to evaluate the analgesic efficacy of intraoperative nefopam on acute and chronic postoperative pain after VATS in lung cancer patients. The primary outcome was total opioid consumption during the first 6 h postoperatively. The secondary outcomes were pain intensities, the time to first request for rescue analgesia, adverse events during the 72 h postoperatively, and the incidence of chronic pain evaluated 3 months after surgery. We hypothesized that intraoperative nefopam would reduce postoperative opioid consumption after VATS for lung cancer.

2. Materials and Methods

2.1. Study Design and Ethical Statements

This prospective, single-blinded, randomized controlled trial was approved by the Institutional Review Board (IRB No: SMC 2020-12-167, approval date: 22 February 2021) and registered with the Korean Clinical Research Information Service (registration No: KCT0006246; principal investigator: Ji Won Choi; date of registration: 11 June 2021; http://cris.nih.go.kr). Screening and enrollment for the study were conducted between March 2021 and September 2021 at a tertiary academic hospital in Seoul, South Korea. Written informed consent was obtained from all participants. This study was performed in accordance with the ethical principles of the 1964 Declaration of Helsinki and its later amendments. The trial was conducted following an original protocol and CONSORT guideline [19].

2.2. Participants

Patients between 20 and 70 years of age with ASA physical statuses I to III who were scheduled for elective VATS lung lobectomy were included. The exclusion criteria were as follows: patient refusal to participate, allergy to nefopam, renal dysfunction (serum creatinine > 1.5 mg/dL), hepatic dysfunction, history of seizure or epilepsy, recent myocardial infarction, current use of monoamine oxidase inhibitor, urinary tract disease causing urinary retention, and closed angle glaucoma.

2.3. Randomization and Blinding Method

Randomization was performed using a computer-generated random permuted block design, with a block size of 4 and 1:1 ratio. Allocation was sequentially numbered and sealed in opaque envelopes by the primary investigator. A study group member (HY) opened the envelope before induction of anesthesia and prepared the study drug according to the group allocation. The patients, outcome investigators, and surgeons were blinded to group assignment.

2.4. Intervention, Anesthesia Protocol, and Perioperative Pain Management

After standard monitoring (non-invasive blood pressure, electrocardiogram, pulse oximetry) and bispectral index monitoring (BIS; Medtronic, Minneapolis, NM, USA), 1.5–2 mg/kg of propofol, 0.8 mg/kg of rocuronium, and 0.05–0.20 μg/kg/min of remifentanil were administered for anesthesia induction. After intubation, anesthesia was maintained using sevoflurane within a BIS level of 40–60. Remifentanil was infused to maintain blood pressure and heart rate within 20% of baseline.

In the nefopam group, 20 mg of nefopam mixed with 100 mL of normal saline was administered intravenously during 15 min immediately after the induction of anesthesia and 15 min before the end of surgery. In the control group, 100 mL of normal saline was administered in the same manner. For postoperative pain control, 0.01 mg/kg of hydromorphone and 1 g of acetaminophen were administered intravenously 20 min before the end of surgery, and intravenous patient-controlled analgesia (IV-PCA; fentanyl 1000 µg diluted with 0.9% saline to make 100 mL of total volume, bolus dose of 1 mL, lockout time of 15 min, and basal infusion rate of 1 mL/h) was also applied for both groups. The tracheal tube was removed after the patient had fully recovered from neuromuscular block and was able to properly obey a command. After extubation, the patient was transferred to the post-anesthesia care unit (PACU) and monitored for approximately 1 h. Pain intensity was measured using a numeric rating scale (NRS; 0 = no pain, 10 = worst pain imaginable), and rescue analgesics (IV hydromorphone 0.01 mg/kg) were allowed with an NRS score $\geq$ 5. If a patient complained of pain with an NRS $\geq$ 5 more than 15 min after receiving rescue medication, more hydromorphone (0.3 mg) was administered intravenously.

Postoperative care was performed in the intensive care unit (ICU) during the first night after surgery, and most patients were then transferred to the general ward on the next day. The patients were routinely given 8 mg of hydromorphone orally beginning on the first postoperative day (POD 1). Intravenous hydromorphone (1 mg) or morphine (5 mg) was administered when the NRS score was $\geq$5. When patients required rescue analgesics more than 3 times per day, ibuprofen, acetaminophen, or tramadol was added orally as routine analgesics. Postoperative nausea and vomiting were treated with 0.3 mg of intravenous ramosetron hydrochloride (Naseron Inj., Boryung Co., Ltd., Seoul, Korea).

2.5. Outcome Measurements

The primary outcome was total morphine equivalent consumption during the first 6 h postoperatively. We also evaluated total opioid consumption (the IV-PCA and all rescue opioids) during the PACU stay and for the first 12, 24, and 72 h postoperatively. The dose of IV-PCA opioid was recorded by the intravenous pump device (Accumate 1200, Woo Young Medical, Jincheon-gun, Chungcheongbuk-do, South Korea). All opioid consumption was converted to the intravenous morphine milligram equivalent dose for comparison. The time to first request for rescue analgesics in the ICU or general ward after surgery was also recorded.

Acute postoperative pain was assessed with the NRS score during the PACU stay (the highest value of pain scores reported) and at 6, 12, 24, and 72 h postoperatively. Chronic postoperative pain was evaluated with the Brief Pain Intensity-short form (BPI-SF) questionnaire and the Neuropathic Pain Questionnaire-short form (NPQ-SF) via a phone call visit 3 months after surgery [20,21].

Adverse events, such as nausea and vomiting, dizziness, respiratory depression, and sedation (Richmond agitation sedation scale score of ≤ -2 during the daytime), were also evaluated during the first 72 h postoperatively. Aspartate aminotransferase (AST) and alanine aminotransferase (ALT) were monitored until POD 3.

2.6. Statistical Analysis

Based on a previous study, we hypothesized that cumulative opioid consumption during the first 6 h postoperatively would be decreased by 20% in the nefopam group [15]. With a two-tailed significance level of 0.05 and a power of 80%, the number of study subjects needed in each group to find statistical differences between the groups was 42. Considering a dropout rate of 15%, 50 patients were included in each group. All patients who were randomized and treated were included in the analysis based on the intention-to-treat principle.

Categorical variables are presented as frequency (percentage), and continuous variables are presented as mean ± standard deviation or median [interquartile range] according to their normality, which we evaluated with the Shapiro–Wilk test. The t-test or the Wilcoxon rank sum test was used to compare continuous variables between two groups, and the chi-square test or Fisher's exact test was used to compare categorical variables. For median differences, 95% confidence intervals (CI) were computed by the 2.5th and 97.5th percentiles of the bootstrap distribution with 1000 bootstrap replications. Bonferroni correction was used for multiple testing. A two-sided, p-value < 0.05 was considered statistically significant, and all statistical analysis were performed using Statistical Analysis System (SAS) version 9.4 (SAS Institute, Cary, NC, USA).

3. Results

A flow diagram of the study is shown in Figure 1. Between March 2021 and September 2021, 118 patients scheduled for elective VATS for lung cancer were assessed for eligibility. Among those 118 patients, 14 patients who refused to participate in the study and four patients diagnosed with benign disease were excluded. Thus, 100 patients were randomly allocated to the control (n = 50) or nefopam (n = 50) group. One patient allocated to the nefopam group dropped out because of withdrawal of consent. The operations of 4 patients were converted to thoracotomy, and 11 patients underwent a wedge resection or segmentectomy due to intraoperative changes in the surgical plan. Those 15 patients are included in the analysis based on the intention-to-treat principle. Therefore, 99 patients completed the 72 h follow-up. Of them, 75 patients (37 from the control group, 38 from the nefopam group) completed the 3-month follow-up measures.

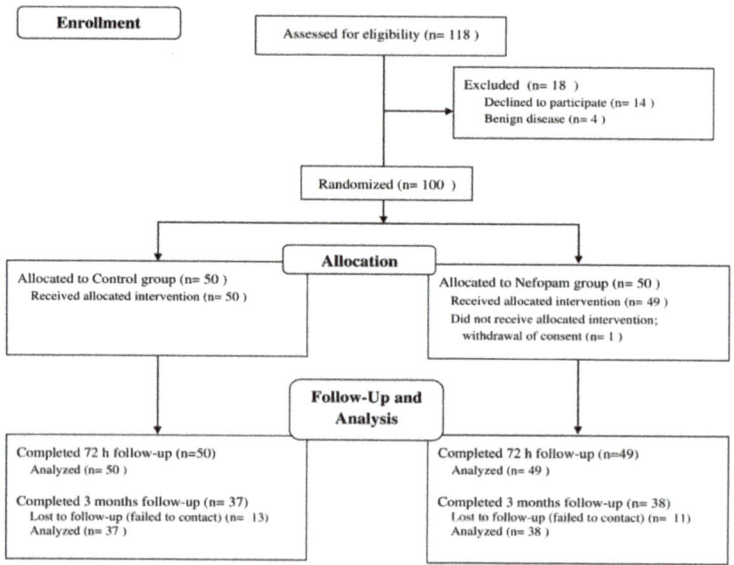

Figure 1. CONSORT flow diagram.

The baseline demographics and intraoperative data were comparable between the groups, except that the infusion dose of intraoperative remifentanil was higher in the nefopam group (0.450 [0.300–0.550] mg vs. 0.300 [0.250–0.450] mg; p = 0.013; Table 1).

Table 1. The baseline characteristics and perioperative clinical data.

	Control Group (n = 50)	Nefopam Group (n = 49)	p-Value
Age, year	59.5 [55.0, 63.0]	59.0 [53.0, 63.0]	0.606
Males/Females, n	17 (34)/33 (66)	21 (43)/28 (57)	0.484
Weight, kg	62.7 [55.0, 67.6]	64.5 [56.5, 69.9]	0.566
Height, cm	160.6 ± 7.8	162.8 ± 8.4	0.181
Body mass index, kg/m^2	24.1 [21.9, 26.4]	24.1 [22.7, 24.9]	0.740
Smoking, n	16 (32)	21 (43)	0.573
Hypertension, n	10 (20)	10 (20)	>0.999
Diabetes mellitus, n	5 (10)	6 (12)	0.972
ASA physical class (I/II/III), n	5/42/3	10/36/3	0.383
Type of surgical incision, n			0.362
VATS	49 (98)	46 (94)	
Thoracotomy	1 (2)	3 (6)	
Type of surgery, n			0.189
Lobectomy	47 (94)	41 (84)	
Wedge resection or Segmentectomy	3 (6)	8 (16)	
Operator (1/2/3/4/5/6/7), n	7/9/5/17/0/1/11	11/11/4/12/2/4/5	0.257
Duration of anesthesia, min	157.5 [135.0, 197.0]	166.0 [143.0, 193.0]	0.669
Duration of operation, min	104.5 [84.0, 145.0]	109.0 [88.0, 148.0]	0.583
Amount of intraoperative remifentanil administration, μg	300.0 [250.0, 450.0]	450.0 [300.0, 550.0]	0.013 [1]

Values are n (%), mean ± standard deviation or median [interquartile range]. [1] p-value < 0.05; ASA: American Society of Anesthesiologists, VATS: video-assisted thoracoscopic surgery.

Total opioid consumption during the first 6 h postoperatively did not differ between the nefopam and control groups (19.8 [13.5–25.3] mg vs. 20.3 [13.9–27.0] mg; median difference: −1.55 mg, 95% CI: −6.64 to 3.69; $p = 0.356$). Opioid consumption during the PACU stay and at 12, 24, and 72 h postoperatively was also comparable between the two groups. These data are shown in detail in Table 2. The time between the end of surgery and the first request for rescue analgesia in the ICU or general ward was likewise comparable between the nefopam and control groups (212.5 [104.0–371.0] min vs. 259.5 [142.0–432.0] min; median difference: −47.0 min, 95% CI: −169.00 to 73.95; $p = 0.302$; Table 2). The NRS pain scores at rest during the first 72 h postoperatively did not differ significantly between the groups at any time (Table 3). Likewise, the incidence of adverse events did not differ significantly between the groups. Changes in AST and ALT between the preoperative value and POD 1 or POD 3 did not differ significantly between the groups. The duration of ICU stay and hospitalization did not differ between the groups either (Table 3).

Table 2. Postoperative analgesic outcomes between the groups.

	Control Group (n = 50)	Nefopam Group (n = 49)	Median Difference 95% CI	p-Value
Total opioid consumption (mg)				
6 h postoperatively [1]	20.3 [13.9, 27.0]	19.8 [13.5, 25.3]	−1.55 [−6.64, 3.69]	0.356
During PACU stay	8.9 [6.9, 10.1]	7.4 [6.1, 9.4]	−1.45 [−2.76, 0.07]	0.196 [2]
12 h postoperatively [3]	31.6 [26.3, 39.7]	31.5 [22.7, 41.0]	−0.04 [−7.93, 8.10]	>0.999 [2]
24 h postoperatively	58.5 [48.8, 78.7]	63.0 [48.8, 83.5]	4.45 [−8.96, 16.29]	>0.999 [2]
72 h postoperatively	120.0 [85.0, 166.4]	130.6 [109.0, 178.0]	10.57 [−9.53, 33.50]	0.618 [2]
Time to first rescue analgesia (min)	259.5 [142.0, 432.0]	212.5 [104.0, 371.0]	−47.00 [−169.00, 73.95]	0.302

Values are presented as morphine milligram equivalent doses and median [interquartile range]. For median difference, 95% CI are computed by the 2.5th and 97.5th percentiles of the bootstrap distribution by 1000 bootstrap replications.; [1] Primary outcome: amount of morphine equivalent consumption includes both IV-PCA and all rescue opioids.; [2] Bonferroni's method was used for multiple comparisons at four time points; during PACU stay, 12, 24 and 72 h postoperatively.; [3] For the postoperative 12 h readings, n = 98 due to 1 follow up loss of PCA data; n = 49 for both groups; CI, confidence interval; PACU, post-anesthesia care unit.

Table 3. NRS pain scores at each time point and postoperative clinical outcomes between the groups.

	Control Group (n = 50)	Nefopam Group (n = 49)	Median/Risk Difference 95% CI	p-Value
NRS pain score during 72 h postoperatively				
PACU stay [1]	6.0 [5.0, 7.0]	5.0 [3.0, 6.0]	−1.0 [−2.0, 0.0]	0.355 [2]
6 h postoperatively	3.0 [3.0, 4.0]	3.0 [3.0, 4.0]	0.0 [−1.0, 1.0]	>0.999 [2]
12 h postoperatively	3.0 [3.0, 5.0]	3.0 [3.0, 4.0]	0.0 [−1.0, 0.0]	>0.999 [2]
24 h postoperatively	3.0 [2.0, 5.0]	3.0 [2.0, 4.0]	0.0 [−1.0, 1.0]	>0.999 [2]
72 h postoperatively	2.0 [2.0, 3.0]	2.5 [1.0, 3.0]	0.5 [0.0, 1.0]	>0.999 [2]
Incidence of adverse events				
PONV	33 (66)	34 (69)	3.4 [−15.0, 21.8]	0.884
Dizziness	24 (48)	19 (39)	−9.2 [−28.7, 10.2]	0.470
Desaturation	8 (16)	8 (16)	0.3 [−14.2, 14.8]	>0.999
Sedation	1 (2)	2 (4)	2.1 [−4.7, 8.9]	0.617
Changes in AST and ALT at POD1 and POD3 [2,3]				
AST POD1	3.0 [0.0, 6.0]	5.0 [0.0, 11.0]	2.0 [−1.0, 7.0]	0.144
AST POD3	0.0 [−3.0, 5.0]	0.5 [−4.5, 4.0]	0.5 [−3.0, 3.0]	>0.999
ALT POD1	−1.0 [−7.0, 1.0]	−1.0 [−5.0, 4.0]	0.0 [−3.0, 4.0]	0.864
ALT POD3	−2.0 [−7.0, 0.0]	−2.0 [−8.0, 3.5]	0.0 [−4.0, 3.0]	>0.999
Duration of ICU stay (min)	1140.0 [1020.0, 1280.0]	1177.0 [1050.0, 1339.0]	37.0 [−35.5, 50.0]	0.283
Duration of hospitalization (day)	6.0 [5.0, 7.0]	6.0 [5.0, 7.0]	0.0 [−1.0, 1.0]	0.904

Values are n (%) or median [interquartile range]. For median difference, 95% CI are computed by the 2.5th and 97.5th percentiles of the bootstrap distribution by 1000 bootstrap replications.; [1] Highest NRS score during PACU stay; [2] Bonferroni's method was used for multiple comparisons.; [3] Changes in AST and ALT were calculated by subtracting the preoperative value from POD1 or POD3 value. CI, confidence interval; NRS, numeric rating scale; PACU, post-anesthesia care unit; PONV, postoperative nausea and vomiting; AST, aspartate aminotransferase; ALT, alanine aminotransferase.; ICU, intensive care unit.

Thirty-seven patients from the control group and thirty-eight patients from the nefopam group responded to a phone call visit 3 months postoperatively. The incidence of chronic pain at 3 postoperative months was 55 and 65% in the nefopam and control groups, respectively ($p = 0.540$). Among the 45 patients who answered that they had persistent pain, the pain scores differed insignificantly between the groups (Table 4). The interference of pain with daily function also differed insignificantly between the groups (online Supporting Information, Table S1).

Table 4. The short form of brief pain inventory on 3 months after surgery.

	Control Group (n = 37)	Nefopam Group (n = 38)	Median Difference 95% CI	p-Value
Presence of pain	24 (65)	21 (55)		0.540
Pain intensity [1]				
Worst pain	3.00 [2.00, 4.00]	2.00 [1.00, 3.00]	−1.0 [−2.0, 1.0]	0.150
Least pain	0.00 [0.00, 0.00]	0.00 [0.00, 0.00]	0.0 [0.0, 0.0]	0.189
Average Pain	1.00 [0.75, 2.00]	1.00 [0.00, 2.00]	0.0 [−2.0, 1.0]	0.299
Current Pain	0.00 [0.00, 1.25]	0.00 [0.00, 0.00]	0.0 [−1.0, 0.0]	0.272
Pain interference with daily activities [2]	0.00 [0.00, 0.00]	0.00 [0.00, 0.00]	0.0 [0.0, 0.0]	NS

Values are n (%) or median [interquartile range]. For median difference, 95% CI are computed by the 2.5th and 97.5th percentiles of the bootstrap distribution by 1000 bootstrap replications.; Each item (except for presence of pain) is rated on a numeric rating scale from 0 (no pain) to 10 (worst) or from 0 (no interference) to 10 (interferes completely). [1] Pain intensity scores and interference items were analyzed only among the patients that they have current pain (control group, $n = 24$; nefopam group, $n = 21$). [2] The median (IQR) value of all interference items was the same as above, and details are attached as supplementary data.; CI, confidence interval; NS: not significant.

In their answers to the NPQ-SF questionnaire, 43 patients (57%) indicated that they had at least one neuropathic pain component, and the incidence of neuropathic pain did not differ significantly between the groups (18/38 [47%] vs. 25/37 [68%], $p = 0.103$). The severity of pain and numbness was also comparable between the groups (online Supporting Information, Table S2).

4. Discussion

In this study, intraoperative nefopam administration did not decrease total opioid consumption or postoperative pain intensity during the first 72 h after VATS for lung cancer. It also did not reduce the incidence of chronic post-surgical pain 3 months after surgery.

Several studies have shown promising results for the multimodal opioid-sparing analgesia of nefopam on acute postoperative pain [15–18,22,23]. In those studies, the nefopam groups required fewer opioids via IV-PCA or rescue analgesics or showed reductions in pain scores compared with the control groups during the postoperative period. As potential causes of its analgesic effects, those authors suggested triple neurotransmitter inhibition, NMDA receptor antagonism, and the modulation of presynaptic glutaminergic transmission [11–14].

However, conflicting results have also been reported, especially in surgeries anticipated to cause moderate to severe pain [24–27]. Cuvillon et al. reported that continuous intravenous infusion of nefopam (120 mg) during the first 48 h after open colectomy did not reduce perioperative opioid consumption and produced no differences in patient satisfaction or adverse events compared with the control group [24]. Eiamcharoenwit et al. administered 30 mg of nefopam before incision, at the end of spine surgery, or at both times and compared the outcomes with placebo. They also found no significant difference in postoperative morphine consumption among the four groups [26]. Other studies have also shown that nefopam had no or limited efficacy on postoperative pain management when it was used as a part of multimodal analgesia [28,29].

Our results are consistent with those studies reporting that the opioid-sparing effect of nefopam is unclear. Many of the studies that demonstrated the analgesic efficacy of nefopam involved surgeries with mild to moderate postoperative pain, such as laparoscopic cholecystectomy, mastectomy, thyroidectomy, and middle ear surgery [22,30–32]. 20 mg of intravenous nefopam is comparable to 6–12 mg of intravenous morphine [33], and the median effective dose (ED50) of nefopam for moderate surgical pain was 21.7–28 mg [34–36]. We administered 20 mg of nefopam twice during surgery. Although that dose was higher than the ED50 found in previous studies, it might still have been insufficient because the ED50 value was not determined based on thoracic surgery. Although post-surgical pain after VATS is less than that after thoracotomy, it is still severe during the acute postoperative period, and the incidence of CPTPS does not differ from that following thoracotomy [3].

Furthermore, no adequate dose, infusion rate, or duration of nefopam administration has yet been established for postoperative pain control. In previous studies, nefopam was administered in three major ways [11,12]. The first is administration before surgical incision and at the end of surgery, as in our study. The second is continuous infusion for 24–48 h beginning at the end of surgery, and the third is continuous infusion during surgery after an initial administration. The dose of nefopam used in previous studies varied from 20 to 120 mg per day, depending on the type of surgery, operation time, and administration method. However, in those studies, the analgesic effects were different, not uniform.

To prevent the development of CPTPS involving a neuropathic pain component, perioperative pain control is very important [1,3–5]. The action of nefopam on the glutaminergic pathway was proven in in vitro studies, and its antiallodynic and antinociceptive effect on neuropathic pain was also demonstrated in in vivo animal studies [37]. Ok et al. reported that additive nefopam in IV-PCA reduced neuropathic pain after percutaneous endoscopic lumbar discectomy [18]. In this study, however, nefopam did not reduce the incidence of acute, chronic or neuropathic pain after VATS for lung cancer. This result could reflect an inadequate dose of nefopam. One study in laparoscopic colectomy also reported that 20 mg of nefopam did not reduce acute or chronic postoperative pain [38]. Those authors suggested that a low dose of nefopam caused negative preemptive analgesic results, which might not be enough to prevent nociceptive transmission and central sensitization for moderate to severe pain [38]. On the other hand, a study in breast surgery reported that 20 mg of nefopam administered before surgical incision reduced the use of rescue analgesics and lowered the incidence of chronic postoperative pain [30].

In this study, five patients who complained of moderate to severe pain (NRS score ≥ 5) 3 months after surgery were all in the control group. Although there was no statistically significant difference between the groups, that result could suggest that nefopam has a potential role in attenuating severe pain in CPTPS. Further studies will be needed to clarify the effect of nefopam on chronic postoperative pain.

A characteristic finding of this study is that the dose of remifentanil infused during surgery was significantly higher in the nefopam group. We attribute that finding to the tachycardia effect of nefopam [11]. However, a study reported that nefopam had analgesic efficacy after laparoscopic gastrectomy and that intraoperative remifentanil consumption was lower in the nefopam group than in the control group [15]. The mean infusion rate of the control group in that study was 0.13 ± 0.06 μg/kg/min. As an explanation for their finding, those authors suggested that nefopam might be an NMDA receptor antagonist and thereby prevent remifentanil-induced hyperalgesia. In our study, on the other hand, the mean infusion rate in the nefopam and control groups was 0.07 ± 0.03 μg/kg/min and 0.05 ± 0.02 μg/kg/min, respectively. Only one patient in the nefopam group was given a dose of remifentanil greater than 0.1 μg/kg/min, which could induce remifentanil-induced hyperalgesia [39]. Therefore, it is unlikely that the difference in remifentanil infusion between the groups affected postoperative opioid consumption.

This study has several limitations. First, the patients in this study were not completely blinded. Although they did not know which group they were in during the acute postoperative period, they could have known their group if they read their medical records later. Second, we only evaluated postoperative pain intensities at rest. Assessing pain scores during coughing or movement would have been more appropriate. Third, we could not evaluate the incidence of tachycardia and sweating during the perioperative period, and they are known to be frequent adverse effects of nefopam. However, it was difficult to evaluate the occurrence of tachycardia during surgery because many factors can induce tachycardia during VATS. Fourth, the chronic pain evaluation was conducted by telephone, rather than in face-to-face interviews. Finally, the sample size of this study was not determined by the incidence of CPTPS. Furthermore, only 37 patients in the control group and 38 patients in the nefopam group were evaluated chronic pain at postoperative 3 months due to the follow-up loss. This sample size was rather small to demonstrate the incidence of chronic pain or compare it between the two groups.

5. Conclusions

In conclusion, intraoperative nefopam administration did not decrease total opioid consumption or postoperative pain intensity during the first 72 h after VATS for lung cancer. It also did not reduce the incidence of chronic post-surgical pain 3 months after surgery, compared with the control group. Further studies are required to elucidate the potential role of nefopam in multimodal analgesia for patients undergoing VATS.

Supplementary Materials: The following supporting information can be downloaded at: https://www.mdpi.com/article/10.3390/jcm11164849/s1, Table S1: The details of Brief pain inventory-short form on 3 months after surgery; Table S2: The short form of neuropathic pain questionnaire on 3 months after surgery.

Author Contributions: Conceptualization, E.J.L. and J.W.C.; methodology, J.W.C., H.J. and E.J.L.; software, H.Y. and S.J.P.; validation, W.S.S., M.Y. and J.A.K.; formal analysis, S.L. and H.J.A.; investigation, H.Y. and S.L.; resources, M.Y. and J.A.K.; data curation, H.Y. and S.J.P.; writing—original draft preparation, H.Y., H.J. and J.W.C.; writing—review and editing, H.J. and J.W.C.; visualization, E.J.L. and H.Y.; supervision, J.W.C., W.S.S. and H.J.A.; project administration, H.Y., E.J.L. and J.W.C. All authors have read and agreed to the published version of the manuscript.

Funding: This research received no external funding.

Institutional Review Board Statement: This study was approved by the Institutional Review Board of Samsung Medical Center (IRB No: SMC 2020-12-167, approval date: 22 February 2021) and was performed in accordance with the ethical principles of the 1964 Declaration of Helsinki and its later amendments. The trial was conducted following an original protocol and CONSORT guideline. This study is registered at the Clinical Trial Registry of Korea (http://cris.nih.go.kr; accessed on 11 June 2021; identifier: KCT0006246).

Informed Consent Statement: Written informed consent was obtained from all individual participants included in the study.

Data Availability Statement: The data presented in this study are available on request from the corresponding author.

Conflicts of Interest: The authors declare no conflict of interest.

References

1. Lederman, D.; Easwar, J.; Feldman, J.; Shapiro, V. Anesthetic considerations for lung resection: Preoperative assessment, intraoperative challenges and postoperative analgesia. *Ann. Transl. Med.* **2019**, *7*, 356. [CrossRef] [PubMed]
2. Gerner, P. Postthoracotomy pain management problems. *Anesthesiol. Clin.* **2008**, *26*, 355–367. [CrossRef] [PubMed]
3. Gotoda, Y.; Kambara, N.; Sakai, T.; Kishi, Y.; Kodama, K.; Koyama, T. The morbidity, time course and predictive factors for persistent post-thoracotomy pain. *Eur. J. Pain* **2001**, *5*, 89–96. [CrossRef] [PubMed]
4. Kampe, S.; Geismann, B.; Weinreich, G.; Stamatis, G.; Ebmeyer, U.; Gerbershagen, H.J. The Influence of Type of Anesthesia, Perioperative Pain, and Preoperative Health Status on Chronic Pain Six Months after Thoracotomy—A Prospective Cohort Study. *Pain Med.* **2017**, *18*, 2208–2213. [CrossRef]
5. Katz, J.; Jackson, M.; Kavanagh, B.P.; Sandler, A.N. Acute pain after thoracic surgery predicts long-term post-thoracotomy pain. *Clin. J. Pain* **1996**, *12*, 50–55. [CrossRef]
6. Bayman, E.O.; Parekh, K.R.; Keech, J.; Selte, A.; Brennan, T.J. A Prospective Study of Chronic Pain after Thoracic Surgery. *Anesthesiology* **2017**, *126*, 938–951. [CrossRef]
7. Manion, S.C.; Brennan, T.J. Thoracic epidural analgesia and acute pain management. *Anesthesiology* **2011**, *115*, 181–188. [CrossRef]
8. Wildsmith, J.A. Continuous thoracic epidural block for surgery: Gold standard or debased currency? *Br. J. Anaesth.* **2012**, *109*, 9–12. [CrossRef]
9. Conacher, I.D. Pain relief after thoracotomy. *Br. J. Anaesth.* **1990**, *65*, 806–812. [CrossRef]
10. Mesbah, A.; Yeung, J.; Gao, F. Pain after thoracotomy. *BJA Educ.* **2015**, *16*, 1–7. [CrossRef]
11. Evans, M.S.; Lysakowski, C.; Tramèr, M.R. Nefopam for the prevention of postoperative pain: Quantitative systematic review. *Br. J. Anaesth.* **2008**, *101*, 610–617. [CrossRef]
12. Girard, P.; Chauvin, M.; Verleye, M. Nefopam analgesia and its role in multimodal analgesia: A review of preclinical and clinical studies. *Clin. Exp. Pharmacol. Physiol.* **2016**, *43*, 3–12. [CrossRef]
13. Tiglis, M.; Neagu, T.P.; Elfara, M.; Diaconu, C.C.; Bratu, O.G.; Vacaroiu, I.A.; Grintescu, I.M. Nefopam and its role in modulating acute and chronic pain. *Rev. Chim.* **2018**, *69*, 2877–2880. [CrossRef]
14. Verleye, M.; Andre, N.; Heulard, I.; Gillardin, J.M. Nefopam blocks voltage-sensitive sodium channels and modulates glutamatergic transmission in rodents. *Brain Res.* **2004**, *1013*, 249–255. [CrossRef]
15. Na, H.S.; Oh, A.Y.; Ryu, J.H.; Koo, B.W.; Nam, S.W.; Jo, J.; Park, J.H. Intraoperative Nefopam Reduces Acute Postoperative Pain after Laparoscopic Gastrectomy: A Prospective, Randomized Study. *J. Gastrointest. Surg.* **2018**, *22*, 771–777. [CrossRef]
16. Mimoz, O.; Incagnoli, P.; Josse, C.; Gillon, M.C.; Kuhlman, L.; Mirand, A.; Soilleux, H.; Fletcher, D. Analgesic efficacy and safety of nefopam vs. propacetamol following hepatic resection. *Anaesthesia* **2001**, *56*, 520–525. [CrossRef]
17. Du Manoir, B.; Aubrun, F.; Langlois, M.; Le Guern, M.E.; Alquire, C.; Chauvin, M.; Fletcher, D. Randomized prospective study of the analgesic effect of nefopam after orthopaedic surgery. *Br. J. Anaesth.* **2003**, *91*, 836–841. [CrossRef]
18. Ok, Y.M.; Cheon, J.H.; Choi, E.J.; Chang, E.J.; Lee, H.M.; Kim, K.H. Nefopam Reduces Dysesthesia after Percutaneous Endoscopic Lumbar Discectomy. *Korean J. Pain* **2016**, *29*, 40–47.
19. Schulz, K.F.; Altman, D.G.; Moher, D. CONSORT 2010 statement: Updated guidelines for reporting parallel group randomised trials. *J. Pharmacol. Pharmacother.* **2010**, *1*, 100–107. [CrossRef]
20. Gjeilo, K.H.; Stenseth, R.; Wahba, A.; Lydersen, S.; Klepstad, P. Validation of the brief pain inventory in patients six months after cardiac surgery. *J. Pain Symptom Manag.* **2007**, *34*, 648–656. [CrossRef]
21. Backonja, M.M.; Krause, S.J. Neuropathic pain questionnaire—Short form. *Clin. J. Pain* **2003**, *19*, 315–316. [CrossRef]
22. Zhao, T.; Shen, Z.; Sheng, S. The efficacy and safety of nefopam for pain relief during laparoscopic cholecystectomy: A meta-analysis. *Medicine* **2018**, *97*, e0089. [CrossRef]
23. Jin, H.S.; Kim, Y.C.; Yoo, Y.; Lee, C.; Cho, C.W.; Kim, W.J. Opioid sparing effect and safety of nefopam in patient controlled analgesia after laparotomy: A randomized, double blind study. *J. Int. Med. Res.* **2016**, *44*, 844–854. [CrossRef]

24. Cuvillon, P.; Zoric, L.; Demattei, C.; Alonso, S.; Casano, F.; L'hermite, J.; Ripart, J.; Lefrant, J.; Muller, L. Opioid-sparing effect of nefopam in combination with paracetamol after major abdominal surgery: A randomized double-blind study. *Minerva Anestesiol.* **2017**, *83*, 914–920. [CrossRef]
25. Koh, H.J.; Joo, J.; Kim, Y.S.; Lee, Y.J.; Yoo, W.; Lee, M.S.; Park, H.J. Analgesic Effect of Low Dose Nefopam Hydrochloride after Arthroscopic Rotator Cuff Repair: A Randomized Controlled Trial. *J. Clin. Med.* **2019**, *8*, 553. [CrossRef]
26. Eiamcharoenwit, J.; Chotisukarat, H.; Tainil, K.; Attanath, N.; Akavipat, P. Analgesic efficacy of intravenous nefopam after spine surgery: A randomized, double-blind, placebo-controlled trial. *F1000Research* **2020**, *9*, 516. [CrossRef]
27. Richebe, P.; Picard, W.; Rivat, C.; Jelacic, S.; Branchard, O.; Leproust, S.; Cahana, A.; Janvier, G. Effects of nefopam on early postoperative hyperalgesia after cardiac surgery. *J. Cardiothorac. Vasc. Anesth.* **2013**, *27*, 427–435. [CrossRef] [PubMed]
28. Remerand, F.; Le Tendre, C.; Rosset, P.; Peru, R.; Favard, L.; Pourrat, X.; Laffon, M.; Fusciardi, J. Nefopam after total hip arthroplasty: Role in multimodal analgesia. *Orthop. Traumatol. Surg. Res.* **2013**, *99*, 169–174. [CrossRef]
29. Chalermkitpanit, P.; Limthongkul, W.; Yingsakmongkol, W.; Thepsoparn, M.; Pannangpetch, P.; Tangchitcharoen, N.; Tanansomboon, T.; Singhatanadgige, W. Analgesic Effect of Intravenous Nefopam for Postoperative Pain in Minimally Invasive Spine Surgery: A Randomized Prospective Study. *Asian Spine J.* **2022**. [CrossRef]
30. Na, H.S.; Oh, A.Y.; Koo, B.W.; Lim, D.J.; Ryu, J.H.; Han, J.W. Preventive Analgesic Efficacy of Nefopam in Acute and Chronic Pain After Breast Cancer Surgery: A Prospective, Double-Blind, and Randomized Trial. *Medicine* **2016**, *95*, e3705. [CrossRef]
31. Kim, B.G.; Moon, J.Y.; Choi, J.Y.; Park, I.S.; Oh, A.Y.; Jeon, Y.T.; Hwang, J.W.; Ryu, J.H. The Effect of Intraoperative Nefopam Administration on Acute Postoperative Pain and Chronic Discomfort After Robotic or Endoscopic Assisted Thyroidectomy: A Randomized Clinical Trial. *World J. Surg.* **2018**, *42*, 2094–2101. [CrossRef] [PubMed]
32. Yoo, J.Y.; Lim, B.G.; Kim, H.; Kong, M.H.; Lee, I.O.; Kim, N.S. The analgesic effect of nefopam combined with low dose remifentanil in patients undergoing middle ear surgery under desflurane anesthesia: A randomized controlled trial. *Korean J. Anesthesiol.* **2015**, *68*, 43–49. [CrossRef] [PubMed]
33. Sunshine, A.; Laska, E. Nefopam and morphine in man. *Clin. Pharmacol. Ther.* **1975**, *18*, 530–534. [CrossRef] [PubMed]
34. Delage, N.; Maaliki, H.; Beloeil, H.; Benhamou, D.; Mazoit, J.X. Median effective dose (ED50) of nefopam and ketoprofen in postoperative patients: A study of interaction using sequential analysis and isobolographic analysis. *Anesthesiology* **2005**, *102*, 1211–1216. [CrossRef]
35. Van Elstraete, A.C.; Sitbon, P. Median effective dose (ED50) of paracetamol and nefopam for postoperative pain: Isobolographic analysis of their antinociceptive interaction. *Minerva Anestesiol.* **2013**, *79*, 232–239.
36. Beloeil, H.; Eurin, M.; Thevenin, A.; Benhamou, D.; Mazoit, J.X. Effective dose of nefopam in 80% of patients (ED80): A study using the continual reassessment method. *Br. J. Clin. Pharmacol.* **2007**, *64*, 686–693. [CrossRef]
37. Kim, K.H.; Abdi, S. Rediscovery of nefopam for the treatment of neuropathic pain. *Korean J. Pain* **2014**, *27*, 103–111. [CrossRef]
38. Lim, H.; Kang, S.; Kim, B.; Ko, S. Comparison Between Preoperative and Intraoperative Administration of Nefopam for Acute and Chronic Postoperative Pain in Colon Cancer Patients: A Prospective, Randomized, Double-Blind Study. *World J. Surg.* **2019**, *43*, 3191–3197. [CrossRef]
39. Kim, S.H.; Stoicea, N.; Soghomonyan, S.; Bergese, S.D. Intraoperative use of remifentanil and opioid induced hyperalgesia/acute opioid tolerance: Systematic review. *Front. Pharmacol.* **2014**, *5*, 108. [CrossRef]

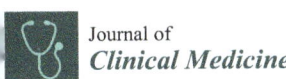

Article

Is the Erector Spinae Plane Block Effective for More than Perioperative Pain? A Retrospective Analysis

Uri Hochberg [1,2,*], Silviu Brill [1,2], Dror Ofir [2,3], Khalil Salame [2,3], Zvi Lidar [2,3], Gilad Regev [2,3] and Morsi Khashan [2,3]

1. Division of Anesthesiology, Institute of Pain Medicine, Tel Aviv Sourasky Medical Center, Tel Aviv 6423906, Israel
2. Sackler School of Medicine, Tel Aviv University, Tel Aviv 6997801, Israel
3. Spine Surgery Unit, Neurosurgical Department, Tel Aviv Medical Center, Tel Aviv 6423906, Israel
* Correspondence: urihochberg@hotmail.com; Tel.: +972-3-6974477

Citation: Hochberg, U.; Brill, S.; Ofir, D.; Salame, K.; Lidar, Z.; Regev, G.; Khashan, M. Is the Erector Spinae Plane Block Effective for More than Perioperative Pain? A Retrospective Analysis. *J. Clin. Med.* **2022**, *11*, 4902. https://doi.org/10.3390/jcm11164902

Academic Editor: Marco Cascella

Received: 19 July 2022
Accepted: 19 August 2022
Published: 21 August 2022

Publisher's Note: MDPI stays neutral with regard to jurisdictional claims in published maps and institutional affiliations.

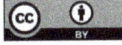

Copyright: © 2022 by the authors. Licensee MDPI, Basel, Switzerland. This article is an open access article distributed under the terms and conditions of the Creative Commons Attribution (CC BY) license (https://creativecommons.org/licenses/by/4.0/).

Abstract: Introduction: The thoracic Erector Spinae Plane Block (ESPB) is an ultrasound-guided block that has gained popularity and is widely used in acute pain setups. However, data regarding its role in chronic and cancer-related pain are anecdotal. **Material and Methods:** The study is a retrospective analysis of patients who underwent ESPB. The cohort was divided into subgroups based on three determinants: etiology, pain type, and chronicity. **Results:** One hundred and ten patients were included, and genders were affected equally. The average age was 61.2 ± 16.1 years. The whole group had a statistically significant reduction in a numerical rating scale (NRS) (7.4 ± 1.4 vs. 5.0 ± 2.6, p-value > 0.001). NRS reduction for 45 patients (41%) exceeded 50% of the pre-procedural NRS. The mean follow-up was 7.9 ± 4.6 weeks. Baseline and post-procedure NRS were comparable between all subgroups. The post-procedural NRS was significantly lower than the pre-procedural score within each group. The proportion of patients with over 50% improvement in NRS was lower for those with symptom duration above 12 months (p-value = 0.02). **Conclusions:** Thoracic ESPB is a simple and safe technique. The results support the possible role of ESPB for chronic as well as cancer-related pain.

Keywords: chronic pain; cancer-related pain; ESP block; pain management; ultrasound-guided

1. Introduction

Chronic pain is a common, complex, and distressing condition that impacts many aspects of patients' health and quality of life. Therefore, it can place a significant burden on patients and on the broader healthcare system. The Global Burden of Disease Study of 2016 reaffirmed that the high prominence of pain and pain-related diseases is the leading cause of disability and disease burden globally [1,2].

The Erector Spinae Plane Block (ESPB) belongs to a growing number of ultrasound-guided blocks that aim to deliver an analgesic solution to the soft tissue, or the interfascial plane, as opposed to the classic method of a direct nerve block. Shortly after its first description, the ESPB was adopted in clinical practice for multiple types of thoracic, abdominal, and extremity surgeries [3]. It is regarded as an effective, safe, and simple method for acute pain management [4]; however, despite its popularity, both the mechanism of the block and the extent of injectate spread are unclear [5].

Thoracic origin chronic pain represents a particular challenge as the interventional aspect requires its own special consideration. As with all neuraxial techniques, thoracic neuraxial procedures have contraindications and limitations (for example, coagulopathies, thoracic spine deformations, patient refusal) and other possible complications with considerable potential morbidity, including pneumothorax and neurovascular damage.

Although the first description of the block was for chronic neuropathic pain, most publications are concerned with acute pain management. The current literature addressing its use for chronic and cancer-related pain is scarce and mostly anecdotal in nature [6–10].

In this paper, we described the outcomes of the ESPB applied to patients at our pain institute, a regional referral center within a tertiary, university-affiliated medical center. We compared outcomes between different groups of patients based on the origin of the pain, type of pain, and symptom duration.

2. Materials and Methods

2.1. Study Design

A retrospective analysis.

2.2. Setting and Study Population

The study was conducted at the Pain Institute Center of the Tel Aviv Souraski Medical Center and was approved by the hospital's ethics committee (No. 0003-20-TLV). A retrospective review was carried out on the medical records of all patients who underwent thoracic ESPB between October 2018 and August 2021.

All participants provided written informed consent prior to undergoing the procedure, similar to other invasive procedures in our center. Inclusion criteria included: age of 18 years or above, diagnosis of thoracic back pain, a numerical rating scale (NRS) for pain ≥ 6, no significant motor weakness, no signs or symptoms of myelopathy, failure of other conservative treatment (i.e., physical therapy and oral analgesics), and at least a one-month post-procedure follow up.

Exclusion criteria: Allergy or hypersensitivity to steroid or amide local anesthetics, pregnancy, and breastfeeding.

2.3. Thoracic ESP Block Technique

The procedure was carried out under ultrasound guidance. The patient was placed in a prone position, and the ultrasound probe was set 2.5–3 cm laterally to the spinous process at the desired thoracic vertebral level on a parasagittal plane. Normally, a high-frequency linear probe was used. In the case of obese patients, a curvilinear (2–5 MHz) probe was used. Under ultrasound guidance, a 22 G needle measuring 50 or 100 mm was then inserted in a craniocaudal direction using the in-plane technique. The injection takes place at the fascial plane, deeper into the erector spinae muscle group. The solution injected was 10 mL of 1% lidocaine with dexamethasone 10 mg for a unilateral injection and 15–20 mL of 1% lidocaine with dexamethasone 10 mg for a bilateral injection.

2.4. Data Collection

Pre-procedural baseline demographic, clinical, and imaging data were collected. Demographic and procedural variables included: age, gender, pre-procedural NRS, and duration of symptoms at the first visit. Procedural variables included the side and level of the injection. Post-procedural variables included post-procedural NRS scores and the total number of ESPBs performed. Adverse effects were also monitored and documented. The data were collected and recorded by the pain physician in charge of the patient at the pain institute.

Thoracic pain was defined as pain experienced in the thoracic area, between the T1 and T12 boundaries, and across the posterior aspect of the trunk [11].

The main outcome measured was the change in pain intensity which was assessed using an 11-point numerical rating scale (NRS), with a range from 0 (no pain) to 10 (worst possible pain). In order to evaluate clinical significance, we used a minimal clinically important change (MCID) of 2.5 [12] for NRS, and we looked at a patient with more than 50% reduction in baseline NRS.

We divided the patients into different groups based on etiology, dominant pain type, and pain chronicity. For etiology, we divided the patients into two groups: one with patients suffering from cancer-related pain and the other with patients suffering from non-cancer-related pain. Cancer-related pain was defined as pain originating directly from a thoracic neoplastic lesion.

Regarding the dominant pain type, we divided the patients again into three groups according to the pain type: nociceptive, neuropathic, and mixed pain. The neuropathic pain type was defined using strict criteria, following the current International Association for the Study of Pain (IASP) definition of "definite neuropathic pain" [13]. In cases where a discrete pathophysiological classification of pain was not either purely neuropathic or purely nociceptive, a "mixed type" diagnosis was given [14].

In order to analyze the effect of chronicity, the cohort was divided into three groups according to the duration of symptoms: up to four months, four to twelve months, and more than twelve months.

The patient clinical assessments were conducted before the procedure and at the post-procedure follow-up appointments. The pre- and post-procedural NRS were compared in the entire group and within each of the sub-groups.

At the post-procedure follow-up, patients with motor neurological deficits were referred for further surgical evaluation. Patients with significant pain (NRS > 6) were offered a second thoracic ESPB. A maximum of three procedures were allowed for each patient. Patients with no significant pain (NRS < 4) at the follow-up visit, were either discharged or offered an additional second follow-up.

2.5. Statistical Analysis

The statistical analysis was performed using SPSS version 19 (IBM Corp., Armonk, NY, USA). Significant differences between the groups were determined using one sample t-test, the X^2 test, and the Fisher exact test to evaluate categorical variables' independence. ANOVA and independent t-test were used to compare NRS values between the symptom duration groups. Pre-procedure to post-Procedure NRS changes within each group were analyzed with paired t-tests. A p-value < 0.05 was considered statistically significant.

3. Results

3.1. Participant Characteristics

One hundred and ten patients underwent the procedure, and both genders were affected equally. The average age was 61.2 ± 16.1. Sixty-one (55%) patients underwent unilateral injections, and 49 (45%) underwent bilateral injections (Table 1). Seventy-two patients (65%) were discharged from the pain clinic after one injection, and 35 (32%) patients were discharged after two injections. The most common level of injection was T3 (26 patients) (Table 2).

Table 1. Demographic and preprocedural variables.

	(A) Etiology			
	Non-Cancer Related	Cancer Related	p-Value	Total
Total	66	44		110
Male	26 (39%)	17 (39%)	0.92	43 (39%)
Age	61.8 ± 16.9	60.4 ± 14.8	0.26	61.2 ± 16.1
Bilateral injection	29 (44%)	20 (45%)	0.91	49 (45%)
Num of injections				
1	46 (70%)	26 (59%)		72 (65%)
2	18 (27%)	17 (39%)		35 (32%)
3	2 (3%)	1 (2%)	0.48	3 (3%)
Follow-up (weeks)	8.1 ± 2.8	7.6 ± 2.2	0.5	7.9 ± 4.6
	(B) Dominant Pain Type			
	Nociceptive	Neuropathic	Mixed	p-Value
Total	55	45	10	
Male	18 (33%)	22 (49%)	3 (30%)	0.223

Table 1. Cont.

	(B) Dominant Pain Type			
	Nociceptive	Neuropathic	Mixed	p-Value
Age	62.4 ± 15.1	59.8 ± 18.3	61.1 ± 9.7	0.710
Bilateral injection	32 (58%)	17 (38%)	0 (0%)	0.003
Num of injections				
1	37 (67%)	26 (58%)	9 (90%)	
2	17 (31%)	17 (38%)	1 (10%)	
3	1 (2%)	2 (4%)	0 (0%)	0.348
Follow-up (weeks)	8.0 ± 4.5	8.1 ± 5.1	6.3 ± 2.6	0.570
	(C) Duration of Pain			
	≤4 Months	4–12 Months	≥12 Months	p-Value
Total	20	22	68	
Male	6 (30%)	12 (55%)	25 (37%)	0.238
Age	68.1 ± 15.5	64.0 ± 12.9	58.3 ± 16.5	0.1
Bilateral injection	5 (25%)	5 (23%)	39 (57%)	0.001
Num of injections				
1	16 (80%)	14 (64%)	42 (62%)	
2	4 (20%)	8 (36%)	23 (34%)	
3	0 (0%)	0 (0%)	3 (4%)	0.568
Follow-up (weeks)	6.5 ± 3.7	7.9 ± 5.5	8.3 ± 4.5	0.37

Table 2. Level of injection.

Level	Number of Injections
Total	110
T2	5 (5%)
T3	26 (24%)
T4	8 (7%)
T5	10 (9%)
T6	13 (12%)
T7	15 (14%)
T8	7 (6%)
T9	5 (5%)
T10	12 (11%)
T11	3 (3%)
T12	6 (5%)

3.2. Demographic and Preprocedural Variables

When observing the etiology groups, no significant difference was found between patients with cancer-related pain and patients with non-cancer pain (Table 1). As for the pain type groups, we found significant differences in the side of injection (Table 1). In the mixed pain group, no patients received bilateral injections (p-value = 0.003). Analysis of pain duration groups showed a significant difference in the distribution of the injection site (p-value < 0.001) (Table 1).

3.3. Average Pain Intensity

A statistically significant reduction in NRS was found when the mean pre- and post-procedural NRS were compared across the entire cohort (p-value > 0.001). In fifty-eight (53%) patients, the NRS improvement exceeded the MCID, and in 45 (41%), it exceeded 50% of the pre-procedural NRS (Table 3).

Table 3. Average pain intensity.

	(A) Etiology			
	Non-Cancer Related	Cancer Related	Total	p-Value
Pre NRS	7.7 ± 1.4	7.1 ± 1.3	7.4 ± 1.4	0.88
Post NRS	5.1 ± 2.8	5.0 ± 2.3	5.0 ± 2.6	0.077
p-values (pre vs. post procedure)	>0.001	>0.001	>0.001	
NRS improved >2.5	37 (56%)	21 (48%)	58 (53%)	0.44
NRS improved >50%	32 (48%)	13 (30%)	45 (41%)	0.051
	(B) Dominant Pain Type				
	Nociceptive	Neuropathic	Mixed	Total	p-Value
Pre NRS	7.6 ± 1.3	7.4 ± 1.4	6.9 ± 1.6	7.4 ± 1.4	0.71
Post NRS	5.0 ± 2.3	5.0 ± 2.5	5.7 ± 4.5	5.0 ± 2.6	0.19
p-values (pre vs. post procedure)	>0.001	>0.001	0.334	>0.001	
NRS improved >2.5	32 (58%)	22 (49%)	4 (40%)	58 (53%)	0.45
NRS improved >50%	24 (44%)	17 (38%)	4 (40%)	45 (41%)	0.92
	(C) Duration of Pain				
	≤4 Months	4–12 Months	≥12 Months	Total	p-Value
Pre NRS	7.1 ± 1.7	7.1 ± 1.1	7.6 ± 1.4	7.4 ± 1.4	0.164
Post NRS	4.7 ± 3.7	4.4 ± 2.4	5.5 ± 2.3	5.0 ± 2.6	0.276
p-values (pre vs. post procedure)	0.01	>0.001	>0.001	>0.001	
NRS improved >2.5	12 (60%)	15 (68%)	31 (46%)	58 (53%)	0.14
NRS improved >50%	12 (60%)	12 (55%)	21 (31%)	45 (41%)	0.02

The etiology group comparison showed comparable pre-procedural NRS. The post-procedural NRS was significantly lower than the pre-procedural score within each etiological group. The proportion of patients who achieved improvement higher than MCID as well as above 50% of the baseline NRS was higher in the non-cancer related group, yet, without statistical significance (p-value = 0.51) (Table 3).

Comparing the pain type groups showed comparable pre- and post-NRS scores. However, in the mixed pain group, the improvement in NRS did not reach statistical significance (p-value = 0.334) (Table 3).

In the pain chronicity groups, the pre- and post-NRS were comparable between the groups, and the improvement in these scores was found to be statistically significant within each group. The proportion of patients with more than 50% improvement in NRS was significantly lower in patients with symptoms duration of more than 12 months (p-value = 0.02) (Table 3).

There were no major adverse effects reported. The main adverse effect was injection site soreness. Other adverse effects reported were systemic response attributed to steroid exposure, none requiring hospitalization.

4. Discussion

Thoracic spine pain is prevalent, affecting about 20% of people in their lifetime. However, research related to thoracic pain is sparse compared to lumbar and cervical spine pain [11].

Thoracic ESPB has gained popularity since its introduction and is being widely used in acute pain setups; however, data regarding its role in chronic pain are mostly anecdotal.

In this work, our purpose was to evaluate the role of ESPB in the management of chronic and cancer-related thoracic pain. We compared the outcomes based on three fundamental determinants: etiology, the dominant pain quality, and the chronicity of pain.

Our results are consistent with those of previously published reports describing the possible benefits of ESPB [6–10]. The mean reduction in NRS in our study was 2.4 points (p-value > 0.001), with 53% reporting NRS improved by more than 2.5 points, and 41% with NRS score improved by more than 50% compared to pre-procedure score. In our study, a successful, clinically meaningful procedure was defined as either a reduction in the NRS score by 2.5 or more points [15] or as a reduction of 50% compared to baseline NRS. This strict threshold, which was also selected by other trials [16,17], was chosen over the more common 30% improvement in NRS score to exclude the potential placebo effect.

Cancer patients frequently suffer from a wide range of other symptoms, and the multi-factorial causes result in a "total pain experience" [18]. As such, an etiology-based sub-group analysis was carried out, comparing patients with cancer-related pain to patients suffering from pain caused by other conditions. The first sub-group included all patients with an active neoplastic disease that causes intractable pain that is refractory to a medical regimen treatment. The proportion of patients who achieved improvement exceeding the 50% of the baseline NRS was higher in the non-oncological patients, showing a strong tendency toward statistical significance (p-value = 0.51).

Of the 66 cases of non-cancer-related pain, 33 were nociceptive (50%), 28 were neuropathic (42.4%), and 5 (7.6%) were mixed pain types. The nociceptive group included pain resulting from vertebral or rib fractures, deformations including kyphosis and scoliosis, soft tissue myofascial pain [19], degenerative changes in the disc and the facet joints, and bones lesions including hemangiomas. Within the 33 cases of the nociceptive group, 11 cases were due to degenerative spinal changes, 7 were myofascial pain, 6 cases were due to pain secondary to osteoporotic thoracic vertebrae fracture, 4 cases were due to consistent pain after the fracturing of ribs, 3 cases were due to pain secondary to traumatic thoracic vertebra fracture, and 2 cases were due to post-operative pain for correction of scoliosis.

These results suggest that although the ESPB analgesic effect may differ slightly, overall, this effect is comparable between patients with pain originating from oncological and non-oncological sources and that ESPB can have a potential role in treating pain with these conditions.

A second subgroup analysis, based on the dominant pain type, did not reveal significant differences in either the pre- or post-pain NRS score nor in the portion of patients who reported more than 50% improvement.

When the pre- and post-NRS scores were compared within the mixed pain [14] group, the improvement did not reach statistical significance (p-value = 0.334). However, due to the small number of patients in this subgroup, this finding should be interpreted carefully, and conclusions should not be drawn.

An analysis of the chronicity of the pain experience duration was also carried out. More than 60% of the study population experienced pain for more than a year prior to the execution of the ESPB. Given that our clinic serves as a tertiary center, often with long waiting times, such a proportion is expected. Although all three subgroups reported statistically significant NRS reduction, the largest proportion of patients with pain reduction of more than 50% was found in the patients with symptom durations of less than four months. These results support previous findings regarding the importance of early treatment and support the recommendation of early referral to a pain specialist for early intervention [20,21].

4.1. Procedure-Related Aspects

As mentioned above, much is yet unknown about thoracic ESPB. Not only regarding its indications and efficacy but also various technical aspects. As the procedure is a single shot, not a continuous infusion, the dosage delivered should not exceed the recommended daily dosage. We use 10 mL of 1% lidocaine with dexamethasone 10 mg for a unilateral injection and 15–20 mL of 1% lidocaine with dexamethasone 10 mg for a bilateral procedure. Corticosteroid has an established role in the management of both neuropathic and cancer pain [22–24]. The choice of Dexamethasone is for two sets of reasons. As a corticosteroid, it has high potency, a long duration of action, and minimal mineralocorticoid effect. Moreover, the solution is non-particulate; hence, it confers a lower risk of vascular damage in the thoracic area and is the recommended corticosteroid for thoracic injection [25].

4.2. Safety Aspects

Most chronic pain patients are treated at an ambulatory outpatient clinic. This should be considered when evaluating the approach and safety aspects of such a procedure.

In the immediate vicinity of the needle performing the block, there are no neurovascular structures at risk. To date, there have been minimal procedure-related complications reported with this block compared to the traditional thoracic neuraxial blocks [8,26,27]. Our data support this notion, as no major adverse effects were recorded. A total of 145 procedures were carried out, of which 45% were in a bilateral manner. The only adverse effects reported were a systemic response to steroids consisting of a mild and expected transient increased level of blood glucose level and increased blood pressure, none of which required further investigation or hospital admission.

The classification of the American Society of Regional Anesthesia (ASRA) for pain procedures considers musculoskeletal injections and thoracic facet medial branch block as procedures with a low risk for bleeding [28,29]. Recent reports also suggest a low risk of bleeding from the ESPB [30]. However, some patients are at higher risk due to various co-morbidities, and hence, we perform a personal stratification of risk for bleeding for each patient before recommending the procedure. Three patients underwent the procedure while treated with Enoxaparin at therapeutic dosage. Those patients were instructed to stay on bed rest for an hour following the procedure and were later discharged without adverse effects.

4.3. Post-Procedure Aspects

All patients undergoing lower thoracic ESPB are tested for motor function following the procedure to screen for any unintended motor weakness. However, we do not carry out sensory tests to evaluate the dermatomal coverage.

We do not perform additional procedures before evaluating the response of the first procedure. A follow-up is routinely scheduled 6–8 weeks after the procedure. A patient that reports a substantial improvement is discharged with a set of recommendations for future maintenance by their primary care physician.

4.4. Limitations

This study is a single-center trial and is limited by its retrospective nature. Part of the challenge associated with retrospective analyses is the possibility that pharmaceutical changes or other manual manipulations unbeknown to the team might affect the outcomes. However, in our pain institute, we avoid the use of pharmaceutical changes following ESP in order to allow for precise estimation of the analgesic effect of the procedure for future reference in cases of additional pain management advice. Even though a substantial percentage presented an NRS improvement exceeding 50%, our results should be interpreted carefully due to the sample size of the study. Another limitation that future studies should address is the long follow-up time, as the positive effect of the block may wane over time. Furthermore, a distinction of possible spinal anatomical structures and mechanisms (i.e., facet joint degeneration, discogenic changes, etc.) is missing and should be explored on a larger scale study.

In summary, thoracic pain is common and could lead to substantial disability and other negative impacts on the patient's life and society. It was argued that thoracic pain should be considered a discrete and important clinical entity, independent of pain experienced in other areas of the spine [31]. This study was conducted with the aim of better understanding and providing pain management for thoracic pain.

5. Conclusions

Thoracic ESPB is a simple and safe technique. The results support the possible role of ESPB for chronic as well as cancer-related pain.

Due to the simplicity of the ESPB, it could potentially be applied in multiple disciplines and setups, such as the emergency department and at an ambulatory practice.

In the future, prospective trials should be carried out to expand our knowledge and determine the proper and safe application of this type of block.

Author Contributions: U.H. and S.B. performed the procedures. All the above authors (U.H., S.B., D.O., K.S., Z.L., G.R. and M.K.) took an active role in creating the concept and design of the study. S.B. and G.R. oversaw the collection and recording of the data. U.H. and M.K. carried out the analysis and interpretation of data. All authors have read and agreed to the published version of the manuscript.

Funding: This research received no external funding.

Institutional Review Board Statement: The study received the approval of the Research Ethics Board of our institution, the Tel-Aviv Souraski Medical Centre. Research, Development, and innovation division, Helsinki committee, Trial registration number: (No. 0003-20-TLV). All the patients in this study gave their written informed consent for the procedure.

Informed Consent Statement: Informed consent was obtained from all subjects involved in the study.

Data Availability Statement: The data presented in this study are available on request from the corresponding author.

Acknowledgments: The authors would like to thank Vivian Serfaty and Basma Fahoum for proof-reading this paper.

Conflicts of Interest: The authors declare no conflict of interest.

References

1. Fayaz, A.; Croft, P.; Langford, R.M.; Donaldson, L.J.; Jones, G.T. Prevalence of chronic pain in the UK: A systematic review and meta-analysis of population studies. *BMJ Open* **2016**, *6*, e010364. [CrossRef] [PubMed]
2. GBD 2017 Disease and Injury Incidence and Prevalence Collaborators. Global, regional, and national incidence, prevalence, and years lived with disability for 354 diseases and injuries for 195 countries and territories, 1990–2017: A systematic analysis for the Global Burden of Disease Study 2017. *Lancet* **2018**, *392*, 1789–1858, Erratum in *Lancet* **2018**, *393*, e44. [CrossRef]
3. Tsui, B.C.; Fonseca, A.; Munshey, F.; McFadyen, G.; Caruso, T.J. The erector spinae plane (ESP) block: A pooled review of 242 cases. *J. Clin. Anesth.* **2019**, *53*, 29–34. [CrossRef]
4. Viderman, D.; Dautova, A.; Sarria-Santamera, A. Erector spinae plane block in acute interventional pain management: A systematic review. *Scand. J. Pain* **2021**, *21*, 671–679. [CrossRef] [PubMed]
5. Schwartzmann, A.; Peng, P.; Maciel, M.A.; Alcarraz, P.; Gonzalez, X.; Forero, M. A magnetic resonance imaging study of local anesthetic spread in patients receiving an erector spinae plane block. *Can. J. Anesth.* **2020**, *67*, 942–948. [CrossRef] [PubMed]
6. Chung, K.; Choi, S.T.; Jun, E.H.; Choi, S.G.; Kim, E.D. Role of erector spinae plane block in controlling functional abdominal pain. *Medicine* **2021**, *100*, e27335. [CrossRef] [PubMed]
7. Urits, I.; Charipova, K.; Gress, K.; Laughlin, P.; Orhurhu, V.; Kaye, A.D.; Viswanath, O. Expanding Role of the Erector Spinae Plane Block for Postoperative and Chronic Pain Management. *Curr. Pain Headache Rep.* **2019**, *23*, 71. [CrossRef]
8. Bharati, S.J.; Sirohiya, P.; Yadav, P.; Sushma, B. Unfolding role of erector spinae plane block for the management of chronic cancer pain in the palliative care unit. *Indian J. Palliat. Care* **2020**, *26*, 142–144. [CrossRef]
9. Hasoon, J.; Urits, I.; Viswanath, O.; Dar, B.; Kaye, A.D. Erector Spinae Plane Block for the Treatment of Post Mastectomy Pain Syndrome. *Cureus* **2021**, *13*, e12656. [CrossRef]
10. Benkli, B.; Ansoanuur, G.; Hernandez, N. Case Report: Treatment of Refractory Post-Surgical Neuralgia With Erector Spinae Plane Block. *Pain Pract.* **2019**, *20*, 539–543. [CrossRef]
11. Briggs, A.M.; Smith, A.J.; Straker, L.M.; Bragge, P. Thoracic spine pain in the general population: Prevalence, incidence and associated factors in children, adolescents and adults. A systematic review. *BMC Musculoskelet. Disord.* **2009**, *10*, 77. [CrossRef] [PubMed]
12. Pool, J.J.M.; Ostelo, R.; Hoving, J.L.; Bouter, L.; De Vet, H.C.W. Minimal Clinically Important Change of the Neck Disability Index and the Numerical Rating Scale for Patients with Neck Pain. *Spine* **2007**, *32*, 3047–3051. [CrossRef] [PubMed]
13. Finnerup, N.B.; Haroutounian, S.; Kamerman, P.; Baron, R.; Bennett, D.L.; Bouhassira, D.; Cruccu, G.; Freeman, R.; Hansson, P.; Nurmikko, T.; et al. Neuropathic pain: An updated grading system for research and clinical practice. *Pain* **2016**, *157*, 1599–1606. [CrossRef] [PubMed]

14. Freynhagen, R.; Rey, R.; Argoff, C. When to consider "mixed pain"? The right questions can make a difference! *Curr. Med. Res. Opin.* **2020**, *36*, 2037–2046. [CrossRef] [PubMed]
15. Bedard, G.; Zeng, L.; Zhang, L.; Lauzon, N.; Holden, L.; Tsao, M.; Danjoux, C.; Barnes, E.; Sahgal, A.; Poon, M.; et al. Minimal Clinically Important Differences in the Edmonton Symptom Assessment System in Patients with Advanced Cancer. *J. Pain Symptom Manag.* **2012**, *46*, 192–200. [CrossRef]
16. Yoon, D.M.; Yoon, K.B.; Baek, I.C.; Ko, S.H.; Kim, S.H. Predictors of analgesic efficacy of neurolytic celiac plexus block in patients with unresectable pancreatic cancer: The importance of timing. *Support. Care Cancer* **2018**, *26*, 2023–2030. [CrossRef] [PubMed]
17. Perez, J.; Olivier, S.; Rampakakis, E.; Borod, M.; Shir, Y. The McGill University Health Centre Cancer Pain Clinic: A Retrospective Analysis of an Interdisciplinary Approach to Cancer Pain Management. *Pain Res. Manag.* **2016**, *2016*, 2157950. [CrossRef]
18. Saunders, C. Introduction: History and challenge. In *The Management of Terminal Malignant Disease*; Saunders, C., Sykes, N., Eds.; Hodder and Stoughton: London, UK, 1993; pp. 1–14.
19. Gerwin, R.D. Diagnosis of Myofascial Pain Syndrome. *Phys. Med. Rehabil. Clin. N. Am.* **2014**, *25*, 341–355. [CrossRef]
20. Hochberg, U.; Minerbi, A.; Boucher, L.M.; Perez, J. Interventional Pain Management for Cancer Pain: An Analysis of Outcomes and Predictors of Clinical Response. *Pain Physician* **2020**, *23*, E451–E460. [CrossRef]
21. Yang, J.; A Bauer, B.; Wahner-Roedler, D.L.; Chon, T.Y.; Xiao, L. The Modified WHO Analgesic Ladder: Is It Appropriate for Chronic Non-Cancer Pain? *J. Pain Res.* **2020**, *ume13*, 411–417. [CrossRef]
22. Tulgar, S.; Ahiskalioglu, A.; De Cassai, A.; Gurkan, Y. Efficacy of bilateral erector spinae plane block in the management of pain: Current insights. *J. Pain Res.* **2019**, *ume12*, 2597–2613. [CrossRef]
23. Pehora, C.; Pearson, A.M.; Kaushal, A.; Crawford, M.W.; Johnston, B. Dexamethasone as an adjuvant to peripheral nerve block. *Cochrane Database Syst. Rev.* **2017**, *2017*, CD011770. [CrossRef] [PubMed]
24. Leppert, W.; Buss, T. The role of corticosteroids in the treatment of pain in cancer patients. *Curr. Pain Headache Rep.* **2012**, *16*, 307–313. [CrossRef] [PubMed]
25. Van Boxem, K.; Rijsdijk, M.; Hans, G.; De Jong, J.; Kallewaard, J.W.; Vissers, K.; Van Kleef, M.; Rathmell, J.P.; Van Zundert, J. Safe Use of Epidural Corticosteroid Injections: Recommendations of the WIP Benelux Work Group. *Pain Pract.* **2018**, *19*, 61–92. [CrossRef]
26. Adhikary, S.D.; Bernard, S.; Lopez, H.; Chin, K.J. Erector Spinae Plane Block Versus Retrolaminar Block: A Magnetic Resonance Imaging and Anatomical Study. *Reg. Anesth. Pain Med.* **2018**, *43*, 756–762. [CrossRef]
27. Yeung, J.H.; Gates, S.; Naidu, B.V.; Wilson, M.J.; Gao Smith, F. Paravertebral block versus thoracic epidural for patients undergoing thoracotomy. *Cochrane Database Syst. Rev.* **2016**, *2*, CD009121. [CrossRef] [PubMed]
28. Warner, N.S.; Hooten, W.M.; Warner, M.A.; Lamer, T.J.; Eldrige, J.S.; Gazelka, H.M.; Kor, D.J.; Hoelzer, B.C.; Mauck, W.D.; Moeschler, S.M. Bleeding and Neurologic Complications in 58,000 Interventional Pain Procedures. *Reg. Anesth. Pain Med.* **2017**, *42*, 782–787. [CrossRef]
29. Narouze, S.; Benzon, H.T.; Provenzano, D.; Buvanendran, A.; De Andres, J.; Deer, T.; Rauck, R.; Huntoon, M.A. Interventional Spine and Pain Procedures in Patients on Antiplatelet and Anticoagulant Medications (Second Edition): Guidelines from the American Society of Regional Anesthesia and Pain Medicine, the European Society of Regional Anaesthesia and Pain Therapy, the American Academy of Pain Medicine, the International Neuromodulation Society, the North American Neuromodulation Society, and the World Institute of Pain. *Reg. Anesth. Pain Med.* **2018**, *43*, 225–262. [CrossRef]
30. Maddineni, U.; Maarouf, R.; Johnson, C.; Fernandez, L.; Kazior, M.R. Safe and Effective Use of Bilateral Erector Spinae Block in Patient Suffering from Post-Operative Coagulopathy Following Hepatectomy. *Am. J. Case Rep.* **2020**, *21*, e921123. [CrossRef]
31. Wedderkopp, N.; Leboeuf-Yde, C.; Andersen, L.B.; Froberg, K.; Hansen, H.S. Back Pain Reporting Pattern in a Danish Population-Based Sample of Children and Adolescents. *Spine* **2001**, *26*, 1879–1883. [CrossRef]

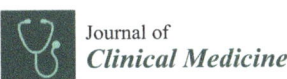

Article

Early Postoperative Pain Trajectories after Posterolateral and Axillary Approaches to Thoracic Surgery: A Prospective Monocentric Observational Study

Pascaline Dorges [1,2], Mireille Michel-Cherqui [1,2], Julien Fessler [1,2], Barbara Székely [1,2], Edouard Sage [2,3], Matthieu Glorion [2,3], Titouan Kennel [4], Marc Fischler [1,2,*], Valeria Martinez [2,5], Alexandre Vallée [4] and Morgan Le Guen [1,2]

[1] Department of Anesthesiology and Pain Management, Hôpital Foch, 92150 Suresnes, France
[2] Université Versailles-Saint-Quentin-en-Yvelines, 78000 Versailles, France
[3] Department of Thoracic Surgery and Lung Transplantation, Hôpital Foch, 92150 Suresnes, France
[4] Department of Research and Innovation, Hôpital Foch, 92150 Suresnes, France
[5] Department of Anesthesiology and Pain Unit, Hôpital Raymond Poincaré, Assistance Publique Hôpitaux de Paris, 92380 Garches, France
* Correspondence: m.fischler@hopital-foch.com

Abstract: Less-invasive thoracotomies may reduce early postoperative pain. The aims of this study were to identify pain trajectories from postoperative days 0–5 after posterolateral and axillary thoracotomies and to identify potential factors related to the worst trajectory. Patients undergoing a posterolateral (92 patients) or axillary (89 patients) thoracotomy between July 2014 and November 2015 were analyzed in this prospective monocentric cohort study. The best-fitting model resulted in four pain trajectory groups: trajectory 1, the "worst", with 29.8% of the patients with permanent significant pain; trajectory 2 with patients with low pain (32.6%); trajectory 3 with patients with a steep decrease in pain (22.7%); and trajectory 4 with patients with a steep increase (14.9%). According to a multinomial logistic model multivariable analysis, some predictive factors allow for differentiation between trajectory groups 1 and 2. Risk factors for permanent pain are the existence of preoperative pain (OR = 6.94, CI 95% (1.54–31.27)) and scar length (OR = 1.20 (1.05–1.38)). In contrast, ASA class III is a protective factor in group 1 (OR = 0.02 (0.001–0.52)). In conclusion, early postoperative pain can be characterized by four trajectories and preoperative pain is a major factor for the worst trajectory of early postoperative pain.

Keywords: lung surgery; pain; trajectory; thoracotomy

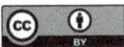

1. Introduction

Effective postoperative analgesia plays a major role in the prevention of major morbidity and mortality [1] and is particularly important after thoracotomy since postoperative pain can increase the risk of respiratory complications, especially by limiting physical activity and physiotherapy [2]. Numerous advances have been made both in the surgical and anesthetic fields to reduce postoperative complications. Surgical techniques have been oriented towards less-damaging incisions (muscle-sparing posterolateral thoracotomy, axillary, or anterior approaches) or mini-invasive procedures (video-assisted thoracic surgery (VATS), and robot-assisted thoracic surgery (RATS) [3,4]. Postoperative analgesia techniques have also progressed with new techniques in loco-regional analgesia, which are substitutes for epidural analgesia (paravertebral nerve block, erector spinae plane block of the spine, cryoanalgesia, etc.) [5,6].

A better understanding of postoperative pain could make it possible to treat or even prevent it and, therefore, improve the postoperative experience [7]. Usually described as individual measurements of pain scores reported for each postoperative day, postoperative pain can also be described using the trajectory method, an original approach proposed by Chapman et al. [8] The pain trajectory is a longitudinal characterization of acute pain as a growth curve, normally resolving in intensity over days. The psychometric goal of growth curve modeling is to estimate the true dynamic course of acute pain resolution in each individual. With this simple linear model, each patient's trajectory has two key features: the intercept or initial pain level, and the slope or the rate of pain resolution [8]. This makes it possible to classify a patient into a specific cluster (resolving pain over time, maintaining a constant level of pain over time, or increasing in pain over time) and to look for predictive factors.

This method was used to identify patient subgroups based on pain in various surgeries and notably after breast cancer surgery [9]. In a recent study, Vasilopoulos et al. identified five distinct postoperative pain trajectories from the data from day 1 to day 7 and characterized each group by age, gender, preoperative anxiety, and preoperative opioid consumption, but the patients enrolled had different surgeries [10].

Having conducted a prospective study regarding the risk of developing chronic pain after the axillary approach, a standard mini-invasive procedure, and posterolateral thoracotomies in thoracic surgery, we used the early postoperative data to establish the trajectories in post-operative pain and to identify their pre- and intraoperative predictive factors.

2. Materials and Methods

2.1. Ethics Approval

The present study reports the postoperative findings of a prospective, observational, single-center study performed in a tertiary care university hospital and was approved by the Ethical Committee Ile-de-France XI (n° 2013-A01641-44; Chairperson M. Catz) on 16 January 2014. The study was designed in accordance with the STROBE Standard for Observational studies) and published on the Clinical.trials.gov (accessed on 12 September 2014) website (NCT02237963).

2.2. Study Subjects

Patients were approached for consent before surgery and gave their written informed consent to participate. To be eligible, patients had to be at least 18 years old; French−speaking; and scheduled for lung surgery with a muscle-sparing posterolateral (PL group) or axillary thoracotomy (AX group) for lobectomy, pneumonectomy, wedge resection, bulla resection, or pneumothorax surgery for cancer or a non-cancer condition. Patients were excluded (a) if the planned procedure was a video-assisted thoracoscopic procedure, a partial or total pulmonary decortication, or a procedure extending to the chest wall; (b) if they had limitations of self-expression or communication by phone, or a severe psychiatric illness; and (c) if they had chronic thoracic pain before surgery (i.e., permanent pain over at least the three preoperative months). Pregnant and lactating women, and other vulnerable persons as defined by French regulation were not eligible.

2.3. Procedures

2.3.1. Surgical Management

For each patient, PL thoracotomy or AX thoracotomy was chosen by the participating surgeons according to their experience.

For patients undergoing PL thoracotomy, the skin incision spanned the width of the latissimus dorsi. The latissimus muscle was completely divided, but the serratus anterior was spared if possible and reflected anteriorly. The chest was opened in the fifth intercostal space, and a rib retractor was systematically used.

The incision for the AX approach extended approximately 7 cm caudal from just below the axillary hairline along the anterior border of the latissimus. The latissimus was completely spared and did not require mobilization. The insertions of the serratus anterior muscle on ribs 4 and 5 were dissected from these ribs, allowing the muscle to be lifted from the chest wall to allow the intercostal incision to be made in the fourth intercostal space. A rib retractor was only used if required by the surgeon.

For both approaches, the intercostal incision was extended far anteriorly and posteriorly beyond the limits of the skin incision.

A small portion of the posterior sixth rib was occasionally resected (shingled) during PL thoracotomy. Both types of incisions were closed with three or four interrupted pericostal or intracostal sutures. A running absorbable suture was used on the muscle, subcutaneous, and skin layers of the PL thoracic incision and on the subcutaneous and skin layers of the axillary thoracic incision.

Postoperative chest tube management was at the discretion of the surgical team.

2.3.2. Anesthetic and Pain Management

Anesthesia and pain management were standardized for all patients.

Anesthesia was total intravenous anesthesia by propofol and remifentanil, the doses of which were titrated according to hemodynamic stability and to maintain a Bispectral Index between 40 and 60, a range corresponding to the desired depth of anesthesia.

The usual pain management was thoracic patient-controlled epidural analgesia associated with co-analgesics (acetaminophen, nefopam, and nonsteroidal anti-inflammatory drugs in the absence of contraindication) given IV first and then orally as soon as possible. The epidural catheter was inserted before surgery at the T5–T6 or T6–T7 level; a first bolus of ropivacaine 0.375% mixed with 5 µg/mL (3 to 5 mL) of sufentanil was administered prior to anesthetic induction and was followed by a 5 mL/h infusion of 0.2% ropivacaine and 0.5 µg/mL of sufentanil. As soon as the patient was able to use the patient-controlled function, 3 mL boluses with a refractory period of 20 min were provided. In the case of contraindication to epidural analgesia (e.g., coagulopathy, systemic infection, or spinal disease), a paravertebral catheter was placed during surgery and allowed for 0.375% (3 to 5 mL/h) ropivacaine infusion. In the case of failure of epidural analgesia despite routine procedures, intravenous morphine patient-controlled analgesia or oral morphine was started. As specified in our institutional protocol, the epidural catheter was removed after the last chest tube was removed, typically on postoperative days 3 to 5, and oral analgesics (opioids and acetaminophen) were used alone.

Post-operative analgesia was given by nurses who specialize in pain management. This allowed for therapeutic adaptation.

2.4. Data Collection and Outcomes

Data were collected at inclusion, during surgery, and during the postoperative period. A complete assessment was performed on the 6th ± 1 postoperative day.

Demographic variables, history of cancer and tobacco use, pain, and anxiety were collected at inclusion. Regarding pain, patients were asked to respond to the question "Do you regularly suffer from pain?". In the case of a positive response, they provided a self-assessment of pain at rest during the visit and the mean value of pain score during the prior week using an 11-point numerical rating scale (NRS) from 0 = no pain to 10 = maximum imaginable pain. They were also asked to locate the pain and to report their painkiller use using the World Health Organization analgesic classification. A neuropathic pain was defined by a DN4 score ≥ 4 [11]. Patients' self-reporting of anxiety also used NRS with 0 = no anxiety and 3 = maximal imaginable anxiety.

The duration of anesthesia and surgery as well as the particularities of the surgical techniques were noted.

Postoperative pain was assessed each day from day 0 (day of surgery) to day 6 ± 1 at rest, when coughing and during ipsilateral shoulder mobilization using NRS [12]. The latter was the main outcome that was used to establish the trajectories of post-operative pain after thoracic surgery regardless of the surgical approach (PL thoracotomy or AX thoracotomy).

In addition, at day 6 ± 1, the postoperative analgesia technique; the DN4 score; the skin anesthesia or hypoesthesia around the scars using a 10 g Von Frey filament on three vertical measures at the midclavicular, midaxillary, and scapular lines; the total length of the scar; and patient satisfaction with pain management using a NRS from 0 = totally disappointed to 10 = totally satisfied were recorded.

Finally, the duration of postoperative stay and postoperative complications were collected using the Clavien classification [13].

2.5. Statistical Analysis

2.5.1. Number of Patients to Be Included

The number of patients to be included was calculated using the occurrence of chronic pain after PL and AX thoracotomies as the main outcome. When planning the study as a randomized controlled trial, the sample size was calculated based on a preliminary report from our group showing a 48% prevalence of chronic pain one year after a posterolateral thoracotomy [14]. It was hypothesized that post-thoracotomy pain syndrome prevalence would be 40% lower after an AX thoracotomy. However, since there were about twice as many surgeons performing posterolateral thoracotomy than surgeons performing AX thoracotomies, it was anticipated that the ratio of patients in the two arms would be about 2 to 1. Based on a 2-sided Fisher's exact test, with an alpha risk of 0.05, group sample sizes of 103 in the smaller group and 206 in the larger one achieve 90% power to detect a 0.60 smaller to larger ratio (i.e., 0.29 for the AX group and 0.48 for the posterolateral group) for the primary outcome. In April 2016, following a modification of our surgical practice, it appears that there were as many AX procedures as PL procedures. We therefore decided to stop our inclusions at 196 patients.

2.5.2. Statistical Methods

All statistical analyses were conducted on an intention-to-treat basis.

Categorical variables are presented as number (proportion); continuous variables are presented as median (25th percentile–75th percentile).

The statistical analysis was carried out in three steps: comparison of patients according to their surgical incision, identification of postoperative pain trajectories, and comparison of patients according to their pain trajectories.

Comparisons of variables between patients who had a PL or an AX thoracotomy used a Chi2 or a Fisher test for categorical variables and a Mann–Whitney test for continuous variables. Mixed model repeated measures were used to compare pain scores at mobilization during the early (day 0 to day 5) postoperative days. The surgery group and the days were used as fixed factors.

In the primary analysis, to identify clusters or subgroups of patients with similar progressions, defining trajectories of pain after surgery (measured from day 1 to day 5), a mixed ascending hierarchical classification was implemented with PROC CLUSTER in SAS software (SAS Institute). Each patient was clustered into the trajectory group to which they had the highest posterior probability of membership. First, a principal component analysis (PCA) was applied on postoperative pain variables. Then, factor axes were used to determine a dendrogram using a mixed ascending hierarchical classification. The dendrogram was cut using the Euclidean distance between each point with the Ward method to identify the best number of subgroups (i.e., trajectories). Comparisons of variables between all trajectories used a Chi2 or a Fisher test for categorical variables and a Kruskal–Wallis test followed by a Dunn's multiple comparisons test. Finally, a multivariable multinomial logistic model was performed to identify risk factors for trajectories. All factors associated with clusters in the univariate analysis with p-values < 0.20 were included in the multivariable model.

All statistics tests were two tailed, and P was considered significant when the p-values < 0.05.

Analyses were performed using SAS 9.4 (SAS Institute Inc., Cary, NC, USA) and R software (version 3.1, R Foundation for Statistical Computing, Vienna, Austria) using the application GMRC Shiny Stat (Strasbourg, France, 2017).

3. Results

3.1. Participants

Two hundred and fifteen patients were approached from July 2014 to November 2015, with one hundred and ninety-six finally included. Ninety-six patients underwent surgery through an AX incision, and one hundred underwent surgery through a PL incision. Initially, 25 patients (13 in the AX group and 12 in the PL group) were excluded from analysis due to missing pain scores. However, after imputation of the missing data, ten patients (six in the AX group and four in the PL group) were retrieved for data analysis. The analysis concerned 89 patients in the AX group and 92 patients in the PL group (Figure 1).

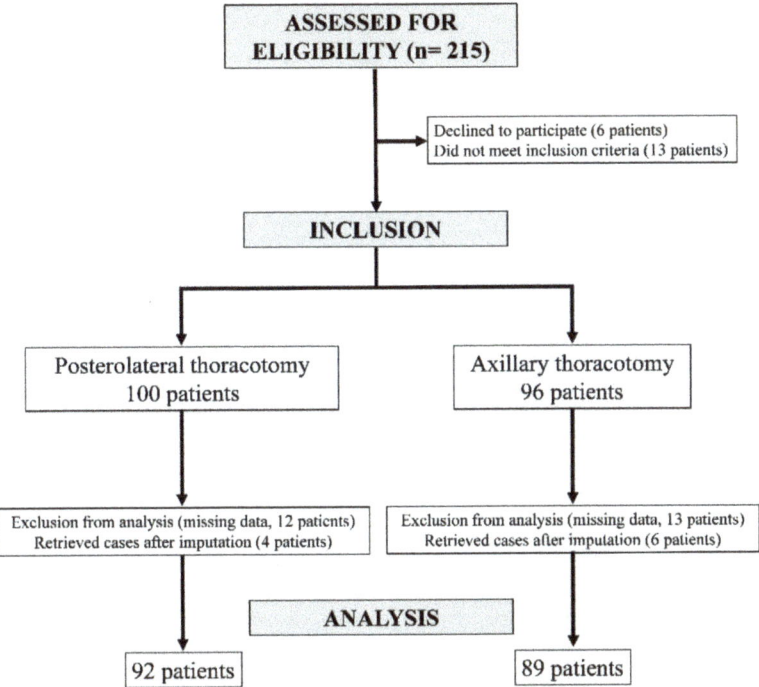

Figure 1. Flowchart.

3.2. Comparison of Variables between the PL Group and the AX Group

There was only one difference between the patient characteristics at inclusion in the AX and in the PL groups; patients in the AX group were younger, with a median age of 62 years old, whereas patients in the PL group had a median age of 66 ($p = 0.041$) (Table 1).

During the intraoperative period, differences between the two groups were related to surgical particularities (surgical retractors and rib fracture more common in the PL group ($p < 0.001$ and $p = 0.004$, respectively), and latissimus dorsi preservation and transcostal suture more frequent in the AX group ($p < 0.001$)) (Table 2).

Table 1. Patient characteristics at inclusion in posterolateral and axillary groups.

	Posterolateral Thoracotomy n = 92	Axillary Thoracotomy n = 89	p Value
Age, years	66 (57–72)	62 (53–69)	0.041
Sex, Male/Female	50 (54.3)/42 (45.7)	42 (47.2)/47 (52.8)	0.374
Body mass index, kg/m^2	25 (22–28)	24 (22–27)	0.227
ASA			0.129
I	5 (5.4)	13 (14.6%)	
II	68 (73.9)	59 (66.3%)	
III	19 (20.6)	17 (19.1%)	
Cancer	74 (80.4)	71 (79.8)	1
History of tobacco use	63 (75.0) {84}	60 (76.9) {78}	0.855
Current anxiety *	64 (69.6)	67 (81.7) {82}	0.079
Painful patients	42 (45.6)	33 (37.1)	0.291
Pain on inclusion day **	1 (0–3) {41}	2 (0–3) {29}	0.997
Mean pain during the prior week **	3 (2–6) {39}	4 (2–5) {28}	0.639
Thoracic location of pain	10 (25.0) {40}	4 (12.9) {31}	0.242
Neuropathic pain ***	8 (12.5) {64}	5 (9.1) {55}	0.769
Analgesic used by all patients ****	{66}	{59}	
At least one	27 (40.9)	17 (28.8%)	0.191
Step 1	24 (36.4)	17 (28.8%)	0.446
Step 2	9 (13.6)	2 (3.4%)	0.058
Step 3	2 (3.0)	0 (0.0%)	0.497

* Current anxiety was evaluated using four levels from 0 (null) to 3 (extreme) and is reported when present (1 or 2 or 3). ** Pain was evaluated using an 11-point numerical rating scale (NRS) from 0 = no pain to 10 = maximum imaginable pain. *** A neuropathic pain was defined by a DN4 score $\geq$ 4 [11]. **** Classification according the World Health Organization analgesic ladder. Number of available data in case of missing data is expressed as {xx}. Values are expressed as median (25th percentile–75th percentile) or n (%) as appropriate.

Table 2. Intraoperative variables in posterolateral and axillary groups.

	Posterolateral Thoracotomy n = 92	Axillary Thoracotomy n = 89	p Value
Duration of anesthesia, minutes	158 (136–195) {85}	166 (139–195) {88}	0.551
Duration of surgery, minutes	103 (78–129) {84}	109 (82–133) {88}	0.623
Surgical procedure			0.153
Lobectomy	57 (62.0)	64 (71.9%)	0.160
Wedge resection	23 (25.0)	19 (21.3%)	0.600
Pneumonectomy	7 (7.6)	1 (1.1%)	0.065
Other procedure	5 (5.4)	5 (5.6%)	1
Right side of surgery	46 (50.0)	52 (58.4)	0.297
Surgical retractors	92 (100.0)	59 (67.8) {87}	<0.0001
Rib fracture	22 (24.7) {89}	7 (8.2) {85}	0.004
Number of pleural drains			0.600
One	23 (25.0)	19 (21.3%)	
Two	69 (75.0)	70 (78.6%)	
Serratus preservation	83 (92.2) {90}	73 (85.9) {85}	0.226
Latissimus dorsi preservation	6 (6.8) {88}	65 (76.5) {85}	<0.0001
Transcostal suture	3 (3.4) {88}	48 (55.8) {86}	<0.0001
Extrapleural detachment	16 (18.0) {89}	7 (8.4) {83}	0.076

Number of available data in case of missing data is expressed as {xx}. Values are expressed as median (25th percentile–75th percentile) or n (%) as appropriate.

Pain scores for mobilization of the ipsilateral shoulder from the day of surgery to postoperative day 5 were similar in both groups (p = 0.83, Figure 2).

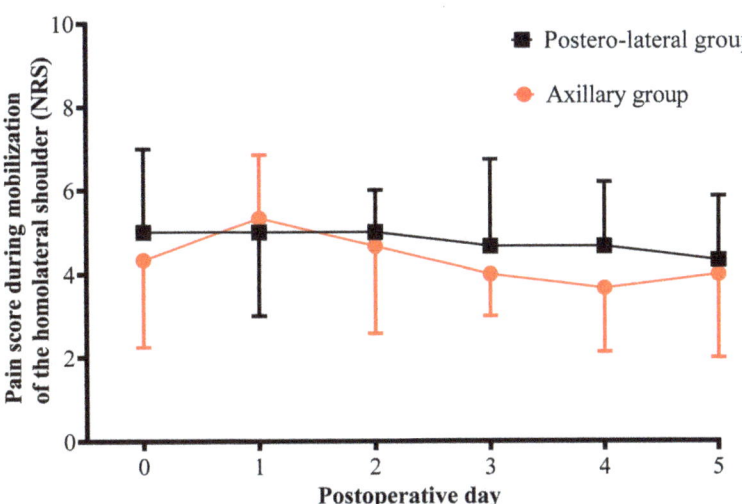

Figure 2. Comparison of pain score for mobilization of the ipsilateral shoulder measured from the day of surgery to postoperative day 5 for each surgical technique. Black boxes represent median NRS in the posterolateral thoracotomy group. Red circles represent median NRS in the axillary thoracotomy group. Pain was evaluated using an 11-point numerical rating scale (NRS) from 0 = no pain to 10 = maximum imaginable pain.

Most patients received thoracic epidural analgesia. Pain scores for cough and pain scores for mobilization of the ipsilateral shoulder were significantly lower in the AX group (respectively, medians of 3 and 2 in the AX group vs. medians of 4 and 3 in the PL group, with $p = 0.019$ and $p = 0.035$, respectively). Height of the hypoesthesia area around the scar was lower in the AX group ($p = 0.016$). Finally, the scar length was significantly greater in the PL group: median size 17 cm vs. 8 cm in the AX group ($p < 0.001$) (Table 3).

Table 3. Postoperative hospital stay variables in posterolateral and axillary groups.

	Posterolateral Thoracotomy n = 92	Axillary Thoracotomy n = 89	p Value
Type of postoperative analgesia			0.101
Thoracic epidural analgesia	82 (89.1)	77 (86.5)	0.591
Paravertebral block	7 (7.6)	3 (3.4)	0.330
No locoregional procedure	3 (3.3)	9 (10.1)	0.078
Chest tube in place at day 6 (±1)	18 (19.6)	21 (23.6)	0.589
Pain at day 6 (±1 day) *			
Pain score at rest	1 (0–2)	1 (0–2)	0.867
Pain score for cough	4 (2–6) {90}	3 (2–5) {87}	0.019
Pain score for mobilization of the ipsilateral shoulder	3 (2–4)	2 (1–4)	0.035
Neuropathic pain **	6 (6.5)	4 (4.5)	0.747
Height of hypoesthesia area around the scar, cm			
On the breast line	0 (0–8)	0 (0–5) {87}	0.722
On the axillary line	0 (0–5)	0 (0–4) {88}	0.354
On the tip of the scapula	0 (0–0) {91}	0 (0–0) {88}	0.016

Table 3. *Cont.*

	Posterolateral Thoracotomy n = 92	Axillary Thoracotomy n = 89	*p* Value
Scar length, cm	17 (14–19) {91}	8 (6–11) {84}	<0.0001
Satisfaction score ***	8 (7–9) {91}	9 (8–10) {87}	0.075
Postoperative complications ≥ IIIa ****	3 (3.3)	6 (6.7)	0.325
Postoperative hospital stay, days (n)	8 (7–12)	8 (7–11)	0.132

* Pain was evaluated using an 11-point numerical rating scale (NRS) from 0 = no pain to 10 = maximum imaginable pain. ** Neuropathic pain was defined by a DN4 score ≥ 4 [11]. *** Satisfaction was evaluated using an 11-point numerical rating scale (NRS) from 0 = totally disappointed to 10 = totally satisfied. **** Classification of postoperative complications according to the Clavien classification [13]. Number of available data in case of missing data is expressed as {xx}. Values are expressed as median (25th percentile–75th percentile) or n (%) as appropriate.

3.3. Pain Trajectories

The best-fitting model included four pain trajectory groups, with a combination of linear and quadratic trajectory groups. Those who partly or fully resolved their pain over five days had negative slopes, and those who demonstrated a pattern of increasing pain over days had positive slopes. Pain trajectory group 1 corresponds to patients with permanent significant pain from day 0 to day 5 (29.8% of the patients), pain trajectory group 2 corresponds to patients with moderate pain from day 0 to day 5 (32.6%), pain trajectory group 3 corresponds to patients with steep decreases in pain across the five days after surgery (22.7%), and pain trajectory group 4 corresponding to patients with steep increases in pain across the 5 days after surgery (14.9%) (Figure 3).

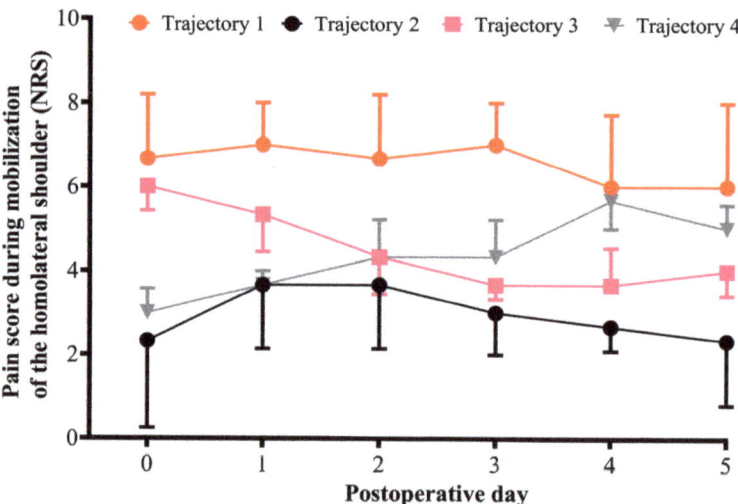

Figure 3. Comparison of pain score for mobilization of the ipsilateral shoulder measured from the day of surgery to postoperative day 5 for each trajectory. For each trajectory the median pain score is represented (numeric rating scale: 11-point scale for patient self-reporting of pain from 0 = no pain to 10 = maximal imaginable pain). The black line represents median pain scores in cluster 1 (permanent significant pain group). The red line represents median pain scores in cluster 2 (permanent moderate pain group). The pink line represents median pain scores in cluster 3 (decreasing pain group). The gray line represents median pain scores in cluster 4 (increasing pain group).

3.4. Comparison of Variables between the Trajectory Groups

Some patient characteristics at inclusion differed between trajectory groups, especially between trajectory group 1 and trajectory group 2: younger patients ($p = 0.031$), more patients with neuropathic pain ($p = 0.013$), and more patients having taken at least one analgesic medication before surgery ($p = 0.022$) in group 1. The percentage of preoperative painful patients was greater in group 1 than in the other groups (Table 4).

Table 4. Patient characteristics at inclusion for each trajectory group.

	Trajectory 1 n = 54	Trajectory 2 n = 59	Trajectory 3 n = 41	Trajectory 4 n = 27	Global p Value	Intergroup p Value
Age, years	60 (51–67)	69 (58–72)	64 (55–71)	64 (56–70)	0.049	T1 vs. T2; p = 0.031
Sex, Male/Female	22 (40.7)/32 (59.3)	35 (59.3)/24 (40.7)	22 (53.7)/19 (46.3)	13 (48.1)/14 (51.9)	0.251	
Body mass index, kg/m²	23 (21–27)	24 (22–27)	25 (22–27)	26 (22–29)	0.442	
ASA					0.073	
I	8 (14.8)	4 (6.8)	3 (7.3)	3 (11.1)		
II	42 (77.8)	37 (62.7)	29 (70.7)	19 (70.4)		
III	4 (7.4)	18 (30.5)	9 (21.9)	5 (18.5)		
Cancer	42 (77.8)	47 (79.7)	33 (80.5)	23 (85.2)	0.917	
History of tobacco use	36 (73.5) {49}	38 (71.7) {53}	30 (85.7) {35}	19 (76.0) {25}	0.479	
Current anxiety *	45 (86.5) {52}	39 (68.4) {57}	28 (71.8) {39}	19 (73.1) {26}	0.131	
Painful patients	33 (61.1)	19 (32.2)	15 (36.6)	8 (29.6)	0.006	T1 vs. T2; p = 0.006 T1 vs. T3; p = 0.049 T1 vs. T4; p = 0.021
Pain on inclusion day **	2 (0–4) {29}	1 (0–2) {18}	2 (0–5) {15}	0 (0,1) {8}	0.306	
Mean pain during the prior week **	4 (3–6) {29}	3 (2–4) {17}	4 (2–4) {13}	4 (1–4) {8}	0.085	
Thoracic pain	7 (23.3) {30}	3 (16.7) {18}	3 (20) {15}	1 (12.5) {8}	0.947	
Neuropathic pain ***	9 (25.0) {36}	1 (2.5) {40}	2 (8.0) {25}	1 (5.6) {18}	0.015	T1 vs. T2; p = 0.013
Analgesic used by all patients ****	{36}	{46}	{27}	{16}		
At least one	19 (52.8)	10 (21.7)	9 (33.3)	6 (37.5%)	0.035	T1 vs. T2; p = 0.022
Step 1	16 (44.4)	10 (21.7)	9 (33.3)	6 (37.5%)	0.166	
Step 2	5 (13.9)	2 (4.3)	2 (7.4)	2 (12.5%)	0.409	
Step 3	1 (2.8)	1 (2.2)	0 (0.0)	0 (0.0%)	1	

* Current anxiety was evaluated using four levels from 0 (null) to 3 (extreme) and is reported when present (1 or 2 or 3). ** Pain was evaluated using an 11-point numerical rating scale (NRS) from 0 = no pain to 10 = maximum imaginable pain. *** A neuropathic pain was defined by a DN4 score ≥ 4 [11]. **** Classification according the World Health Organization analgesic ladder. Number of available data in case of missing data is expressed as {xx}. Values are expressed as median (25th percentile–75th percentile) or n (%) as appropriate.

Intraoperative variables were similar regardless of trajectory group (Table 5).

Table 5. Intraoperative variables for each trajectory group.

	Trajectory 1 n = 54	Trajectory 2 n = 59	Trajectory 3 n = 41	Trajectory 4 n = 27	Global p Value
Axillary approach	24 (44.4)	32 (54.2)	20 (48.8)	13 (48.1)	0.781
Duration of anesthesia, minutes	162 (129–189) {52}	156 (134–198) {57}	166 (149–199) {39}	168 (135–214) {25}	0.502
Duration of surgery, minutes	102 (77–127) {52}	109 (76–130) {57}	107 (89–134) {38}	111 (79–152) {25}	0.825
Surgical procedure					
Lobectomy	35 (64.8)	39 (66.1)	29 (70.7)	18 (66.7)	0.940
Wedge resection	11 (20.4)	17 (28.8)	8 (19.5)	6 (22.2)	0.679
Pneumonectomy	3 (5.6)	1 (1.7)	3 (7.3)	1 (3.7)	0.513
Other procedure	5 (9.3)	2 (3.4)	1 (2.4)	2 (7.4)	0.444
Right side of surgery	29 (53.7)	32 (54.2)	23 (56.1)	14 (51.8)	0.993
Surgical retractors	48 (88.9)	46 (80.0)	33 (82.5) {40}	24 (92.3) {26}	0.283
Rib fracture	8 (14.8)	10 (17.9) {56}	3 (7.9) {38}	8 (30.8) {26}	0.121
Number of pleural drains					0.884
One	12 (22.2)	15 (25.4)	8 (19.5)	7 (25.9)	
Two	42 (77.8)	44 (74.6)	33 (80.5)	20 (74.1)	
Serratus preservation	47 (88.7) {53}	51 (87.9) {58}	36 (94.7) {38}	22 (84.6) {26}	0.595
Latissimus dorsi preservation	19 (36.5) {52}	28 (48.3) {58}	17 (45.9) {37}	7 (26.9) {26}	0.244

Table 5. Cont.

	Trajectory 1 n = 54	Trajectory 2 n = 59	Trajectory 3 n = 41	Trajectory 4 n = 27	Global p Value
Transcostal suture	13 (25.5) {51}	21 (36.2) {58}	14 (35.9) {39}	3 (11.5) {26}	0.082
Extrapleural detachment	7 (13.5) {52}	7 (12.3) {57}	6 (16.2) {37}	3 (11.5) {26}	0.947

Number of available data in case of missing data is expressed as {xx}. Values are expressed as median (25th percentile–75th percentile) or n (%) as appropriate.

Of interest, scar lengths did not differ from one group to another (Table 6).

Table 6. Postoperative hospital stay variables for each trajectory group.

	Trajectory 1 n = 54	Trajectory 2 n = 59	Trajectory 3 n = 41	Trajectory 4 n = 27	Global p Value	Intergroup p Value
Type of postoperative analgesia					0.788	
Thoracic epidural analgesia	48 (88.9)	52 (88.1)	34 (82.9)	25 (92.6)	0.707	
Paravertebral block	4 (7.4)	2 (3.4)	3 (7.3)	1 (3.7)	0.736	
No locoregional procedure	2 (3.7)	5 (8.5)	4 (9.8)	1 (3.7)	0.615	
Chest tube in place at day 6 (±1)	13 (24.1)	13 (22.0)	7 (17.1)	6 (22.2)	0.880	
Pain at day 6 (±1 day) *						
Pain score at rest	2 (0–3)	0 (0,1)	1 (0–2)	1 (0–3)	<0.0001	T1 vs. T2; $p < 0.0001$ T2 vs. T4; $p = 0.024$
Pain score for cough	5 (4–7) {51}	2 (1–3)	4 (2–5)	5 (3–6) {26}	<0.0001	T1 vs. T2; $p < 0.0001$ T1 vs. T3; $p = 0.005$ T2 vs. T3; $p = 0.034$ T2 vs. T4; $p < 0.0001$
Pain score for mobilization of the ipsilateral shoulder	4 (2–6)	2 (1–3)	3 (2–4)	4 (2–4)	<0.0001	T1 vs. T2; $p < 0.0001$ T2 vs. T4; $p = 0.018$
Neuropathic pain **	5 (9.3)	1 (1.7)	2 (4.9)	2 (7.4)	0.296	
Height of hypoesthesia area around the scar, cm						
On the breast line	1.5 (0–7.7) {54}	0 (0–4) {58}	0 (0–7) {41}	0 (0–8.5) {26}	0.353	
On the axillary line	0 (0–3) {54}	0 (0–5) {58}	0 (0–5) {41}	3 (0–5.5) {27}	0.413	
On the line tip of the scapula	0 (0–0) {54}	0 (0–0) {57}	0 (0–0) {41}	0 (0–0) {27}	0.674	
Scar length, cm	15 (9–19) {54}	12 (7–16) {54}	12 (8–17) {41}	14 (13–18) {26}	0.047	ns
Satisfaction score ***	9 (8,9) {53}	9 (8–10) {58}	8 (7–10) {40}	9 (6–10) {27}	0.183	
Postoperative complications ≥ IIIa ****	2 (3.7)	1 (1.7)	4 (9.8)	2 (7.4)	0.247	
Postoperative hospital stay, days (n)	8 (7–13)	9 (7–11)	9 (6–13)	8 (7–11)	0.840	

* Pain was evaluated using an 11-point numerical rating scale (NRS) from 0 = no pain to 10 = maximum imaginable pain. ** Neuropathic pain was defined by a DN4 score ≥ 4 [11]. *** Satisfaction was evaluated using an 11-point numerical rating scale (NRS) from 0 = totally disappointed to 10 = totally satisfied. **** Classification of postoperative complications according to the Clavien classification [13]. Number of available data in case of missing data is expressed as {xx}. Values are expressed as median (25th percentile–75th percentile) or n (%) as appropriate. ns = not statistically significant.

3.5. Predictive Factors of Pain Trajectories

Variables in the multinomial logistic regression were age, preoperative state of health qualified by the ASA score, presence of preoperative pain, use of at least one pain medication, and preoperative anxiety. Three entities relevant to thoracic surgery were also analyzed: rib fractures, transcostal suture, and scar length. This corresponds to the variables reaching the defined threshold for inclusion ($p < 0.20$). The preoperative neuropathic component of pain was not included in the analysis because of the large number of missing values. The permanent non-significant pain trajectory group (group 2) is the reference group for multinomial logistic regression.

Some predictive factors allow for differentiation between trajectory groups 1 and 2. Risk factors for permanent pain are the existence of preoperative pain (OR = 6.94, 95% CI (1.54–31.27)) and scar length (OR = 1.20 (95% CI (1.05–1.38))). In contrast, ASA class III is a protective factor in group 1 (OR = 0.02, 95% CI (0.001–0.52)) (Table 7).

Table 7. Multivariable analysis of factors linked to pain trajectories (trajectory group 2 as reference).

	Trajectory Group 1 OR (CI95%)		Trajectory Group 3 OR (CI95%)		Trajectory Group 4 OR (CI95%)	
Age	0.96	(0.91–1)	0.99	(0.94–1.03)	0.98	(0.93–1.04)
ASA class						
II	0.15	(0.01–2.36)	0.57	(0.03–13.01)	0.21	(0.01–6.07)
III	0.02	(0.001–0.52)	0.51	(0.02–13.78)	0.06	(0.001–2.48)
Anxiety	4.75	(0.90–25.14)	0.75	(0.21–2.59)	1.91	(0.38–9.64)
Preoperative pain	6.94	(1.54–31.27)	1.46	(0.40–5.34)	0.78	(0.13–4.56)
At least one analgesic	1.58	(0.39–6.44)	1.85	(0.46–7.48)	2.58	(0.40–16.72)
Rib fracture	0.86	(0.15–4.78)	0.13	(0.01–1.33)	2.51	(0.49–12.85)
Transcostal suture	0.59	(0.14–2.54)	1.49	(0.39–5.73)	0.32	(0.05–2.08)
Scar length	1.20	(1.05–1.38)	1.11	(0.98–1.27)	1.12	(0.96–1.31)

OR (CI95%): odds ratios and 95% confidence intervals.

No predictive factor could allow for differentiation between trajectory group 2 and groups 3 or 4.

4. Discussion

4.1. Main Results of Our Study

To our knowledge, this is the first description of pain trajectories during the early postoperative period after lung surgery. For patients operated by PL or AX approaches using a mini-invasive technique like video-assisted thoracoscopic surgery, in terms of early complications, pain, performance status, and quality of life [15], four pain trajectories can be identified after lung surgery: constantly high, constantly low, decreased, and increased pain trajectories over time. Moreover, we identified two risk factors (preoperative pain and scar length) and a protective factor (ASA class III) for the worst pain trajectory when compared to the best one.

4.2. Interpretation

Defining acute postoperative pain as a trajectory rather than as one or more simple point estimates of intensity increases the information yield of pain assessment and improves measurement precision [8,16]. Thus, it must be underlined that a high percentage of patients experience pain during the early postoperative period despite the analgesic techniques put in place and followed-up by nurses who specialize in pain management. This percentage is 44.7% when adding patients with permanent significant pain from day 0 to day 5 (group 1) and patients with steep increases in pain over these days (group 4). Few authors have reported early postoperative pain trajectories. Althaus et al. pooled data of patients having undergone orthopedic surgery, general surgery, visceral surgery, and neurosurgery and reported three types of pain trajectory: little initial pain on the first postoperative day with further pain resolution (57% of the patients), severe pain with a high rate of pain resolution (30%), and permanent high pain intensity (13%) [17]. Five trajectory groups were reported by Vasilopoulos et al. after pooling data of patients having undergone major orthopedic, urologic, colorectal, pancreatic/biliary, thoracic, or spine surgery. Four trajectories identified patients with low (7% of the patients), moderate-to-low (24%), moderate-to-high (46%), and high pain (17%) over time; one trajectory corresponded to patients with drastically decreasing postoperative pain (6%) [10]. It is difficult to compare the distribution of patients according to trajectories between this study and ours. Thus, as in our study, Vasilopoulos et al. found that approximately one in two patients can be categorized as having a painful experience despite the use of many preoperative nerve blocks. However, postoperative pain treatment is not detailed, as pointed out by Kehlet and Foss [18].

There are numerous studies of the risk factors of postoperative pain using pain as the main outcome. Ip et al., studying 48 eligible studies with 23,037 patients, identified preoperative pain, anxiety, age, and type of surgery, but not gender, as significant predictors for postoperative pain [19]. A similar study by Gerbershagen et al. reported that female gender, younger age, and preoperative chronic pain are associated with higher postoperative pain in a large multicenter cohort of patients having had heterogeneous surgical procedures [20]. More recently, a systematic review and meta-analysis identified nine predictors of poor postoperative pain control, with odds ratios ranging from 1.02 to 2.32: younger age, female gender, smoking, depression, anxiety, sleep difficulties, high body mass index, presence of preoperative pain, and use of preoperative analgesics [21].

Regarding the specific question of postoperative pain after lung surgery, the work carried out by Kwon et al. must be underlined since it compared pain after robotic, video-assisted thoracoscopic surgery and open anatomic pulmonary resection and reported that female gender, younger age, and baseline narcotic use were associated with acute postoperative pain [22].

Replacing the measurement of postoperative pain with the determination of pain trajectories has little effect on the determination of risk factors. Thus, Vasilopoulos et al. also reported that risk factors for the stable moderate-to-high and high pain groups are female gender and young age while preoperative high anxiety and depression and greater pain behaviors and pain catastrophizing were linked to the stable high group [10]. After lung surgery, we found dissimilar predictive factors, preoperative pain and scar length, for painful trajectories and a protective factor, ASA class III. We did not find an association between female gender and increased postoperative pain intensity, as previously shown across a variety of surgical procedures [20,23,24], but as we have seen above, other studies did not find this factor [19]. Similarly, we did not find that young age is linked to increased postoperative pain, as previously reported [10,19,20,22], although van Dijk et al. reported in a large and heterogenous international cohort that postoperative pain decreases with increasing age, but these authors qualified this relation as small and of questionable clinical significance [25].

Among behavioral factors that have been reported as strongly associated with acute postoperative pain intensity, preoperative anxiety is highlighted [10,19,21]. This point is unfortunately not confirmed in our study, perhaps because more than two thirds of the patients were anxious preoperatively. This underscores the importance of studying risk factors in a homogeneous patient population with respect to their pathology and surgical procedure.

4.3. Strength and Limitations of the Study

The strength of our study is that it was conducted under real-life conditions, with the data collected reflecting the vagaries of management, including the successes and failures of surgical procedures and analgesia techniques.

On the other hand, our study suffers from several important limitations.

As specified before, this study is an ancillary study from another that studied the development of chronic pain after PL and AX approaches for thoracic surgery.

This study established four clusters describing postoperative pain by mixing patients operated on by PL thoracotomy or by AX thoracotomy. Posterolateral thoracotomy is increasingly being replaced by video-assisted thoracoscopic surgery and robot-assisted thoracic surgery, which result in less acute pain [22]. On the other hand, AX thoracotomy is rarely performed at present but represents a model of mini-invasive surgery. Numerous patients received thoracic epidural postoperative analgesia, preventing an analysis of the role of this technique in the prevention of postoperative pain.

Our study did not include randomization for the choice of approach because the surgeons considered it unethical to use approaches they were unfamiliar with. It was decided that participating surgeons would use the approach they routinely used and were familiar with. Such conduct is usual since most studies comparing PL thoracotomy and VATS do not include randomization.

Our preoperative screening of potential factors linked to postoperative pain was obviously incomplete. The evaluation of anxiety was rather short, and we did not evaluate psychological factors such as depression, pain coping and catastrophism, and sleep disorders. A genetic study is also missing.

4.4. Generalizability

Our study combined patients having had a large surgical approach and a mini-invasive one. These two approaches are being progressively discarded and replaced by video-assisted thoracoscopic surgery and robot-assisted thoracic surgery; our results cannot be generalized to the whole lung surgical population.

Moreover, most of our patients benefited from a thoracic epidural postoperative analgesia. This was the choice of our team at the time of this study, but this strategy has evolved towards less-invasive techniques [5,6].

5. Conclusions

In conclusion, we identified four trajectories for early postoperative pain after lung surgery performed by posterolateral and axillary approaches. The major risk factor for permanent pain trajectory is preoperative pain, which should lead to a more aggressive pre-operative management unless it represents a constitutive factor, perhaps genetic. We confirmed the benefit of mini-invasive surgery since scar length is also reported as a risk factor for postoperative pain. On the other hand, it is difficult to explain why ASA class III is a strong protective factor unless it is related to more careful management.

Author Contributions: Conceptualization, M.M.-C., M.F. and V.M.; methodology, M.M.-C. and M.F.; validation, P.D., M.M.-C. and M.F.; formal analysis, T.K. and A.V.; investigation, P.D., M.M.-C., J.F., B.S., E.S., M.G. and M.L.G.; data curation, M.M.-C. and M.F.; writing—original draft preparation, P.D., M.M.-C. and M.F.; writing—review and editing, P.D., M.M.-C., J.F., B.S., E.S., M.G., T.K., M.F., V.M., A.V. and M.L.G.; supervision, M.F.; project administration, M.F. All authors have read and agreed to the published version of the manuscript.

Funding: This research received no external funding.

Institutional Review Board Statement: The present study reports the postoperative findings of a prospective, observational, single-center study and was approved by the Ethics Committee of Ile-de-France XI (n° 2013-A01641-44; Chairperson M. Catz) on 16 January 2014. The study was designed in accordance with the STROBE Standard for Observational studies).

Informed Consent Statement: Informed consent was obtained from all subjects involved in the study.

Data Availability Statement: Data supporting the reported results are available on the Dryad website open-access repository (https://doi:10.5061/dryad.f4qrfj6zp, accessed on 26 August 2022).

Acknowledgments: The authors thank Virginie Vaillant, Margot Ribeiro, and Amélie Schmidt for their help in collecting clinical data, B. Lefebvre for her help in collecting and organizing data, and Polly Gobin for her linguistic assistance.

Conflicts of Interest: The authors declare no conflict of interest.

References

1. Pöpping, D.M.; Elia, N.; Van Aken, H.K.; Marret, E.; Schug, S.A.; Kranke, P.; Wenk, M.; Tramèr, M.R. Impact of epidural analgesia on mortality and morbidity after surgery: Systematic review and meta-analysis of randomized controlled trials. *Ann. Surg.* **2014**, *259*, 1056–1067. [CrossRef] [PubMed]
2. Agostini, P.J.; Naidu, B.; Rajesh, P.; Steyn, R.; Bishay, E.; Kalkat, M.; Singh, S. Potentially modifiable factors contribute to limitation in physical activity following thoracotomy and lung resection: A prospective observational study. *J. Cardiothorac. Surg.* **2014**, *9*, 128. [CrossRef] [PubMed]
3. Ismail, N.A.; Elsaegh, M.; Dunning, J. Novel Techniques in Video-assisted Thoracic Surgery (VATS) Lobectomy. *Surg. Technol. Online* **2015**, *26*, 206–209.

4. Guo, F.; Ma, D.; Li, S. Compare the prognosis of Da Vinci robot-assisted thoracic surgery (RATS) with video-assisted thoracic surgery (VATS) for non-small cell lung cancer: A Meta-analysis. *Medicine* **2019**, *98*, e17089. [CrossRef]
5. Gupta, R.; Van de Ven, T.; Pyati, S. Post-Thoracotomy Pain: Current Strategies for Prevention and Treatment. *Drugs* **2020**, *80*, 1677–1684. [CrossRef]
6. Humble, S.R.; Dalton, A.J.; Li, L. A systematic review of therapeutic interventions to reduce acute and chronic post-surgical pain after amputation, thoracotomy or mastectomy. *Eur. J. Pain* **2015**, *19*, 451–465. [CrossRef]
7. Willingham, M.D.; Vila, M.R.; Ben Abdallah, A.; Avidan, M.S.; Haroutounian, S. Factors Contributing to Lingering Pain after Surgery: The Role of Patient Expectations. *Anesthesiology* **2021**, *134*, 915–924. [CrossRef]
8. Chapman, C.R.; Donaldson, G.W.; Davis, J.J.; Bradshaw, D.H. Improving Individual Measurement of Postoperative Pain: The Pain Trajectory. *J. Pain* **2011**, *12*, 257–262. [CrossRef]
9. Okamoto, A.; Yamasaki, M.; Yokota, I.; Mori, M.; Matsuda, M.; Yamaguchi, Y.; Yamakita, S.; Ueno, H.; Sawa, T.; Taguchi, T.; et al. Classification of acute pain trajectory after breast cancer surgery identifies patients at risk for persistent pain: A prospective observational study. *J. Pain Res.* **2018**, *11*, 2197–2206. [CrossRef]
10. Vasilopoulos, T.; Wardhan, R.; Rashidi, P.; Fillingim, R.B.; Wallace, M.R.; Crispen, P.L.; Parvataneni, H.K.; Prieto, H.A.; Machuca, T.N.; Hughes, S.J.; et al. Patient and Procedural Determinants of Postoperative Pain Trajectories. *Anesthesiology* **2021**, *134*, 421–434. [CrossRef]
11. Bouhassira, D.; Attal, N.; Alchaar, H.; Boureau, F.; Brochet, B.; Bruxelle, J.; Cunin, G.; Fermanian, J.; Ginies, P.; Grun-Overdyking, A.; et al. Comparison of pain syndromes associated with nervous or somatic lesions and development of a new neuropathic pain diagnostic questionnaire (DN4). *Pain* **2005**, *114*, 29–36. [CrossRef] [PubMed]
12. Jonsson, M.; Hurtig-Wennlöf, A.; Ahlsson, A.; Vidlund, M.; Cao, Y.; Westerdahl, E. In-hospital physiotherapy improves physical activity level after lung cancer surgery: A randomized controlled trial. *Physiotherapy* **2019**, *105*, 434–441. [CrossRef] [PubMed]
13. Dindo, D.; Demartines, N.; Clavien, P.A. Classification of surgical complications: A new proposal with evaluation in a cohort of 6336 patients and results of a survey. *Ann. Surg.* **2004**, *240*, 205–213. [CrossRef] [PubMed]
14. Mongardon, N.; Pinton-Gonnet, C.; Szekely, B.; Michel-Cherqui, M.; Dreyfus, J.F.; Fischler, M. Assessment of chronic pain after thoracotomy: A 1-year prevalence study. *Clin. J. Pain* **2011**, *27*, 677–681. [CrossRef]
15. Erus, S.; Tanju, S.; Kapdağlı, M.; Özkan, B.; Dilege, Ş.; Toker, A. The comparison of complication, pain, quality of life and performance after lung resections with thoracoscopy and axillary thoracotomy. *Eur. J. Cardio-Thorac. Surg.* **2014**, *46*, 614–619. [CrossRef]
16. Bayman, E.O.; Oleson, J.J.; Rabbitts, J.A. AAAPT: Assessment of the Acute Pain Trajectory. *Pain Med.* **2021**, *22*, 533–547. [CrossRef]
17. Althaus, A.; Becker, O.A.; Moser, K.-H.; Lux, E.A.; Weber, F.; Neugebauer, E.; Simanski, C. Postoperative Pain Trajectories and Pain Chronification—an Empirical Typology of Pain Patients. *Pain Med.* **2018**, *19*, 2536–2545. [CrossRef]
18. Kehlet, H.; Foss, N.B. Acute Postoperative Pain Trajectory Groups: Comment. *Anesthesiology* **2021**, *135*, 547. [CrossRef]
19. Ip, H.Y.; Abrishami, A.; Peng, P.W.; Wong, J.; Chung, F. Predictors of postoperative pain and analgesic consumption: A qualitative systematic review. *Anesthesiology* **2009**, *111*, 657–677. [CrossRef]
20. Gerbershagen, H.J.; Pogatzki-Zahn, E.; Aduckathil, S.; Peelen, L.M.; Kappen, T.; van Wijck, A.J.M.; Kalkman, C.; Meissner, W. Procedure-specific Risk Factor Analysis for the Development of Severe Postoperative Pain. *Anesthesiology* **2014**, *120*, 1237–1245. [CrossRef]
21. Yang, M.M.H.; Hartley, R.L.; Leung, A.; Ronksley, P.E.; Jetté, N.; Casha, S.; Riva-Cambrin, J. Preoperative predictors of poor acute postoperative pain control: A systematic review and meta-analysis. *BMJ Open* **2019**, *9*, e025091. [CrossRef] [PubMed]
22. Kwon, S.T.; Zhao, L.; Reddy, R.M.; Chang, A.C.; Orringer, M.B.; Brummett, C.M.; Lin, J. Evaluation of acute and chronic pain outcomes after robotic, video-assisted thoracoscopic surgery, or open anatomic pulmonary resection. *J. Thorac. Cardiovasc. Surg.* **2017**, *154*, 652–659. [CrossRef] [PubMed]
23. Bartley, E.J.; Fillingim, R.B. Sex differences in pain: A brief review of clinical and experimental findings. *Br. J. Anaesth.* **2013**, *111*, 52–58. [CrossRef] [PubMed]
24. Tighe, P.J.; Riley, J.L., III; Fillingim, R.B. Sex differences in the incidence of severe pain events following surgery: A review of 333,000 pain scores. *Pain Med.* **2014**, *15*, 1390–1404. [CrossRef] [PubMed]
25. van Dijk, J.F.; Zaslansky, R.; van Boekel, R.L.; Cheuk-Alam, J.M.; Baart, S.J.; Huygen, F.J.; Rijsdijk, M. Postoperative pain and age: A retrospective cohort association study. *Anesthesiology* **2021**, *135*, 1104–1119. [CrossRef]

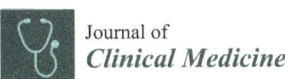

Article

The Analgesic Efficacy of the Single Erector Spinae Plane Block with Intercostal Nerve Block Is Not Inferior to That of the Thoracic Paravertebral Block with Intercostal Nerve Block in Video-Assisted Thoracic Surgery

Sujin Kim [1], Seung Woo Song [1], Hyejin Do [1], Jinwon Hong [1], Chun Sung Byun [2] and Ji-Hyoung Park [1,*]

1 Department of Anesthesiology and Pain Medicine, Wonju College of Medicine, Yonsei University, Wonju 26426, Korea
2 Department of Thoracic and Cardiovascular Surgery, Wonju College of Medicine, Yonsei University, Wonju 26426, Korea
* Correspondence: killerjhjh@yonsei.ac.kr; Tel.: +82-33-741-1536

Citation: Kim, S.; Song, S.W.; Do, H.; Hong, J.; Byun, C.S.; Park, J.-H. The Analgesic Efficacy of the Single Erector Spinae Plane Block with Intercostal Nerve Block Is Not Inferior to That of the Thoracic Paravertebral Block with Intercostal Nerve Block in Video-Assisted Thoracic Surgery. *J. Clin. Med.* **2022**, *11*, 5452. https://doi.org/10.3390/jcm11185452

Academic Editor: Marco Cascella

Received: 28 July 2022
Accepted: 13 September 2022
Published: 16 September 2022

Publisher's Note: MDPI stays neutral with regard to jurisdictional claims in published maps and institutional affiliations.

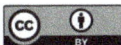

Copyright: © 2022 by the authors. Licensee MDPI, Basel, Switzerland. This article is an open access article distributed under the terms and conditions of the Creative Commons Attribution (CC BY) license (https://creativecommons.org/licenses/by/4.0/).

Abstract: This monocentric, single-blinded, randomized controlled noninferiority trial investigated the analgesic efficacy of erector spinae plane block (ESPB) combined with intercostal nerve block (ICNB) compared to that of thoracic paravertebral block (PVB) with ICNB in 52 patients undergoing video-assisted thoracic surgery (VATS). The endpoints included the difference in visual analog scale (VAS) scores for pain (0–10, where 10 = worst imaginable pain) in the postanesthetic care unit (PACU) and 24 and 48 h postoperatively between the ESPB and PVB groups. The secondary endpoints included patient satisfaction (1–5, where 5 = extremely satisfied) and total analgesic requirement in morphine milligram equivalents (MME). Median VAS scores were not significantly different between the groups (PACU: 2.0 (1.8, 5.3) vs. 2.0 (2.0, 4.0), $p = 0.970$; 24 h: 2.0 (0.8, 3.0) vs. 2.0 (1.0, 3.5), $p = 0.993$; 48 h: 1.0 (0.0, 3.5) vs. 1.0 (0.0, 5.0), $p = 0.985$). The upper limit of the 95% CI for the differences (PACU: 1.428, 24 h: 1.052, 48 h: 1.176) was within the predefined noninferiority margin of 2. Total doses of rescue analgesics (110.24 ± 103.64 vs. 118.40 ± 93.52 MME, $p = 0.767$) and satisfaction scores (3.5 (3.0, 4.0) vs. 4.0 (3.0, 5.0), $p = 0.227$) were similar. Thus, the ESPB combined with ICNB may be an efficacious option after VATS.

Keywords: video-assisted thoracic surgery; erector spinae plane block; paravertebral block; intercostal nerve block

1. Introduction

Although it is less invasive and damaging to tissue, video-assisted thoracic surgery (VATS) still causes moderate to severe postoperative pain [1]. Postoperative pain is an independent predictor of mortality and morbidity [2]. In addition, acute pain after thoracic surgery is associated with chronic pain; therefore, postoperative pain control is a main goal [3]. The thoracic epidural block (TEB) is the standard procedure for a regional block in thoracotomy; however, the paravertebral block (PVB) is known to show equipotent efficacy [4]. These are also widely used in VATS procedures. The erector spinae plane block (ESPB) is a simple fascial plane block that serves as an alternative to an epidural block, with fewer side effects [5]. It appears to be an effective analgesic technique at many levels and functions as an alternative when the PVB or epidural block is contraindicated [6]. However, some clinical trials have shown that ESPB has a lesser analgesic effect than PVB [7]; thus, no consensus has been reached. The intercostal nerve block (ICNB) is a multimodal analgesia technique following thoracic surgery, and its analgesic efficacy has been proven [8]. However, no study has compared the analgesic effects of ESPB and PVB when combined with ICNB.

We hypothesized that the ESPB would not be less effective than the PVB for attenuating pain when combined with ICNB after VATS. The primary outcome of this monocentric, single-blinded, randomized controlled noninferiority trial was the median difference in postoperative pain scores between the groups. The secondary outcomes were the cumulative postoperative analgesic consumption (calculated as oral morphine milligram equivalents, MME) and patient satisfaction scores.

2. Materials and Methods

2.1. Study Population

The study trial was approved by the Institutional Review Board of Yonsei University Wonju College of Medicine, Wonju, Korea, and the participants are listed at https://cris.nih.go.kr (accessed on 18 May 2021, KCT 0006271). We enrolled 52 patients with American Society of Anesthesiologists physical status I, II, or III, aged 19–80 years, who had undergone VATS between June 2021 and January 2022. Patients were excluded from the study for cognitive impairment, anticoagulant administration, coagulopathy, antiplatelet drug administration within 48 h, double antiplatelet therapy, surgical site infection, refusal of procedure, allergic reaction to local anesthetic, requiring therapeutic anticoagulant therapy after surgery, or pregnancy. Patients with comorbid diseases were excluded according to the judgment of the anesthesiologist (sepsis, anatomical thoracic deformity, empyema, increased intracranial pressure, etc.). Patients were randomly and evenly assigned to either the PVB with ICNB group or the ESPB with ICNB group by a computer-generated randomization table. Blinding of the group designation was maintained for the patients and attending anesthesiologists, except one practitioner (J.-H.P.) who performed the PVB or ESPB.

2.2. Perioperative Management

Anesthesia was induced by a bolus of propofol (1.5–2 mg/kg) and remifentanil (1 mcg/kg). Rocuronium (0.6 mg/kg) was used for tracheal intubation. The remifentanil infusion rate was adjusted by the attending anesthesiologist according to the overall hemodynamic data and the suggested intensity of surgical stimuli. The fraction of inhaled anesthetics was administered under BIS guidance. The surgeon performed the ICNB and placed a chest tube during the surgery. At the end of the surgery, the ESPB or PVB was performed in the lateral position. One anesthesiologist (J.-H.P.) performed the PVB and ESPB. The same experienced surgeon (C.S.B.) performed the ICNB. The intravenous patient-controlled analgesia (PCA) was used at the discretion of the anesthesiologist, and the dose was recorded in terms of morphine milligram equivalents (MME). The patients were extubated and transported to the postanesthetic care unit (PACU). The standard analgesic algorithm in PACU was intravenous nonopioid analgesics for visual analog scale pain scores of 4–6 [1] and intravenous fentanyl (50 μg) for VAS pain scores >6 [2]. The postoperative pain in the ward was controlled by the primary physician. Administered analgesic drugs were converted into MME and recorded in case record forms. The analgesics used in the ward were intravenous tramadol, intramuscular or subcutaneous meperidine, oral Ultracet® (tramadol 37.5 mg/acetaminophen 325 mg), and transdermal fentanyl patch.

2.3. Paravertebral Block

After surgery, each patient was placed in the lateral decubitus position, and skin preparation was performed. The patient was palpated at the T5 level, and the linear transducer was positioned in a vertical plane approximately 2.5 cm lateral to the palpated spinous process, obtaining a sagittal plane of the transverse process, superior costovertebral ligament, intertransverse ligaments, desired paravertebral space, pleura, and lung tissue. The paravertebral space was bordered by the vertebral body, intervertebral foramen, parietal pleura, and costovertebral ligament. A 21-gauge, 10 cm echogenic needle (Vygon SA; Ecouen, France) was placed in the paravertebral space using an in-plane approach to confirm that there was no blood aspiration. A small amount of local anesthetic was then injected into the test dose in real time to reduce the anterior displacement of the pleura and spine. Ropivacaine (0.375%, 20 cc) was injected with aspiration every 5 cc to prevent intravascular injection.

2.4. Erector Spinae Plane Block

At the T5 level, the linear transducer was moved slowly from the midline to the lateral, and the transducer was moved approximately 3 cm until a transverse projection was observed. It was distinguishable from the ribs at that level: the transverse process is shallow and wide, whereas the ribs are deep and thin. The trapezius, rhomboid, and erector spinae muscles were then identified. An echogenic needle was inserted from the head to the foot, using an in-plane approach, and advanced toward the transverse process through the trapezius, rhomboid, and erector spinae muscles under ultrasound guidance. A small amount of local anesthetic was administered when the needle tip was located below the erector spinae muscle. The correct position of the needle was verified by visually confirming that the erector spinae muscle was separated from the transverse process. Ropivacaine (0.375%, 20 cc) was injected with aspiration every 5 cc to prevent intravascular injection.

2.5. Intercostal Nerve Block

At the end of the surgical procedure, a total of 10 cc of ropivacaine (2 cc per space) was injected into the intercostal space until swelling of the intercostal nerve at the T4–T8 levels occurred.

2.6. Outcome Measures

The primary endpoint of the present study was to assess the analgesic efficacy of ESPB compared with that of PVB when combined with ICNB by measuring the median differences between the groups in the VAS of pain at the PACU, as well as 24 and 48 h after surgery. The secondary endpoints were to investigate the total amount of analgesics administered to the patients in MME and the satisfaction score of patients using a five-point rating scale.

2.7. Sample Size Calculation

The standard deviation for PVB with ICNB in the pilot study was 2.29, and no significant difference was observed in the variance between the ESPB and PVB in a previous study [9]. When the noninferiority margin (delta value) was set to 2, it was determined based on the opinion of colleagues and a previous study [10]. The significance level was set to 0.05, and the power was set to 0.9; accordingly, the estimated number of patients required in each group was 23. Accounting for a dropout rate of 10%, we decided to enroll 26 patients in each group.

2.8. Statistical Analysis

All statistical analyses were performed using the IBM SPSS statistical software package (IBM SPSS Statistics for Windows, version 25, IBM Corporation, Armonk, NY, USA). Distribution of continuous variables was assessed using the Shapiro–Wilk test. Intergroup comparisons of the non-normally distributed variables were performed using the Mann–Whitney U test and are reported as the median (interquartile range). Intergroup comparisons of other variables that showed a normal distribution were tested using an independent t-test and are reported as the mean ± standard deviation (SD). For pain scores assessed at three timepoints, a post hoc Bonferroni correction was applied to adjust for multiple comparisons.

3. Results

In total, 52 patients were screened, and all of them were enrolled and assigned to the two groups. There was no dropout among the enrolled patients. Hence, all 52 patients were included in the final analysis.

The patient characteristics and types and durations of the surgeries were similar between the groups (Table 1).

Table 1. Patient characteristics and surgery details.

	PVB-ICNB (n = 26)	ESPB-ICNB (n = 26)	p-Value
Female (%)	9 (34.6)	13 (50.0)	
Age	62.42 ± 13.11	60.31 ± 15.43	0.597
Height	161.09 ± 11.33	161.01 ± 10.14	0.978
Weight	62.34 ± 10.43	60.18 ± 10.72	0.464
BSA	1.66 ± 0.18	1.63 ± 0.17	0.591
Diabetes mellitus	11 (42.3)	6 (23.1)	0.143
Preoperative analgesics	3 (11.5)	3 (11.5)	1.000
Operation Type			
Lobectomy	12 (46.2)	13 (50.0)	
Segmentectomy	3 (11.5)	0 (0.0)	
Wedge resection	10 (38.5)	13 (50.0)	
Mediastinal mass	1 (3.8)	0 (0.0)	
OP time (min)	85.96 ± 48.48	97.69 ± 55.38	0.420

Values are displayed as the mean ± SD or n (%). PVB: paravertebral block, ESPB: erector spinae plane block, ICNB: intercostal nerve block, BSA: body surface area, OP: operation.

The visual analog scale (VAS) scores for each timepoint were not significantly different between the ESPB and PVB groups. The higher limit of the 95% CI for this difference (1.428 at PACU, 1.052 at 24 h, 1.176 at 48 h) was within the predefined noninferiority margin of 2 (delta). The total doses of rescue analgesics (110.24 ± 103.64 vs. 118.40 ± 93.52 MME, p = 0.767), the number of rescue analgesic events (5.88 ± 1.56 vs. 5.50 ± 1.45, p = 0.361), and satisfaction scores (3.5 (3.0, 4.0) vs. 4.0 (3.0, 5.0), p = 0.227) were not significantly different between the two groups (Figure 1). There were no significant differences in the intraoperative dose of remifentanil or the frequency of hypotension, bradycardia, or pleural puncture that occurred during the operation after the block (Table 2). The number of patients with moderate (VAS > 3) or severe (VAS > 6) pain was also similar between the two groups. We continuously identified the needle-tip position with ultrasound during the block. However, in the PVB-ICNB group, we recognized the pleural puncture, which was confirmed by the spread of the local analgesics into the pleura in two cases. The placement of the chest tube after the VATS procedure was performed as standard of care [11]. In both cases, the chest tube was removed and discharged without pneumothorax or other complications.

The hemodynamic data, including heart rate and mean arterial blood pressure during surgery, were also similar between the groups (Figure 2).

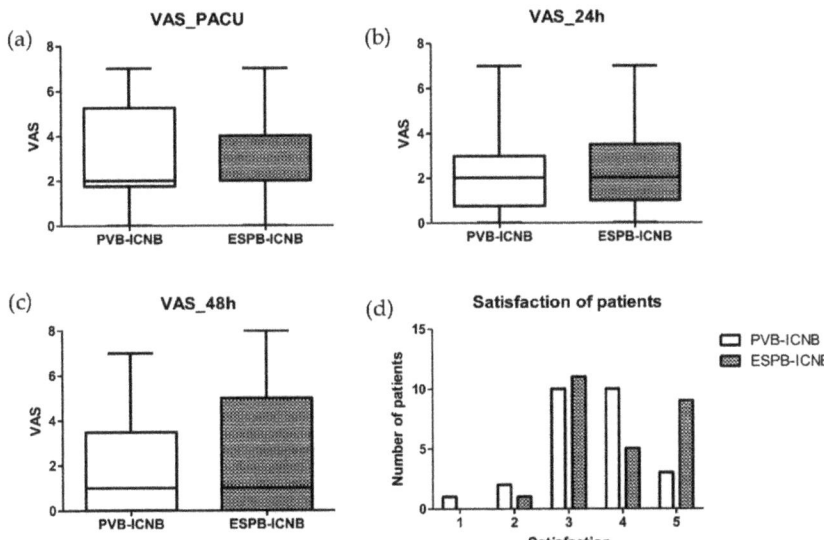

Figure 1. Visual analog scale (VAS) and satisfaction of patients: (**a**) VAS at PACU; (**b**) VAS at 24 h postoperatively; (**c**) VAS at 48 h postoperatively; (**d**) Satisfaction scores of patients. PACU: postanesthetic care unit, PVB: paravertebral block, ESPB: erector spinae plane block, ICNB: intercostal nerve block.

Table 2. Outcome measures.

	PVB-ICNB (n = 26)	ESPB-ICNB (n = 26)	95% CI	p-Value
Primary Endpoint				
VAS PACU	2.0 (1.8, 5.3)	2.0 (2.0, 4.0)	(−0.890, 1.428)	0.970
VAS 24 h	2.0 (0.8, 3.0)	2.0 (1.0, 3.5)	(−1.283, 1.052)	0.993
VAS 48 h	1.0 (0.0, 3.5)	1.0 (0.0, 5.0)	(−1.637, 1.176)	0.985
Above Moderate Pain (VAS > 3)				
VAS PACU	8 (30.8)	7 (26.9)		0.762
VAS 24 h	5 (19.2)	6 (23.1)		0.737
VAS 48 h	6 (23.1)	8 (30.8)		0.536
Above Severe Pain (VAS > 6)				
VAS PACU	4 (15.4)	2 (7.7)		0.390
VAS 24 h	1 (3.8)	2 (7.7)		0.556
VAS 48 h	1 (3.8)	2 (7.7)		0.556
Secondary Endpoints				
Rescue Analgesics (MME)	110.24 ± 103.64	118.40 ± 93.52		0.767
Number of Rescue Analgesic Events	5.88 ± 1.56	5.50 ± 1.45		0.361
Satisfaction of Patients	3.5 (3.0, 4.0)	4.0 (3.0, 5.0)		0.227
Remifentanil (μg)	511.62 ± 205.51	547.42 ± 224.35		0.551
Antiemetics				
Dose	1.59 ± 0.63	1.44 ± 0.67		0.408
Hypotension	2 (7.7)	4 (15.4)		0.390
Bradycardia	0 (0)	2 (3.8)		0.153
Pleural Puncture	2 (3.8)	0 (0)		0.153
Hospital Day	9.04 ± 4.20	9.27 ± 3.77		0.836

Values are displayed as the mean ± SD, n (%), or median (interquartile range). The pain score was assessed using a visual analog scale (VAS) (0 = no pain, 10 = worst imaginable pain). The rescue analgesic requirement was calculated in morphine milligram equivalents (MME). The satisfaction score was assessed using a five-point numerical scale (1 = extremely dissatisfied, 5 = extremely satisfied). VAS: visual analog scale, PACU: postanesthetic care unit, PVB: paravertebral block, ESPB: erector spinae plane block, ICNB: intercostal nerve block, SD: standard deviation, CI: confidence interval.

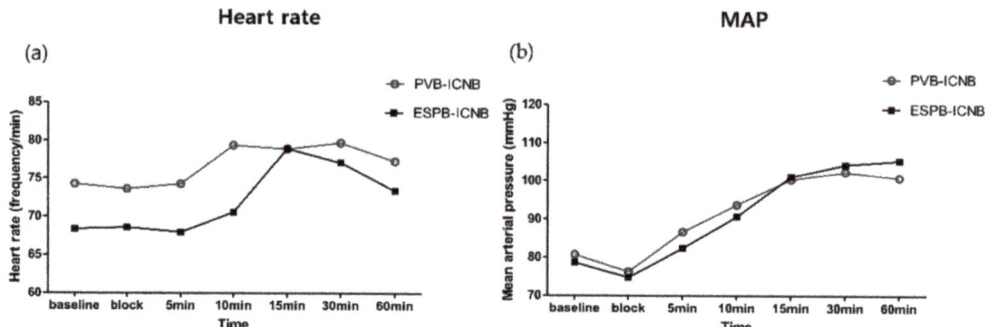

Figure 2. Hemodynamic data: (**a**) Heart rate; (**b**) Mean arterial pressure.

4. Discussion

The results of the present trial suggest that ESPB was not inferior in analgesic efficacy to PVB when combined with ICNB for attenuating surgery-related pain. Moreover, this combination block was similar in terms of patient satisfaction, analgesic requirement, and the frequency of hemodynamic perturbations. In addition, although the difference was not significant, pleural puncture was absent in the ESPB-ICNB group but present in two cases in the PVB-ICNB group.

VATS is a minimally invasive procedure that results in minimal tissue trauma. Nevertheless, it also causes significant and intense acute pain, which may lead to post-thoracotomy pain syndrome [12]. The scope manipulation and use of rib retractors in VATS may cause intercostal nerve injury [13]. In addition, multiple muscle incisions and pleural irritation from chest tubes can cause moderate to severe pain [1].

TEB has long been the standard procedure for pain control after thoracotomy. However, side effects such as hypotension, bradycardia, and pruritus are common, and analgesic failure often occurs because of an incorrect target position. In addition, catastrophic side effects, such as epidural hematoma, require close attention [14]. A previous meta-analysis showed that PVB has an equipotent analgesic effect after thoracotomy compared with TEB [15]. However, the paravertebral space is narrow, and pleural puncture risks are possible [16].

ESPB involves the injection of local anesthetics into the fascial plane between the transverse process and erector spinae muscle [17]. In the case of VATS, the ports are positioned in the intercostal space of the mid-clavicular and post-scapular line, and an incision measuring 4–5 cm is positioned in the mid-axillary line [18]. Mostly, the intercostal nerves originating from the anterior rami of spinal nerves are responsible for sensory innervation [19]. However, since adjacent nerves branch out and perform various anastomoses with each other, sensory innervation is not well-associated with the segment level [20]. Therefore, it is important that the analgesics spread not only to the pathway of the intercostal nerve but also to adjacent segments. A previous literature review reported that the injectates spread to the ventral rami in 13 out of 16 cadaveric studies and to the paravertebral space in 12 studies through the thoracic ESPB. In all 16 studies, craniocaudal spread over three levels was observed [21]. In previous analyses, ESPB showed comparable efficacy to PVB in terms of opioid consumption and pain scores [22,23]. Controversial results indicating that PVB is superior to ESPB in terms of pain scores and opioid consumption have been reported [7,24].

Although there is no consensus on the analgesic effect, ESPB has several advantages over PVB. Firstly, it is technically easier to contact the transverse process than it is to fix a needle tip in the relatively narrow paravertebral space. Therefore, high skill is not required for the practitioners, and the difference in efficacy was shown to be little among the practitioners [19]. Moreover, since the paravertebral space is adjacent to the pleura, the puncture risk in PVB is higher than that in ESPB [19]. Thirdly, in terms of anticoagulation, ESPB has an advantage over PVB, which is considered a neuraxial block. Furthermore, the paravertebral space is a noncompressible area, but the target of the ESPB is compressible.

However, unpredictable spread of injectates in ESPB was reported in some trials [25,26]. Therefore, the use of ICNB in conjunction with ESPB may enhance the analgesic effect. ICNB can be easily performed without complications while directly observing the spread. However, PVB provides better analgesic efficacy than ICNB [27]. In the present study, single ESPB combined with ICNB was not inferior to PVB combined with ICNB in terms of analgesic efficacy and opioid consumption. This combination block can be an effective and safe option to control pain after thoracoscopic surgery.

Our study had several limitations. Firstly, the analgesic effect was compared using a subjective index. However, there is no objective indicator that measures the pain index, and several previous trials have used the NRS as an effective tool for evaluating analgesic efficacy [28,29]. Secondly, we did not study patients for a long duration. According to the literature, moderate to severe pain is maintained postoperatively in approximately 10% of patients at 52 weeks [30]. Therefore, if we evaluated the patients for a longer period, the analgesic efficacy between the groups might have been better exhibited. Thirdly, our single-center setting and small sample size may have been insufficient for validating the secondary endpoints of the study. Fourthly, since both procedures were performed under general anesthesia, examination of the dermatomal level for analgesia, such as the pinprick test, could not be performed. Fifthly, the total dose and number of rescue analgesics exceeded those commonly used in VATS. This may have been a confounding factor in comparing the efficacy between the groups. However, in the previous study, 56% of patients complained of moderate to severe pain when only intravenous PCA was used [31]. Reducing the prevalence of moderate to severe pain and the VAS pain score in the present study showed the advantage of the combined block in both groups. Lastly, we did not include a control group of patients that only received ICNB. Therefore, it is difficult to determine to what extent the combination of regional block techniques in VATS is really advantageous.

In conclusion, the present study is the first trial to compare the effects of ESPB and PVB with ICNB. Both groups provided an adequate analgesic effect in VATS. However, compared to PVB, ESPB is easier to implement and has advantages in terms of safety due to no adjacent vulnerable structures. The present study provided evidence that ESPB with ICNB may be an efficacious analgesic option in VATS.

Author Contributions: Conceptualization, S.K. and J.-H.P.; methodology, S.K. and J.-H.P.; software, S.W.S. and J.-H.P.; validation, S.K., S.W.S., H.D. and J.-H.P.; formal analysis, H.D.; investigation, S.K.; resources, S.W.S., J.H. and C.S.B.; data curation, J.H.; writing—original draft preparation, S.K. and J.-H.P.; writing—review and editing, J.-H.P.; visualization, H.D.; supervision, J.-H.P.; project administration, C.S.B. and J.-H.P. All authors read and agreed to the published version of the manuscript.

Funding: This research received no external funding.

Institutional Review Board Statement: This study was conducted in accordance with the Declaration of Helsinki and approved by the Institutional Review Board of Yonsei University Wonju College of Medicine (IRB No. CR321026 on 18 May 2021).

Informed Consent Statement: Informed consent was obtained from all subjects involved in the study.

Data Availability Statement: The data presented in this study are available upon request from the corresponding author.

Conflicts of Interest: The authors declare no conflict of interest.

References

1. Sun, K.; Liu, D.; Chen, J.; Yu, S.; Bai, Y.; Chen, C.; Yao, Y.; Yu, L.; Yan, M. Moderate-severe postoperative pain in patients undergoing video-assisted thoracoscopic surgery: A retrospective study. *Sci. Rep.* **2020**, *10*, 795. [CrossRef] [PubMed]
2. Kehlet, H. Postoperative pain, analgesia, and recovery-bedfellows that cannot be ignored. *Pain* **2018**, *159*, S11–S16. [CrossRef] [PubMed]
3. Bayman, E.O.; Parekh, K.; Keech, J.; Selte, A.; Brennan, T. A Prospective Study of Chronic Pain after Thoracic Surgery. *Anesthesiology* **2017**, *126*, 938–951. [CrossRef] [PubMed]
4. Steinthorsdottir, K.; Wildgaard, L.; Hansen, H.J.; Petersen, R.H.; Wildgaard, K. Regional analgesia for video-assisted thoracic surgery: A systematic review. *Eur. J. Cardiothorac. Surg.* **2014**, *45*, 959–966. [CrossRef]

5. Elsabeeny, W.Y.; Ibrahim, M.A.; Shehab, N.N.; Mohamed, A.; Wadod, M.A. Serratus Anterior Plane Block and Erector Spinae Plane Block Versus Thoracic Epidural Analgesia for Perioperative Thoracotomy Pain Control: A Randomized Controlled Study. *J. Cardiothorac. Vasc. Anesth.* **2021**, *35*, 2928–2936. [CrossRef]
6. Kot, P.; Rodriguez, P.; Granell, M.; Cano, B.; Rovira, L.; Morales, J.; Broseta, A.; De Andrés, J. The erector spinae plane block: A narrative review. *Korean J. Anesthesiol.* **2019**, *72*, 209–220. [CrossRef]
7. Turhan, O.; Sivrikoz, N.; Sungur, Z.; Duman, S.; Özkan, B.; Şentürk, M. Thoracic Paravertebral Block Achieves Better Pain Control Than Erector Spinae Plane Block and Intercostal Nerve Block in Thoracoscopic Surgery: A Randomized Study. *J. Cardiothorac. Vasc. Anesth.* **2021**, *35*, 2920–2927. [CrossRef]
8. Guerra-Londono, C.E.; Privorotskiy, A.; Cozowicz, C.; Hicklen, R.S.; Memtsoudis, S.G.; Mariano, E.R.; Cata, J.P. Assessment of Intercostal Nerve Block Analgesia for Thoracic Surgery: A Systematic Review and Meta-analysis. *JAMA Netw. Open* **2021**, *4*, e2133394. [CrossRef]
9. Gürkan, Y.; Aksu, C.; Kuş, A.; Yörükoğlu, U.H. Erector spinae plane block and thoracic paravertebral block for breast surgery compared to IV-morphine: A randomized controlled trial. *J. Clin. Anesth.* **2020**, *59*, 84–88. [CrossRef]
10. Gutierrez, J.J.P.; Ben-David, B.; Rest, C.; Grajales, M.T.; Khetarpal, S.K. Quadratus lumborum block type 3 versus lumbar plexus block in hip replacement surgery: A randomized, prospective, non-inferiority study. *Reg. Anesth. Pain Med.* **2020**, *46*, 111–117. [CrossRef]
11. Imperatori, A.; Rotolo, N.; Gatti, M.; Nardecchia, E.; De Monte, L.; Conti, V.; Dominioni, L. Peri-operative complications of video-assisted thoracoscopic surgery (VATS). *Int. J. Surg.* **2008**, *6*, S78–S81. [CrossRef]
12. Gerner, P. Postthoracotomy Pain Management Problems. *Anesthesiol. Clin.* **2008**, *26*, 355–367. [CrossRef]
13. Kirby, T.J.; Mack, M.J.; Landreneau, R.J.; Rice, T.W. Lobectomy—Video-assisted thoracic surgery versus muscle-sparing thoracotomy: A randomized trial. *J. Thorac. Cardiovasc. Surg.* **1995**, *109*, 997–1001; discussion 1001–1002. [CrossRef]
14. Horlocker, T.T.; Vandermeuelen, E.; Kopp, S.L.; Gogarten, W.; Leffert, L.R.; Benzon, H.T. Regional Anesthesia in the Patient Receiving Antithrombotic or Thrombolytic Therapy: American Society of Regional Anesthesia and Pain Medicine Evidence-Based Guidelines (Fourth Edition). *Reg. Anesth. Pain Med.* **2018**, *43*, 263–309. [CrossRef]
15. Yeung, J.; Gates, S.; Naidu, B.V.; Wilson, M.J.A.; Smith, F.G. Paravertebral block versus thoracic epidural for patients undergoing thoracotomy. *Cochrane Database Syst. Rev.* **2016**, *2*, CD009121. [CrossRef]
16. Ardon, A.E.; Lee, J.; Franco, C.D.; Riutort, K.T.; Greengrass, R.A. Paravertebral block: Anatomy and relevant safety issues. *Korean J. Anesthesiol.* **2020**, *73*, 394–400. [CrossRef]
17. Chin, K.J. Thoracic wall blocks: From paravertebral to retrolaminar to serratus to erector spinae and back again—A review of evidence. *Best Pract. Res. Clin. Anaesthesiol.* **2019**, *33*, 67–77. [CrossRef]
18. Kim, H.K. Video-Assisted Thoracic Surgery Lobectomy. *J. Chest Surg.* **2021**, *54*, 239–245. [CrossRef]
19. Chin, K.J.; Versyck, B.; Pawa, A. Ultrasound-guided fascial plane blocks of the chest wall: A state-of-the-art review. *Anaesthesia* **2021**, *76*, 110–126. [CrossRef]
20. Chin, K.J.; Pawa, A.; Forero, M.; Adhikary, S. Ultrasound-Guided Fascial Plane Blocks of the Thorax: Pectoral I and II, Serratus Anterior Plane, and Erector Spinae Plane Blocks. *Adv. Anesth.* **2019**, *37*, 187–205. [CrossRef]
21. Chin, K.J.; El-Boghdadly, K. Mechanisms of action of the erector spinae plane (ESP) block: A narrative review. *Can. J. Anaesth.* **2021**, *68*, 387–408. [CrossRef] [PubMed]
22. Jo, Y.; Park, S.; Oh, C.; Pak, Y.; Jeong, K.; Yun, S.; Noh, C.; Chung, W.; Kim, Y.-H.; Ko, Y.K.; et al. Regional analgesia techniques for video-assisted thoracic surgery: A frequentist network meta-analysis. *Korean J. Anesthesiol.* **2022**, *75*, 231–244. [CrossRef] [PubMed]
23. Lin, J.; Liao, Y.; Gong, C.; Yu, L.; Gao, F.; Yu, J.; Chen, J.; Chen, X.; Zheng, T.; Zheng, X. Regional Analgesia in Video-Assisted Thoracic Surgery: A Bayesian Network Meta-Analysis. *Front. Med.* **2022**, *9*, 842332. [CrossRef] [PubMed]
24. Sertcakacilar, G.; Pektas, Y.; Yildiz, G.O.; Isgorucu, O.; Kose, S. Efficacy of ultrasound-guided erector spinae plane block versus paravertebral block for postoperative analgesia in single-port video-assisted thoracoscopic surgery: A retrospective study. *Ann. Palliat. Med.* **2022**, *11*, 1981–1989. [CrossRef]
25. Zhang, J.; He, Y.; Wang, S.; Chen, Z.; Zhang, Y.; Gao, Y.; Wang, Q.; Xia, Y.; Papadimos, T.J.; Zhou, R. The erector spinae plane block causes only cutaneous sensory loss on ipsilateral posterior thorax: A prospective observational volunteer study. *BMC Anesthesiol.* **2020**, *20*, 88. [CrossRef]
26. Dautzenberg, K.H.W.; Zegers, M.J.; Bleeker, C.P.; Tan, E.C.T.H.; Vissers, K.C.P.; van Geffen, G.-J.; van der Wal, S.E.I. Unpredictable Injectate Spread of the Erector Spinae Plane Block in Human Cadavers. *Anesth. Analg.* **2019**, *129*, e163–e166. [CrossRef]
27. Huan, S.; Deng, Y.; Wang, J.; Ji, Y.; Yin, G. Efficacy and safety of paravertebral block versus intercostal nerve block in thoracic surgery and breast surgery: A systematic review and meta-analysis. *PLoS ONE* **2020**, *15*, e0237363. [CrossRef]
28. Borys, M.; Gawęda, B.; Horeczy, B.; Kolowca, M.; Olszówka, P.; Czuczwar, M.; Woloszczuk-Gebicka, B.; Widenka, K. Erector spinae-plane block as an analgesic alternative in patients undergoing mitral and/or tricuspid valve repair through a right mini-thoracotomy—An observational cohort study. *Wideochir Inne Tech Maloinwazyjne* **2020**, *15*, 208–214. [CrossRef]
29. Liu, L.; Ni, X.-X.; Zhang, L.-W.; Zhao, K.; Xie, H.; Zhu, J. Effects of ultrasound-guided erector spinae plane block on postoperative analgesia and plasma cytokine levels after uniportal VATS: A prospective randomized controlled trial. *J. Anesth.* **2021**, *35*, 3–9. [CrossRef]

30. Bendixen, M.; Jørgensen, O.D.; Kronborg, C.; Andersen, C.; Licht, P.B. Postoperative pain and quality of life after lobectomy via video-assisted thoracoscopic surgery or anterolateral thoracotomy for early stage lung cancer: A randomised controlled trial. *Lancet Oncol.* **2016**, *17*, 836–844. [CrossRef]
31. Bayman, E.O.; Parekh, K.R.; Keech, J.; Larson, N.; Weg, M.V.; Brennan, T.J. Preoperative Patient Expectations of Postoperative Pain Are Associated with Moderate to Severe Acute Pain After VATS. *Pain Med.* **2019**, *20*, 543–554. [CrossRef]

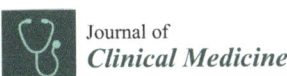

Article

Different Machine Learning Approaches for Implementing Telehealth-Based Cancer Pain Management Strategies

Marco Cascella [1,2,*], Sergio Coluccia [3], Federica Monaco [1], Daniela Schiavo [1], Davide Nocerino [1], Mariacinzia Grizzuti [1], Maria Cristina Romano [1] and Arturo Cuomo [1]

1. Department of Anesthesia and Critical Care, Istituto Nazionale Tumori—IRCCS, Fondazione Pascale, 80100 Naples, Italy
2. Department of Electrical Engineering and Information Technologies—DIETI, University Federico II, 80138 Naples, Italy
3. Epidemiology and Biostatistics Unit, Istituto Nazionale Tumori—IRCCS, Fondazione Pascale, 80100 Naples, Italy
* Correspondence: m.cascella@istitutotumori.na.it; Tel.: +39-0815903221

Abstract: Background: The most effective strategy for managing cancer pain remotely should be better defined. There is a need to identify those patients who require increased attention and calibrated follow-up programs. Methods: Machine learning (ML) models were developed using the data prospectively obtained from a single-center program of telemedicine-based cancer pain management. These models included random forest (RF), gradient boosting machine (GBM), artificial neural network (ANN), and the LASSO–RIDGE algorithm. Thirteen demographic, social, clinical, and therapeutic variables were adopted to define the conditions that can affect the number of teleconsultations. After ML validation, the risk analysis for more than one remote consultation was assessed in target individuals. Results: The data from 158 patients were collected. In the training set, the accuracy was about 95% and 98% for ANN and RF, respectively. Nevertheless, the best accuracy on the test set was obtained with RF (70%). The ML-based simulations showed that young age (<55 years), lung cancer, and occurrence of breakthrough cancer pain help to predict the number of remote consultations. Elderly patients (>75 years) with bone metastases may require more telemedicine-based clinical evaluations. Conclusion: ML-based analyses may enable clinicians to identify the best model for predicting the need for more remote consultations. It could be useful for calibrating care interventions and resource allocation.

Keywords: telemedicine; telehealth; teleconsultations; predictive models; machine learning; cancer pain; random forest; gradient boosting machine; artificial neural network; LASSO–RIDGE algorithm

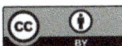

1. Introduction

Managing cancer-related pain typically requires a complex and multimodal approach [1]. One of the main challenges concerns the development of a useful pathway for addressing the multiple problems that can occur during the disease course [2–4].

Given that a model of care based on face-to-face visits requires an important commitment of resources, innovative strategies must be evaluated. Telemedicine may offer a variety of applications to re-evaluate pathways of care, including cancer pain management [5]. In this context, telemedicine-based strategies can have a paramount economic and organizational impact on healthcare systems [6], enhancing the quality of the care provided. A recent evidence-based analysis demonstrated that eHealth interventions are effective in improving pain management [7]. Although during the COVID-19 pandemic, different telemedicine approaches have been proposed [8], there is a need for establishing pathways that are valid beyond the emergency and routinely applied to clinical practice [9,10].

On the other hand, lacking the literature data from large-scale clinical experiences and precise directives from scientific societies, it is difficult to establish a model that provides for the integration of telemedicine in the treatment process. Consequently, a proper strategy for the management of cancer pain through telemedicine should be fully designed.

The use of predictive models represents an important opportunity in medicine. The benefits of artificial intelligence (AI) and its branches such as machine learning (ML) are intended to enhance patient care, but also involve organizational processes and healthcare systems [11]. In the planning of care pathways, AI represents a valuable helpful resource to improve hospital workflows, identifying the activities that require priority and providing an adequate service to the patient's needs. Recently, for example, it was demonstrated that AI strategies such as natural language processing models can be a reliable guide to trigger early access for uncontrolled pain and other symptoms in palliative care [12].

In a recent cross-sectional investigation, we proposed a model of care and evaluated adherence to the telemedicine pathway [13]. This "hybrid" model provides for scheduled remote visits, but the patient can require other consultations. Additionally, in-person access is provided for emergencies or for diagnostic or clinical aims. For each patient, the number of telemedicine visits can vary depending on an unspecified number of reasons, and we have noticed that some patients required a greater number of remote consultations. On these premises, the purpose of this study is the development of data-driven predictive models for identifying those patients who may require more remote consultations. In the context of precision medicine for cancer pain management, we implemented ML algorithms to better customize treatment strategies. As pieces of evidence are needed to establish the most appropriate telemedicine pathways, the recognition of those patients who require a greater number of remote visits can stimulate the planning of ad hoc processes for managing multiple care needs and calibrating resource allocation.

2. Materials and Methods

2.1. Study Population

The study population included adult patients treated for cancer pain at the Istituto Nazionale Tumori, Fondazione Pascale, Italy.

A hybrid model of care was implemented. After the first in-person visit for a complete clinical and instrumental evaluation and for addressing legal and regulatory issues (consent acquisition), data collection, and training, a synchronous real-time video consultation was scheduled according to the clinical need. Further remote controls were programmed or required by the patients. Moreover, face-to-face visits were allowed to carry out minimally invasive procedures, for diagnosis, acute clinical motivations (e.g., drug side effects), or if requested by the patient [13].

The local Medical Ethics Committee approved this study (protocol code 41/20 Oss; date of approval, 26 November 2020), and all patients provided written informed consent. The investigation was conducted in accordance with the Declaration of Helsinki.

2.2. Data Collection

For each patient, 13 demographic, clinical, and therapeutic variables were collected to investigate the potential causes that may affect the number of remote consultations (Table 1). All the data were reported on a prospectively filled database and then registered on Zenodo [14]. The duration of the study was considered the time interval between the first and last remote consultations. The death of the patient and the occurrence of in-person visits or hospitalization were assumed as the conditions for the end of the observation period for data acquisition. The lack of further remote consultations for a two-month period was another condition for considering the observation closed.

The univariate analysis was performed to detect the main associations of selected features with the outcome variable (remote consultations: one or more).

Table 1. Data collection and variables.

Data Collected	Variable(s)
Demographic and Social Information	Age Gender Working status (Y/N) Living with a partner * (Y/N) Education level
Clinical Data	Type of primary tumor Bone metastases ECOG-PS
Pain Therapy	MED Drugs for NP ROOs PAMORAs IV-Morphine
Remote Visits	Number

Abbreviations: ECOG-PS, Eastern Cooperative Oncology Group Performance Status; MED, morphine-equivalent dose; NP, neuropathic pain; ROOs, rapid-onset opioids; PAMORAs, peripherally acting μ-opioid receptor antagonists; IV-Morphine, intravenous morphine. Legend: * including cohabitation and marriage.

2.3. Predictive Analysis

2.3.1. Preprocessing and Exploratory Data Analysis

After the loading, normalization, and standardization of the dataset (preparation process or preprocessing), as well as an exploratory data analysis aimed at discovering trends, the variables were selected. The expectation–maximization (EM) algorithm was used for the imputation of the missing data [15]. To facilitate model implementations and the interpretation of results, three age groups were obtained by categorizing the variable "age": ≤55 years old (called "younger patients"), 56–75 years old, and >75 years old ("older patients").

2.3.2. Machine Learning Algorithms

Four ML-based algorithms were adopted as follows:

- LASSO–RIDGE regression (elastic model): This is a generalized linear regression model that penalizes a loss function through regressor resizing (16 in all). Most of them are made small or led to zero if not important to explain the dependent variable. This approach reduces model complexity and prevents the over-fitting phenomena [16];
- Random forest (RF) algorithm: This algorithm can be used for both regression and classification. It is one of the most popular ML methods, belonging to the specific category of bagging methods. RF works on various overall models (decision trees) to improve the performance of each of them individually. The output is the whole contribution from all of them [17];
- Gradient boosting machine (GBM) is aimed at optimizing previsions by operating on the previous tree regression or classification error and reducing the error function (boosting method). In this way, the succeeding one can improve the prevision skills let by its preceding tree [18];
- Single hidden layer artificial neural network (ANN): This strategy can minimize a loss function by acting on some weights which tune connections between two neurons of two adjoining layers [19].

We chose these four ML-based prediction models for implementing different methods for regression or classification, such as bagging and boosting (RF and GMB, for additive regression models), and a strong learning method to compare different numerical approaches (LASSO–RIDGE, a binary regression model); ANN is one of the function algorithms that are largely used for classification (and regression) problems.

2.3.3. Model Processing and Evaluation

Since a predictive analysis was performed in order to predict which cancer patient should need to have more than one remote consultation, the outcome variable was "the number of remote consultations" as dichotomized. Each classifier was optimized by repeated cross-validation (RCV) methods to focus on the best guess through the K-fold mean error calculus and to determine the hyperparameters that support the best guess and identify its structure. The sample was split into a training set (80% of the total size) to identify the hyperparameters and a test set for testing the models (20% of the total size).

A wide choice of hyperparameters was given to every algorithm to finally evaluate the best performance. In particular, each combination of hyperparameters was inserted as input for the algorithm. An 8-fold 5-repeated cross-validation method was adopted to find the best one, so the dataset was divided into 8 parts (20 individuals for any time), and the training and test parts were performed for each combination and for 5 times; the misclassification error rate was calculated upon 5 attempts (for a more precise managing of results). For each algorithm, the following features were applied:

- GBM: The number of sequential trees from 20 to 100 by 10, tree depth from 2 to 5 shrinkage parameter (regularizing the error function) from 0.01 to 0.1 by 0.01, and a minimum observation-in-a-leaf from 10 to 20 for a total of 3960 were assessed;
- RF: Only the number of splitting variables was required, which was from 3 to 13;
- LASSO–RIDGE: Regression alpha and beta were, respectively, given as from 0 to 1 by 0.05 and 0 to 10 by 0.1, for a total of 2121 trials;
- ANN: This layer was made from 1 to 12 neurons and the decay (a regularization parameter to avoid the over-fitting of weights) ranged from 0.01 to 0.2 by 0.01, for a total of 240 trials.

Comparisons were assessed through these models by calculating the accuracy and area under the receiver operating characteristic (ROC) curve (AUC). The AUC represents the sensibility (i.e., TP/(TP+FN)) and 1-specificity (1-FP/(TN+FP)) ratio. The AUC can easily be approximated with the measure of accuracy in the case of equidistribution between the modalities of the employee, but it is also suitable for solving problems of poorly distributed modalities. Each member is comparable to the observed value conditional correct classification rates, respectively. In other words, the AUC is equivalent to the probability that a random positive response is classified with respect to a random negative one. Another adopted goodness-of-prevision statistic parameter was the F1 score:

$$F1 = 2 * (precision * recall)/(precision + recall) \quad (1)$$

This measure considers the precision and recall of the test; precision is the number of true positives divided by the number of all the positive results, while recall is the number of true positives divided by the number of all the tests that should have been positive (i.e., true positives plus false negatives). The values of F1 scores range from 0 to 1.

Finally, Mathew's correlation coefficients (MCC) were calculated (from the confusion matrix) for each model, for obtaining a broad view of their predictive power and robustness (TP, true positive; TN, true negative; FP, false positive; FN, false negative):

$$MCC = \frac{TP * TN - FP * FN}{\sqrt{(TP+FP)(TP+FN)(TN+FP)(TN+FN)}} \quad (2)$$

2.3.4. Risk Analysis

Based on the ML processes, the risk analysis for an increased number (>1) of remote consultations was assessed. We used an odds-ratio-like analysis that we indicated as the simulated odds ratios (SORs). Simulations were assessed in order to evaluate the risk of more consultations in target individuals. In particular, approximately 500 simulations were performed 150 times for creating a classification rate for the cases (target individuals) and control individuals. Subsequently, we calculated the odds ratio as the ratio of the effective odds for each individual typology and 95% credibility intervals (95% CIs) as the effective 2.5 and 97.5 percentiles for the SOR samples. Although wide possibilities were possible, the following four standard clinical conditions (targets) were established:

- Condition 1: Young patients (≤55 years old) with bone metastases and rapid-acting oral and nasal transmucosal fentanyl formulation (ROO) use (morphine-equivalent dose, MED > 60 mg) for breakthrough cancer pain (BTcP);
- Condition 2: Older cancer patients (>75 years old), with and without bone metastases;
- Condition 3: Male and female young patients (≤55 years old) with bone metastases;
- Condition 4: Younger (≤55 years old) vs. older (>75 years old) patients with bone metastases with gender differences.

2.4. Algorithmic Toolkit

The data were analyzed using the *R* software version 4.1.3 (R Core Teams, R Foundation for Statistical Computing, Vienna, Austria). The toolkit included the mice package [20] for the imputation of the missing data. Caret was the main suite used for the implementation (creation, training) and evaluation (testing) of the classifiers [21]. Moreover, purr, pROC, and pRROC [22] were adopted for the construction and visualization of the ROC curves. The graphics packages included ggplot, ggpubr, and cowplot.

3. Results

A total of 267 patients were evaluated for cancer pain management through remote consultations between March 2021 and February 2022. Of these patients, 109 were excluded for not being available or having incomplete data; finally, the data from 158 patients were used for the descriptive and predictive analyses (Figure 1).

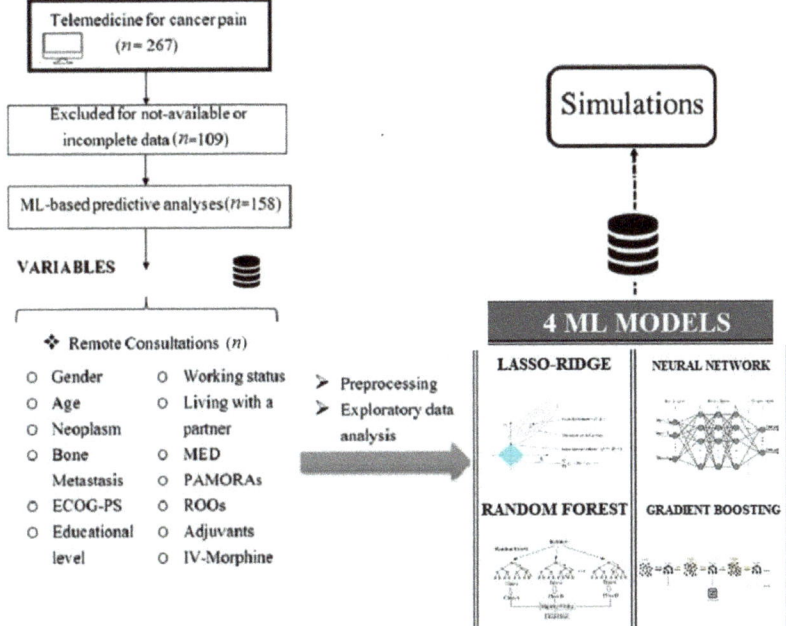

Figure 1. Flowchart of the study. Abbreviations: ML, machine learning; ECOG-PS, Eastern Cooperative Oncology Group Performance Status; MED, morphine-equivalent dose; PAMORAs, peripherally acting μ-opioid receptor antagonists; ROOs, rapid-onset opioids; IV-Morphine, intravenous morphine. Legend: the category "living with a partner" includes cohabitation and marriage.

3.1. Descriptive Analysis

The median age was 63 years old. Fifty-one percent were female. Just over half of the patients (53%) had more than one visit. The average number of visits was 2.27, with a standard deviation of 2.05 (Table 2).

The reasons for interruption of the telemedicine pathway (dropouts) were the patient's death ($n = 63$, 39.9%), the need for an invasive procedure ($n = 15$, 9.5%) or an in-person clinical assessment ($n = 14$, 8.9%). Six patients (3.8%) requested an in-person visit. Unplanned hospital admissions occurred in seven patients (4.4%). About a third of the patients ($n = 53$, 33.5%) were not evaluated (in person or remotely) for at least two months. These patients were contacted (email and telephone), and about half ($n = 28$) did not provide an answer; the remainder ($n = 25$) said they did not need further visits for cancer pain (Figure 2).

The univariate analysis was performed for evaluating the differences between the cohort of patients who underwent one remote consultation and those who received more telemedicine evaluations (Table 3).

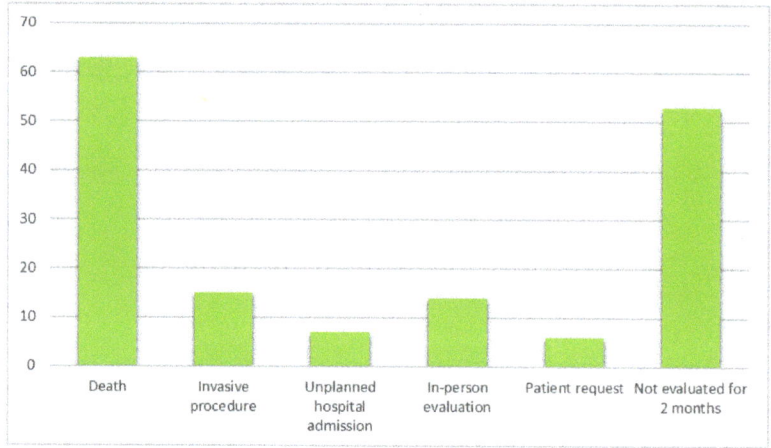

Figure 2. Reasons for interruption of the telemedicine pathway ($n = 158$).

3.2. Predictive Analysis

Table 4 summarizes the results of the implemented ML methods. In our analyses, the accuracy, that is the proportion of the well-ranked parameters, relative to the training set, reached almost 100% for the RF and ANN algorithms. Nevertheless, the accuracy of the ANN on the test set was reduced by almost 50 percentage points. By contrast, RF showed an acceptable classification level (70% accuracy in the test) ($p = 0.05$) with an F1 score of 0.71.

The overall performance of a classifier, summarized over all the possible thresholds, is given by the area under the ROC curve (AUC). An ideal ROC curve will hug the top left corner: the larger the area under the curve, the better the classifier. Reducing the false-positive rate (FPR) and, at the same time, increasing the true-negative rate (TNR) is like finding a trade-off cut point between the error rates. A classifier that performs worse than a random classification has an AUC statistic of 0.5. Thus, an AUC value closer to 1 indicates a more adequate classification and a lower level of error: Its value is theoretically almost 1 as it is built. The AUC performances of the considered classifiers are reported in Figure 3.

Table 2. Data from the considered variables.

Variable	n = 158 *
Age (years)	
Mean (SD)	63 (13)
Median (IQR)	65 (55, 72)
Class of Age (years old)	
≤55	43 (27%)
56–75	86 (54%)
>75	29 (18%)
Gender	
Female	81 (51%)
Male	77 (49%)
Working Status (n = 153)	
Not Working	110 (72%)
Working	43 (28%)
Education Level (n = 146)	
Secondary School	41 (28%)
High School	68 (47%)
Bachelor's or Higher Degrees	37 (25%)
Living with a Partner (n = 153)	
Yes	107 (70%)
No	46 (30%)
Neoplasm	
Lung	22 (14%)
Colorectal	39 (25%)
Breast	21 (13%)
Others	76 (48%)
Bone metastases (n = 156)	
No	72 (46%)
Yes	84 (54%)
ECOG-PS	
ECOG-PS <3	84 (53%)
ECOG-PS = 3	74 (47%)
MED	
≤60 mg	64 (41%)
>60 mg	94 (59%)
Assuming ROOs	
No	114 (72%)
Yes	44 (28%)
Assuming PAMORAs	
No	125 (79%)
Yes	33 (21%)
Assuming drugs for NP	
No	78 (49%)
Yes	80 (51%)
Assuming IV-morphine	
No	146 (92%)
Yes	12 (7.6%)
Remote consultations (n = 158)	
Mean (SD)	2.27 (2.05)
Median (IQR)	2 (1, 3)
Min–Max for Patient	1–16
Remote consultations (categories)	
1	74 (47%)
>1	84 (53%)

Abbreviations: * n (%); ECOG-PS, Eastern Cooperative Oncology Group Performance Status; MED, morphine-equivalent dose; ROOs, rapid-onset opioids; PAMORAs, peripherally acting µ-opioid receptor antagonists; NP, neuropathic pain; IV-Morphine, intravenous morphine.

Table 3. Univariate analysis for data exploration.

	Remote Consultations		
Variable	one, n = 74 *	≥2, n = 84 *	p-value ^
Age (years)			0.019
n	74	84	
Mean (SD)	65 (13)	61 (13)	
Median (IQR)	68 (57, 75)	62 (53, 70)	
Class of Age (years old)			0.030
≤55	13 (18%)	30 (36%)	
56–75	44 (59%)	42 (50%)	
>75	17 (23%)	12 (14%)	
Gender			0.537
Female	36 (49%)	45 (54%)	
Male	38 (51%)	39 (46%)	
Working Status			0.987
No	51 (72%)	59 (72%)	
Yes	20 (28%)	23 (28%)	
(Missing)	3	2	
Education Level			0.374
Secondary School	22 (33%)	19 (24%)	
High School	31 (46%)	37 (47%)	
Graduation	14 (21%)	23 (29%)	
(Missing)	7	5	
Cohabiting/Marriage			0.711
Yes	50 (71%)	57 (69%)	
No	20 (29%)	26 (31%)	
(Missing)	4	1	
Cancer Type			0.516
Lung	8 (11%)	14 (17%)	
Colorectal	19 (26%)	20 (24%)	
Breast	8 (11%)	13 (15%)	
Others	39 (53%)	37 (44%)	
Bone Metastases			0.458
No	36 (49%)	36 (43%)	
Yes	37 (51%)	47 (57%)	
(Missing)	1	1	
ECOG-PS			0.396
<3	42 (57%)	42 (50%)	
=3	32 (43%)	42 (50%)	
MED			
<60 mg	33 (45%)	31 (37%)	
>60 mg	41 (55%)	53 (63%)	
Assuming ROOs			0.829
No	54 (73%)	60 (71%)	
Yes	20 (27%)	24 (29%)	
Assuming PAMORA			0.831
No	58 (78%)	67 (80%)	
Yes	16 (22%)	17 (20%)	
Assuming anti-NP Drugs			0.269
No	40 (54%)	38 (45%)	
Yes	34 (46%)	46 (55%)	
Assuming IV-Morphine			0.115
No	71 (96%)	75 (89%)	
Yes	3 (4.1%)	9 (11%)	

Legend: * n (%); ^ Wilcoxon rank-sum test; Pearson's chi-squared test; significance at 95%. Abbreviations: ECOG-PS, Eastern Cooperative Oncology Group Performance Status; MED, morphine-equivalent dose; ROOs, rapid-onset opioids; PAMORAs, peripherally acting μ-opioid receptor antagonists; NP, neuropathic pain; IV-Morphine, intravenous morphine.

Table 4. Performance comparison of the different classifiers for the developed machine learning models.

Classifier	AUC	ACC (tr)	ACC (tst)	L	U	p	Sens (tst)	Spec (tst)	F1 Score	MCC
GBM	0.59	0.58	0.5	0.31	0.69	0.71	0.69	0.29	0.59	−0.03
RF	0.98	1	0.7	0.51	0.85	0.05	0.69	0.71	0.71	0.40
LASSO	0.5	0.53	0.53	0.34	0.72	0.57	1	0	0.7	-
ANN	0.95	1	0.57	0.37	0.75	0.43	0.5	0.64	0.55	0.14

Abbreviations: GBM, gradient boosting machine; RF, random forest; LASSO, LASSO–RIDGE regression; ANN, artificial neural network; AUC, area under the receiver operating characteristic curve; ACC (tr), accuracy on training; ACC (tst), accuracy on test set; L and U, 95%CI lower and upper limits of test set accuracy statistic; p, accuracy on the test set and relative test for significance; Sens (tst), sensibility on the test; Spec (tst), specificity on the test. MCC, Mathew's Correlation Coefficient.

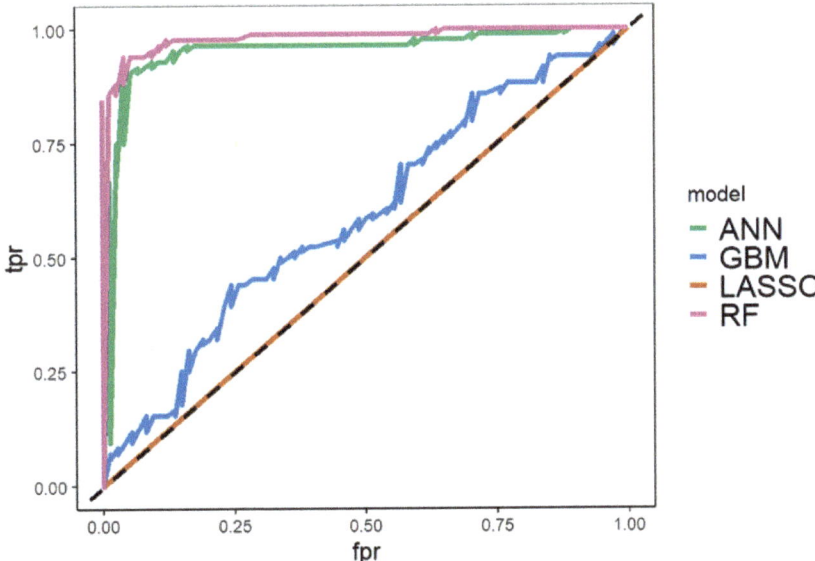

Figure 3. The area under the receiver operating characteristic (ROC) curve (AUC) of the considered models. False-positive rate (fpr) and true-negative rate (tpr) were considered. The plot shows the ROC curves calculated for each classifier over the entire dataset. RF and NN offer the best performance. Abbreviations: LASSO, LASSO–RIDGE regression; GBM, gradient boosting machine; ANN, artificial neural network; RF, random forest.

The confusion matrix for the two best models (RF and ANN) during the training phase is shown in Table 5.

Table 5. Comparison (confusion matrix) for the two best models.

	RF		ANN	
	One	≥2	One	≥2
One	10	5	9	8
≥2	4	11	5	8

Legend: one or more consultations were considered. Abbreviations: RF, random forest; ANN, artificial neural network.

3.3. Risk Analysis

The model with the best performance (i.e., RF) was implemented for assessing the risk analysis in different scenarios.

Condition 1: We calculated the risk of having repeated remote consultations for different cancer types. The other features were kept as randomly chosen. For those with lung neoplasm, there was a probability of 93.4% (92.6%, 94.2%) to receive multiple consultations and a higher risk (+172.2%, 95% CI = +70%, +301.1%) than cancer patients with no bone metastases; for those patients with colorectal neoplasm, the percentage was 88.8% (88%, 89.7%), and this risk was +92.2% (95%CI = +40.4%, +156.4%). For those affected by other cancers, the percentage was 71.9% (70.6%, 73.3%), and the risk was +55.5% (95%CI = +19.2%, +106.9%). For breast neoplasm with bone metastases, 90.1% (89.2%, 91.2%) of the patients were predicted to have multiple consultations, and +90.6% (95%CI = +32.5%, +158%) was their predicted risk for multiple consultations, compared with those without bone metastasis (Figure 4).

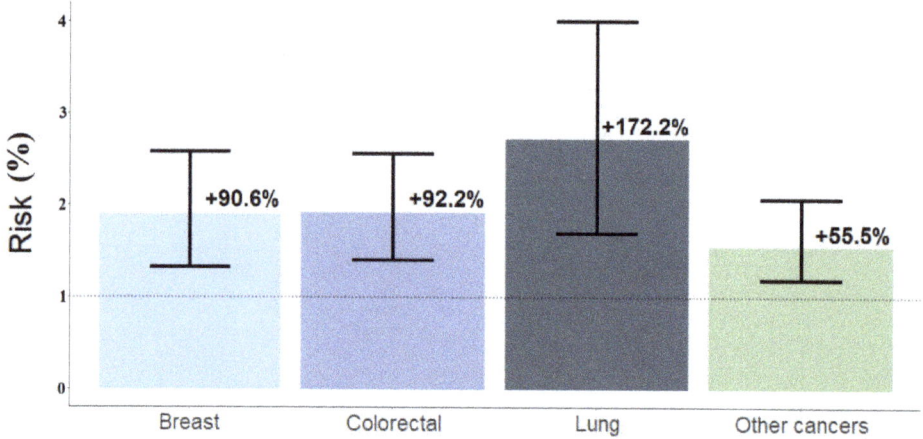

Figure 4. Simulation 1 refers to simulated odds ratios (SORs); percentages are labeled. This was performed for young patients (≤55 years old) with bone metastases and ROO use and young patients with bone metastases vs. those with no bone metastases. SORs for lung cancer were 2.72 (95%CI = 1.70–4.01); colorectal cancer 1.92 (95%CI = 1.40–2.56); other cancers 1.55 (95%CI = 1.19–2.07); breast cancer 1.91 (95%CI = 1.32, 2.58).

Condition 2: The same analysis was performed for older cancer patients (>75 years old), with and without bone metastases. For those patients affected by lung neoplasm, the risk for multiple remote consultations was 4.4 times (+335.5%, 95%CI = +209%, +529.6%) more than those with no bone metastasis, 2.9 times (+189.4%, 95%CI = +117.6%, +276.9%) for colorectal neoplasm, and 4.6 times (+357.9%, 95%CI = +252.6%, +495.5%) for other types of cancer. The expected probabilities were 88.7% (87.6%, 89.6%) for lung cancer, 82.9% (81.6%, 84%) for colorectal cancer, and 69.4% (68.0%, 70.8%) for other cancers. For those with breast neoplasm with bone metastasis, the simulated percentage of multiple remote consultations was 88.7% (87.8%, 89.6%) with a higher risk (+82.3%, 95%CI = +31.6%, +146.8%) of multiple remote evaluations than those without bone metastases (Figure 5).

Condition 3: The model demonstrated that male cancer patients can have an 11 times higher risk to receive multiple remote consultations than female cancer patients. The SORs were 11.3 (95%CI = 4.6, 24.1) for lung neoplasm and 11.1 (95%CI = 5.9, 20.6) for colorectal neoplasm. No statistical significance was found for other cancers (SOR = 0.97, 95%CI = 0.76, 1.23) (Figure 6).

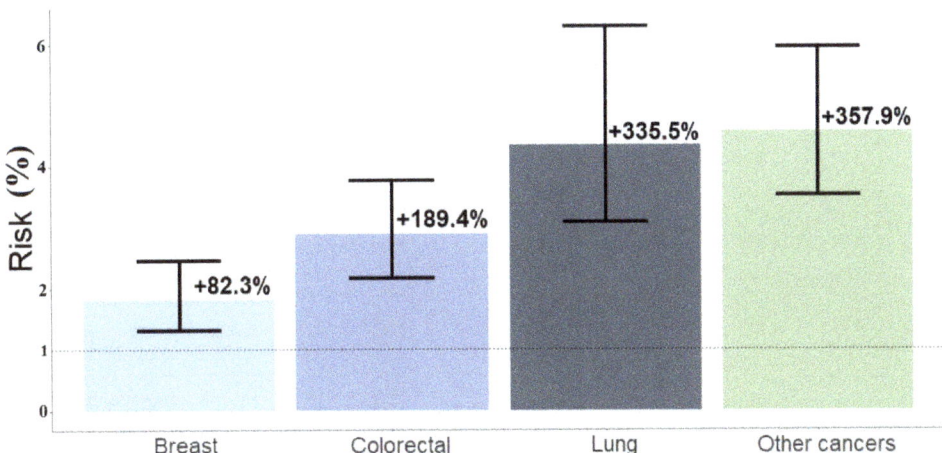

Figure 5. Simulation 2 refers to simulated odds ratios (SORs); percentages are labeled. This was performed for older patients (>75 years old) with bone metastases vs. patients without bone metastases. SORs for lung cancer were 4.35 (95%CI = 3.90–6.30); colorectal cancer 2.89 (95%CI = 2.18–3.77); other cancers 4.58 (95%CI = 3.53–5.95); breast cancer 1.82 (95%CI = 1.32, 2.47).

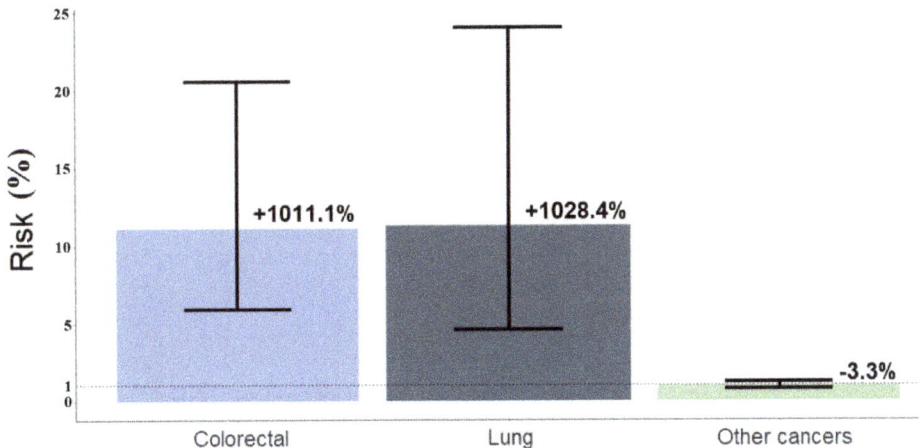

Figure 6. Simulation 3 refers to simulated odds ratios (SORs); percentages are labeled. It was performed for young individuals (≤55 years old) with bone metastases: male vs. female SORs. Young male patients had a significantly higher risk to receive multiple remote consultations when affected by lung cancer (SOR = 11.30, 95%CI = 4.60, 24.10) and colorectal cancer (SOR = 11.1, 95%CI = 5.90, 20.60). No statistical significance was found for other cancers (SOR = 0.97, 95%CI = 0.76, 1.23).

Condition 4: An overall higher risk of having multiple telemedicine visits was found for young cancer patients than for male cancer patients, with SORs of +88.9% (95%CI = +16%, +182%) for lung cancer; +70.1% (95%CI = +24.1%, +143.3%) for colorectal cancer; and +16.5% (95%CI = −0.9%, +51.9%) for other cancers. Compared with older patients, for young female breast cancer patients, no significant risk was found (+19.5%, 95%CI = −20%, +65.2%) (Figure 7).

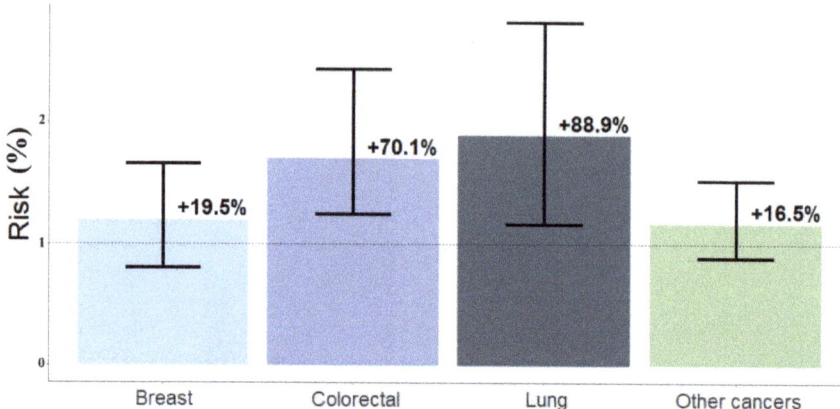

Figure 7. Simulation 4 refers to simulated odds ratios (SORs); percentages are labeled. This was performed for younger vs. older patients with bone metastases. Young patients had a significantly higher risk to receive multiple remote consultations for lung cancer. SORs were 1.89, 95%CI = 1.16, 2.82 for lung cancer and 1.70, 95%CI = 1.24, 2.43 for colorectal cancer. No statistical significance was found for other cancers (SOR = 1.16, 95%CI = 0.91, 1.52) and breast cancer (SOR = 1.19, 95%CI = 0.80, 1.65).

4. Discussion

In the setting of patients suffering from cancer pain, the applications of telemedicine strategies can enhance the effectiveness of clinical management [13] and lead to the optimization of resources [23]. Nevertheless, despite the growing use of telehealth methods, scientific evidence is still scarce to design care pathways.

Previously, we evaluated patient satisfaction with telemedicine and found high satisfaction rates with the care provided and the platform used. The dropout from the telemedicine pathway was investigated, and we found that approximately 10% of patients leave the telemedicine process due to unplanned clinic or hospital readmission or the need for non-pharmacological treatments [13]. Therefore, in this clinical setting, the development of telemedicine-based programs must consider multiple factors. The proposed model of care provides for a variable number of telemedicine visits by combining scheduled consultations and patient requests. In-person visits can be required to carry out minimally invasive procedures, diagnoses, or for other purposes. Furthermore, access to the hospital is provided for acute clinical conditions. Nevertheless, by following this approach, clinical practice has suggested that the careful planning of controls and the design of a safety pathway is a fundamental preliminary phase for validating our telemedicine-based model of care. The aim is to design a model of care that is generalizable while guaranteeing a patient-centered treatment.

In the clinical practice through telemedicine, we observed that many cancer patients had just one consultation. However, some individuals required a large number of closely remote visits. Consequently, we decided to evaluate the typology of cancer patients who may require more than one remote consultation. We searched for a more suitable strategy useful for achieving internal and external validation and translating the chosen model into the clinic [24]. For this aim, we adopted different ML models and decided to categorize the number of remote consultations as "one" or "more than one" remote consultation. Furthermore, the prediction of the number of remote consultations for new patients can involve several practical implications, including the design of personalized paths and optimal resource allocation. An increased number of remote consultations for cancer pain management may also reflect on ad hoc public or private healthcare/insurance health programs. For example, in Italy, the Ministry of Health released guidelines for the provision of telemedicine services, stimulating the design of paths for different care needs [25].

In ML analyses, preprocessing and exploratory data analysis (EDA) are the key elements of the process and take a large part of the time used for the whole analysis. The variable analysis is a crucial point for the modeling: It is part of the data quality and has a significant influence on the model's predictive power, robustness, and confidence. During these phases, it emerged that the variable "age" offered useful information for the model construction and understanding. This variable was categorized into three age groups (younger, mean age, and older patients). Consequently, in the univariate analysis, it was found that younger patients underwent more visits (p = 0.03). These data were used in the predictive analysis (simulations) for assessing, in target individuals, the risk of having multiple remote consultations. For example, the application of the chosen model (RF) showed that younger patients ($\leq$55 years old) with bone metastases and ROO administration for BTcP treatment have an increased risk for more consultations, especially if affected by lung cancer. These data confirm what we previously highlighted in an analysis focused on the BTcP phenomenon. In a hierarchical classification, the worst phenotype of cancer pain patients was characterized by the presence of BTcP, younger age, and lung cancer [26].

In patients of advanced age (>75 years), the variable "bone metastasis" affected the prediction of the number of visits. Although this finding was confirmed above all for lung cancer, it concerns all cancer types. The combination of age and bone metastases identifies a particular class of fragile patients. These patients should be given greater attention by planning closer evaluations, also through telehealth strategies.

Male and female young patients ($\leq$55 years old) with bone metastases were evaluated for their risk of needing multiple remote visits. The RF model showed that male patients had an 11 times higher risk to need multiple remote consultations for pain management than female patients, especially for lung and colorectal cancers. These data must be interpreted very carefully and not only based on the possible gender/age differences in pain perception [27]. This is probably due to the low sample size. The ongoing creation of a larger dataset will allow us to carry out multivariate analyses and define whether other variables such as the differences in the type and stage of the tumor, the impact of the disease on functionality, psychosocial aspects, any comorbidities, as well as the associated anticancer therapies, may influence the data. Based on the results of this predictive analysis, we will develop more accurate pathways for addressing the multiple management problems of cancer pain. The proposed model of care, in fact, also provides for a multidisciplinary approach with the simultaneous involvement of different professionals, such as psychologists, physical therapists, surgeons, general practitioners, etc.

This study has several limitations. The small size of the dataset is the most important limitation. With a higher sample size, some variables could be more representative within the predictive processes. Nevertheless, since not many predictors were present in the models, analyses could be performed despite the limited number of patients.

Numerical variables contain more information than their categorial transformations. For example, the ROO variable could be used as discrete. For these reasons, we chose to categorize the cancer patients' age into three categories (younger, middle-aged, and elderly patients). Another important limitation concerns the number of consultations per patient who is squeezed into the unit. Therefore, with a different distribution and the variables kept as numerical, better results would have been obtained.

The variables we adopted reflect our clinical practice. For example, although several opioids can be used for BTcP management [28], we usually prefer ROOs as the formulations licensed for this aim [29]. Moreover, this set of variables is not exhaustive. In cancer patients, for example, pain may not come from bone metastasis but often derives from invasion or abdominal metastasis, such as the peritoneal metastasis of colon cancer, and other causes. Probably, other variables such as cancer stage (e.g., TNM classification) should have been considered. In this regard, an improved dataset is planned in terms of its sample size and features. This will allow us to implement more sophisticated algorithms. The data from this study, however, can be useful for providing guidance for research in a field (telemedicine for cancer pain management) that is yet to be fully explored. The intervals between remote consultations, the needs for physical examinations, and the approaches for disease progression, as well as a careful definition of the process of early and simultaneous palliative care, are just some of the problems to be faced.

The methodological approach used in the simulations (i.e., SORs) has important potential that the clinician can exploit in predicting the outcome. On the other hand, SORs and simulations are obviously penalized by the sample size. In our analysis, the comparison between genders is an example of this gap. We highlight that their interpretation makes a practical and clinically useful sense if they are assessed through a good classifier.

Finally, we carried out only a few simulations as an example of the application of the evaluated model. The model, indeed, can be applied to a very large series of combinations of variables. Consequently, upon request, the dataset and model are available for further investigation.

5. Conclusions

The application of ML in telemedicine for pain management can enable physicians to make effective, real-time, and data-driven choices. This approach can be a key component in generating a better patient experience and improving health outcomes. A methodological approach to predictive analysis has great potential and could allow clinicians to provide important information to predict the outcome. Despite the important limitations of this study, in our analysis, the outcome (the number of remote consultations) was influenced by the selected variables such as the patient's age, the cancer type, and the occurrence of bone metastases. Further studies are needed to design and refine this model of care for cancer pain patients.

Author Contributions: Conceptualization, M.C. and S.C.; methodology, F.M.; software, SC.; validation, A.C., M.C.R. and D.N.; formal analysis, M.G.; investigation, F.M.; resources, D.S.; data curation, F.M.; writing—original draft preparation, M.C.; writing—review and editing, M.C.; visualization, D.N.; supervision, A.C.; project administration, A.C. All authors have read and agreed to the published version of the manuscript.

Funding: This research received no external funding.

Institutional Review Board Statement: The study was conducted in accordance with the Declaration of Helsinki and approved by the Ethics Committee of the Istituto Nazionale Tumori, Fondazione Pascale of Naples, Italy (protocol code 41/20 Oss; date of approval, 26 November 2020).

Informed Consent Statement: Informed consent was obtained from all the subjects involved in this study.

Data Availability Statement: All data were reported on a prospectively filled database and then registered on Zenodo [13].

Acknowledgments: We acknowledge Valeria Vicario, engineer of the Istituto Nazionale Tumori, Fondazione Pascale of Naples, Italy for her valuable advice.

Conflicts of Interest: The authors declare no conflict of interest.

References

1. Fallon, M.; Giusti, R.; Aielli, F.; Hoskin, P.; Rolke, R.; Sharma, M.; Ripamonti, C.I. ESMO Guidelines Committee. Management of cancer pain in adult patients: ESMO Clinical Practice Guidelines. *Ann. Oncol.* **2018**, *29*, iv166–iv191. [CrossRef]
2. Farquhar-Smith, P. Clinical practice guidelines for cancer pain: Problems and solutions. *Curr. Opin. Support. Palliat. Care* **2021**, *15*, 84–90. [CrossRef]
3. Hill, B.; Moulin, D.; Sanatani, M. Follow-up Visits and Changes in Pain Scores Reported by Oncology Outpatients after Initial Presentation with Severe Pain. *Cureus* **2017**, *9*, e965. [CrossRef]
4. Cascella, M.; Marinangeli, F.; Vittori, A.; Scala, C.; Piccinini, M.; Braga, A.; Miceli, L.; Vellucci, R. Open Issues and Practical Suggestions for Telemedicine in Chronic Pain. *Int. J. Environ. Res. Public Health* **2021**, *18*, 12416. [CrossRef]
5. Coyne, C.J.; Reyes-Gibby, C.C.; Durham, D.D.; Abar, B.; Adler, D.; Bastani, A.; Bernstein, S.L.; Baugh, C.W.; Bischof, J.J.; Grudzen, C.R.; et al. Cancer pain management in the emergency department: A multicenter prospective observational trial of the Comprehensive Oncologic Emergencies Research Network (CONCERN). *Support. Care Cancer* **2021**, *29*, 4543–4553. [CrossRef]

6. Bramati, P.S.; Amaram-Davila, J.S.; Reddy, A.S.; Bruera, E. Reduction of Missed Palliative Care Appointments after the Implementation of Telemedicine. *J. Pain Symptom Manag.* **2022**, *63*, e777–e779. [CrossRef]
7. Li, J.; Zhu, C.; Liu, C.; Su, Y.; Peng, X.; Hu, X. Effectiveness of eHealth interventions for cancer-related pain, fatigue, and sleep disorders in cancer survivors: A systematic review and meta-analysis of randomized controlled trials. *J. Nurs. Scholarsh.* **2022**, *54*, 184–190. [CrossRef]
8. Rahman, S.; Speed, T.; Xie, A.; Shechter, R.; Hanna, M.N. Perioperative Pain Management during the COVID-19 Pandemic: A Telemedicine Approach. *Pain Med.* **2021**, *22*, 3–6. [CrossRef]
9. Cascella, M.; Miceli, L.; Cutugno, F.; Di Lorenzo, G.; Morabito, A.; Oriente, A.; Massazza, G.; Magni, A.; Marinangeli, F.; Cuomo, A.; et al. A Delphi Consensus Approach for the Management of Chronic Pain during and after the COVID-19 Era. *Int. J. Environ. Res. Public Health* **2021**, *18*, 13372. [CrossRef]
10. Cascella, M.; Del Gaudio, A.; Vittori, A.; Bimonte, S.; Del Prete, P.; Forte, C.A.; Cuomo, A.; De Blasio, E. COVID-Pain: Acute and Late-Onset Painful Clinical Manifestations in COVID-19—Molecular Mechanisms and Research Perspectives. *J. Pain Res.* **2021**, *14*, 2403–2412. [CrossRef]
11. Noorbakhsh-Sabet, N.; Zand, R.; Zhang, Y.; Abedi, V. Artificial Intelligence Transforms the Future of Health Care. *Am. J. Med.* **2019**, *132*, 795–801. [CrossRef]
12. DiMartino, L.; Miano, T.; Wessell, K.; Bohac, B.; Hanson, L.C. Identification of Uncontrolled Symptoms in Cancer Patients Using Natural Language Processing. *J. Pain Symptom Manag.* **2022**, *63*, 610–617. [CrossRef]
13. Cascella, M.; Coluccia, S.; Grizzuti, M.; Romano, M.C.; Esposito, G.; Crispo, A.; Cuomo, A. Satisfaction with Telemedicine for Cancer Pain Management: A Model of Care and Cross-Sectional Patient Satisfaction Study. *Curr. Oncol.* **2022**, *29*, 5566–5578. [CrossRef]
14. Cascella, M. PainDatafor_Telemedicine_ML [Data set]. *Zenodo* **2022**. [CrossRef]
15. Hu, H.; Yao, W.; Wu, Y. The Robust EM-type Algorithms for Log-concave Mixtures of Regression Models. *Comput. Stat. Data Anal.* **2017**, *111*, 14–26. [CrossRef]
16. Tibshirani, R. Regression shrinkage and selection via the lasso. *J. R. Stat. Soc.* **1996**, *58*, 267–288. [CrossRef]
17. Breiman, L. Random Forests. *Mach. Learn.* **2001**, *45*, 5–32. [CrossRef]
18. Natekin, A.; Knoll, A. Gradient boosting machines, a tutorial. *Front. Neurorobot.* **2013**, *7*, 21. [CrossRef]
19. Tian, Y.; Shu, M.; Jia, Q. Artificial Neural Network. In *Encyclopedia of Mathematical Geosciences. Encyclopedia of Earth Sciences Series*; Daya Sagar, B., Cheng, Q., McKinley, J., Agterberg, F., Eds.; Springer: Cham, Switzerland, 2021. [CrossRef]
20. Li, Y.; Ji, L.; Oravecz, Z.; Brick, T.R.; Hunter, M.D.; Chow, S.M. dynr.mi: An R Program for Multiple Imputation in Dynamic Modeling. *World Acad. Sci. Eng. Technol.* **2019**, *13*, 302–311. [CrossRef]
21. Kuhn, M. Building Predictive Models in R Using the caret Package. *J. Stat. Softw.* **2008**, *28*, 1–26. [CrossRef]
22. Robin, X.; Turck, N.; Hainard, A.; Tiberti, N.; Lisacek, F.; Sanchez, J.C.; Müller, M. pROC: An open-source package for R and S+ to analyze and compare ROC curves. *BMC Bioinform.* **2011**, *7*, 77. [CrossRef] [PubMed]
23. Calton, B.; Abedini, N.; Fratkin, M. Telemedicine in the Time of Coronavirus. *J Pain Symptom Manage.* **2020**, *60*, e12–e14. [CrossRef] [PubMed]
24. Ghassemi, M.; Oakden-Rayner, L.; Beam, A.L. The false hope of current approaches to explainable artificial intelligence in health care. *Lancet Digit Health* **2021**, *3*, e745–e750. [CrossRef]
25. Health Resources & Services Administration Telehealth Programs. Available online: https://www.hrsa.gov/rural-health/telehealth (accessed on 26 August 2022).
26. Cascella, M.; Crispo, A.; Esposito, G.; Forte, C.A.; Coluccia, S.; Porciello, G.; Amore, A.; Bimonte, S.; Mercadante, S.; Caraceni, A.; et al. Multidimensional Statistical Technique for Interpreting the Spontaneous Breakthrough Cancer Pain Phenomenon. A Secondary Analysis from the IOPS-MS Study. *Cancers* **2021**, *13*, 4018. [CrossRef]
27. Ahmed, Y.; Popovic, M.; Wan, B.A.; Lam, M.; Lam, H.; Ganesh, V.; Milakovic, M.; DeAngelis, C.; Malek, L.; Chow, E. Does gender affect self-perceived pain in cancer patients? -A meta-analysis. *Ann. Palliat. Med.* **2017**, *6*, S177–S184. [CrossRef]
28. Davies, A.N.; Elsner, F.; Filbet, M.J.; Porta-Sales, J.; Ripamonti, C.; Santini, D.; Webber, K. Breakthrough cancer pain (BTcP) management: A review of international and national guidelines. *BMJ Support. Palliat. Care* **2018**, *8*, 241–249. [CrossRef]
29. Cuomo, A.; Cascella, M.; Forte, C.A.; Bimonte, S.; Esposito, G.; De Santis, S.; Cavanna, L.; Fusco, F.; Dauri, M.; Natoli, S.; et al. Careful Breakthrough Cancer Pain Treatment through Rapid-Onset Transmucosal Fentanyl Improves the Quality of Life in Cancer Patients: Results from the BEST Multicenter Study. *J. Clin. Med.* **2020**, *9*, 1003. [CrossRef]

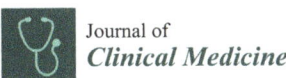

Article

Erector Spinae Plane Block Decreases Chronic Postoperative Pain Severity in Patients Undergoing Coronary Artery Bypass Grafting

Marcin Wiech [1], Sławomir Żurek [2], Arkadiusz Kurowicki [2], Beata Horeczy [3], Mirosław Czuczwar [1], Paweł Piwowarczyk [1], Kazimierz Widenka [2] and Michał Borys [1,*]

[1] Second Department of Anesthesia and Intensive Therapy, Medical University of Lublin, Staszica 16, 20-081 Lublin, Poland
[2] Department of Cardiac Surgery, Medical Faculty, University of Rzeszow, Lwowska 60, 35-301 Rzeszow, Poland
[3] Pro-Familia Hospital, Medical College of Rzeszow University, Witolda 6B, 35-302 Rzeszow, Poland
* Correspondence: michalborys@umlub.pl; Tel.: +48-81-532-2713; Fax: +48-81-532-2712

Abstract: Up to 56% of patients develop chronic postsurgical pain (CPSP) after coronary artery bypass grafting (CABG). CPSP can affect patients' moods and decrease daily activities. The primary aim of this study was to investigate CPSP severity in patients following off-pump (OP) CABG using the Neuropathic Pain Symptom Inventory (NPSI). This was a prospective cohort study conducted in a cardiac surgery department of a teaching hospital. Patients undergoing OP-CABG were enrolled in an erector spinae plane block (ESPB) group (n = 27) or a control (CON) group (n = 24). Before the induction of general anesthesia, ESPB was performed on both sides under ultrasound guidance using 0.375% ropivacaine. The secondary outcomes included cumulative oxycodone consumption, acute pain intensity, mechanical ventilation time, hospital length of stay, and postoperative complications. CPSP intensity was lower in the ESPB group than in the CON group 1, 3, and 6 months post-surgery ($p < 0.001$). Significant between-group differences were also observed in other outcomes, including postoperative pain severity, opioid consumption, mechanical ventilation time, and hospital length of stay, in favor of the ESPB group. Preemptive ESPB appears to decrease the risk of CPSP development in patients undergoing OP-CABG. Reduced acute pain severity and shorter mechanical ventilation times and hospital stays should improve patients' satisfaction and reduce perioperative complications.

Keywords: chronic postoperative pain; erector spinae plane block; coronary artery bypass grafting; Neuropathic Pain Symptom Inventory

1. Introduction

Coronary artery bypass grafting (CABG) is one of the common types of cardiac surgeries performed worldwide, with 44 procedures per 100,000 individuals completed annually [1]. Up to 56% of patients develop chronic postsurgical pain (CPSP) after CABG [2,3]. CPSP following CABG surgery can lower patients' moods and decrease performance of daily activities [3]. A Cochrane meta-analysis found that thoracic epidural analgesia (TEA) could prevent CPSP in patients following thoracic surgery [4]. In our previous study, we showed that continuous paravertebral block lowered CPSP severity and reduced the incidence of CPSP after thoracic surgery [5]. However, not much is known about the use of regional anesthesia techniques in the prevention of CPSP in cardiac surgery.

Erector spinae plane block (ESPB) is a relatively new regional anesthesia technique described by Forero [6]. In the years since its introduction, ESPB has been used in different types of surgical procedures, including cardiac surgery [7–9]. In previous research, we described this type of fascial block in patients undergoing mitral and/or tricuspid valve repair via a right mini-thoracotomy and off-pump CABG (OP-CABG) [10,11]. However, we did not evaluate the incidence of CPSP in the months following patient discharge. This study aimed to assess the severity and incidence of CPSP in patients undergoing OP-CABG via sternotomy with preemptive, bilateral ESPB.

2. Materials and Methods

This was a prospective cohort study conducted in a cardiac surgery department of a teaching hospital. The study protocol was approved by the Bioethics Committee of the Medical University of Lublin, Lublin, Poland (permit number KE-0254/219/2018). Informed consent was obtained from the patients, and the study was conducted in accordance with the tenets of the Declaration of Helsinki for medical research involving human subjects.

2.1. Participants

Patients undergoing an OP-CABG procedure were enrolled in an ESPB group or a control (CON) group. Patients were enrolled consecutively. The same two surgeons performed each surgery. First, we recruited patients to the CON group, then to the ESPB group. The inclusion criteria were adult patients (≥ 18 years) scheduled for elective surgery. Patients with chronic pain at admission, a history of alcohol or recreational drug abuse, known bleeding disorders, allergies to the drugs used during the study, antidepressant or epileptic drug treatment, and chronic use of painkillers were excluded.

2.2. General Anesthesia

For induction of general anesthesia, the following was used: 0.2–0.4 mg/kg of etomidate, 2–4 µg/kg of fentanyl, and 0.6 mg of rocuronium. Fentanyl infusion was continued at a flow of 25–100 µg/hour, and sevoflurane (0.5–1.0 minimal alveolar concentration) was administered for anesthesia maintenance. The patients received additional doses of rocuronium every 30–40 min and norepinephrine or nitroglycerine as required. The physicians who anesthetized the patient adjusted hemodynamic parameters within 25% of the patient's baseline using anesthetics and vasopressors.

2.3. Regional Block and Postoperative Care

In the ESPB group, before the induction of general anesthesia, single-shot bilateral ESPB was performed under ultrasound guidance, as described in our previous studies [10,11]. On each side, $0.2 \text{ mL} \cdot \text{kg}^{-1}$ of 0.375% ropivacaine (Ropimol, Molteni, Italy) was administered. The total volume of local anesthetic solution did not exceed 40 mL per patient.

About 20–30 min before the end of the surgery, the patients received 0.1 mg per kg of oxycodone hydrochloride (up to 10 mg) intravenously (i.v.) and acetaminophen (1.0 g i.v.). Each patient was then transferred to the Intensive Care Unit (ICU). In each case, extubation and weaning from mechanical ventilation were performed according to the attending physician's discretion. The attending physician measured acute postoperative pain intensity using the Numerical Rating Scale (NRS, 0–10) immediately after extubation. The attending nurse then assessed pain severity every 6 h.

The mechanical ventilation time was defined as a period from the end of anesthesia to extubation. Each patient was transferred to the Intensive Care Unit (ICU). Then, an attending anesthesiologist assessed the possibility of extubating the patient in the ICU. The ventilatory settings were continuous positive pressure or pressure support ventilation with positive end-expiratory pressure below 7 mbar, pressure support below 3 mbar, and the fraction of inspired oxygen not exceeding 30%. The suggested respiratory parameters for extubation were respiratory rate below 20/min, tidal volume over 6 mL of the patient's ideal body weight, and oxygen saturation (SpO_2) > 93%, or similar to the patient's basal SpO_2 before preoxygenation. The patient's heart rate and systolic blood pressure should not have exceeded 25% of the basal measurements obtained before the induction of anesthesia. Moreover, the patient should have responded to questions addressed by a physician. If the patient had not been extubated, an attending physician continued ventilation under sedation with propofol and fentanyl. The second attempt for extubation was done the next day. The patient received a bolus of oxycodone (0.1 mg/kg) when sedation was stopped. Then, the next attempt for extubating was performed.

Standard pain treatment included oxycodone administered i.v. via a patient-controlled analgesia pump (1 mg/mL, 1 mL bolus, 5 min refraction time). In addition, the patients received 1.0 g of acetaminophen every 6 h, 100 mg of ketoprofen i.v. twice daily, and ondansetron i.v. (4 mg twice daily) as nausea and vomiting prophylaxis. In cases of severe pain (i.e., exceeding 4 on the NRS), the attending nurse was permitted to administer a bolus of oxycodone (5 mg).

2.4. Persistent Postoperative Pain

For the assessment of persistent postoperative pain, we used the Neuropathic Pain Symptom Inventory (NPSI) developed by Bouhassira et al. [12], as employed in our previous studies [13,14]. All patients were interviewed via telephone 1, 3, and 6 months post-surgery.

2.5. Outcomes

The primary outcome was CPSP severity 1, 3, and 6 months surgery. The secondary outcomes included the cumulative oxycodone dose, acute pain intensity on the NRS, mechanical ventilation time, hospital length of stay, and postoperative complications. Patients without NPSI results were excluded from further analysis.

2.6. Statistics

The Student's *t*-test was used to analyze parametric data. The data are presented as means and 95% confidence intervals. Nonparametric data were calculated using the Mann–Whitney *U* test and are presented as medians and interquartile ranges. Categorical variables were analyzed using Fisher's exact test. Multivariate logistic regression was used to reveal the parameters that affect CPSP occurrence. The odds ratio (OR) was used to describe the predictors that were included in the model. The receiver operating characteristic (ROC) curve was calculated for the best model. All measurements were performed using Statistica 13.1 software (Stat Soft. Inc., Tulsa, OK, USA).

3. Results

The study was conducted from March 2019 to April 2020. In total, 74 patients were enrolled. Overall, 23 patients were lost to follow-up. The final study comprised data from 51 patients: 24 in the CON group and 27 in the ESP group (Figure 1). Patient demographics, time of mechanical ventilation, length of hospital stay, and preoperative results of the ASA scoring systems are presented in Table 1.

Table 1. Patient demographics.

Parameters	ESPB	CON	*p* Value
Number of patients	27	24	
Male (%)	24 (88.9)	22 (91.7)	1.0
Age (years)	64.7 (62.0–67.4)	67.1 (63.4–70.7)	0.28
Weight (kg)	85.2 (80.4–90.0)	83.7 (77.9–89.4)	0.68
Height (cm)	171.1 (167.7–174.5)	170.6 (167.1–174.1)	0.85
BMI	29.1 (27.8–30.3)	28.6 (27.1–30.1)	0.65
ASA	3 (2–3)	3 (3–3)	0.45
Anesthesia time (minutes)	194 (174–215)	201 (141–185)	0.63
Surgery time (minutes)	159 (140–179)	163 (177–225)	0.79
Intraoperative fentanyl (mcg)	381 (359–404)	499 (463–535)	<0.001

Patient age, weight, height, BMI, surgery and anesthesia times, and intraoperative fentanyl are presented as means and confidence intervals. ASA is presented as a median and interquartile range. ASA, American Society of Anesthesiologists; BMI, body mass index; ESPB, erector spinae plane block group; CON, control group.

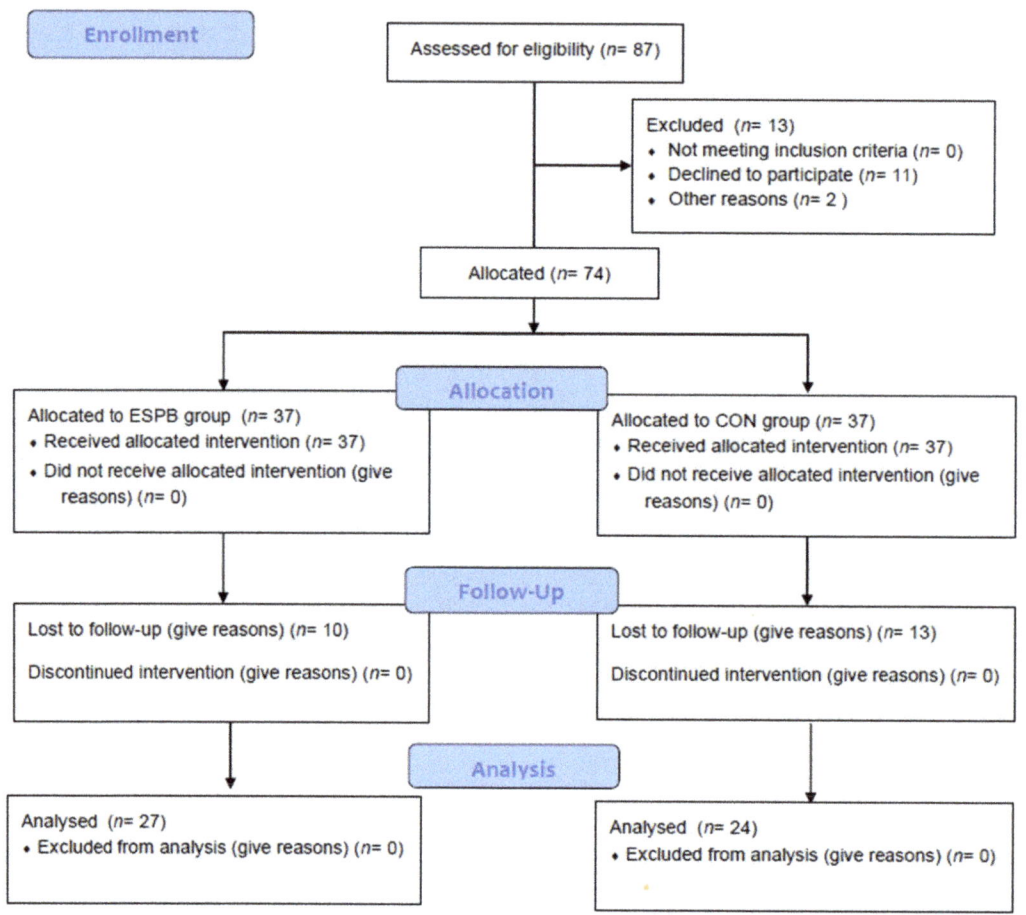

Figure 1. Study flow diagram. ESPB, erector spinae plane block group; CON, control group.

3.1. Primary Outcome

CPSP severity was significantly higher in the CON group than in the ESPB group 1, 3, and 6 months after OP-CABG surgery (Table 2). As presented in Table 3, fewer patients in the ESPB group showed signs of persistent pain.

Table 2. Severity of persistent postoperative pain.

After Discharge	ESPB	CON	p Value
1 month	1 (0–2) *	4 (3–6)	<0.001
3 months	0 (0–1) *	4 (2–6)	<0.001
6 months	0 (0–0) *	2 (14)	<0.001

The severity of post-thoracotomy pain syndrome was detected with the NPSI (0–100). Data are shown as medians (interquartile ranges). * Denotes a significant between-group difference. ESPB, erector spinae plane block group; CON, control group.

Table 3. Incidence of chronic postsurgical pain (CPSP).

After Discharge	Number of Patients (%)		p Value
	ESPB	CON	
1 month	17 (63) *	23 (96)	<0.01
3 months	8 (30) *	23 (96)	<0.001
6 months	6 (22) *	22 (92)	<0.001

* Denotes a significant between-group difference. ESPB, erector spinae plane block group; CON, control group.

Table 3 shows the number of patients who experienced CPSP 1, 3, and 6 months post-surgery.

3.2. Secondary Outcomes

Acute pain severity was significantly lower in the ESPB group than in the CON group (Table 4). The patients in the ESPB group used less oxycodone via PCA than the CON group (4 [2–8] vs. 25 [20–25] mg, $p < 0.001$) (Figure 2). Moreover, patients in the CON group received more rescue doses of oxycodone than the ESPB group (5 [0–5] vs. 0 [0–0], $p = 0.0012$).

Table 4. Acute pain severity.

Hours after Extubation	ESPB	CON	p Value
0	3.0 (2.0–4.5) *	5.0 (4.0–5.8)	<0.001
6	2.5 (2.0–4.0) *	4.5 (3.5–5.0)	<0.001
12	3.0 (2.0–3.5) *	4.0 (3.0–4.0)	<0.01
18	2.0 (0.0–3.0) *	3.0 (2.0–4.0)	<0.01
24	0.0 (0.0–1.5) *	3.0 (1.0–3.5)	<0.001

Data are shown as medians (interquartile ranges). * Denotes a significant between-group difference. ESPB, erector spinae plane block group; CON, control group.

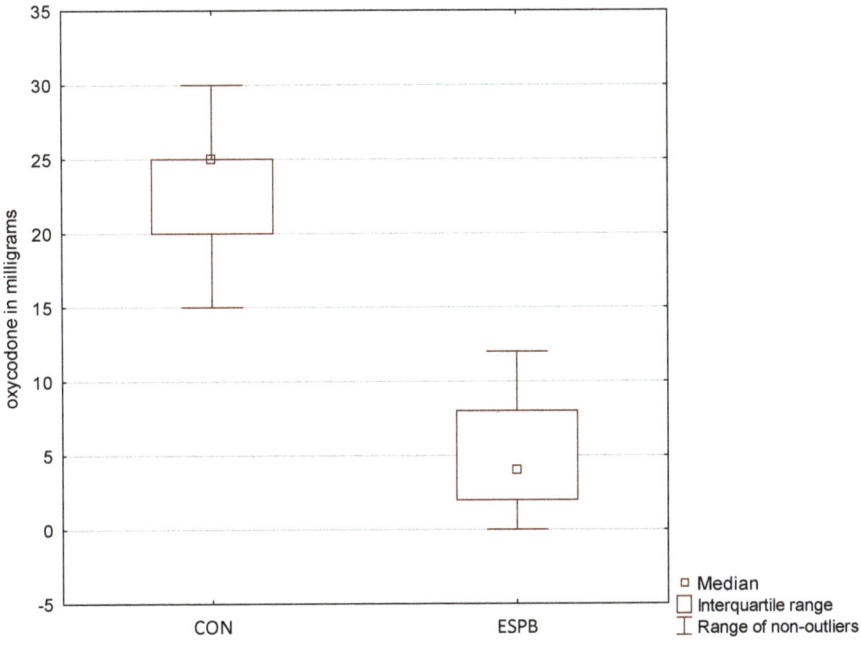

Figure 2. Oxycodone consumption. ESPB, erector spinae plane block group; CON, control group.

The mechanical ventilation time was shorter in the ESPB group than in the CON group (2 [1–3] vs. 10.5 [8–13.25] h, $p < 0.001$). Moreover, the length of hospital stay was shorter in the ESPB group than in the CON group (7 [6–9] vs. 10 [8–12] days, $p < 0.001$). There was no between-group difference in postoperative complications. Figure 1 presents postoperative oxycodone consumption administered via PCA.

We found three variables associated with CPSP occurrence at month 6. The best model was found using stepwise logistic regression. The area under the ROC curve was 0.899 for this model. Two variables positively associated with CPSP occurrence were additional doses of oxycodone and the mechanical ventilation time, which were positively associated with OR 1.65 (1.164–2.339, $p = 0.005$) and 1.303 (1.053–1.614, $p = 0.015$). The anesthesia time was negatively associated with CPSP incidence at month 6 (0.989 (0.982–0.996), $p = 0.002$).

4. Discussion

Our results suggest that preemptive ESPB can alleviate CPSP severity months after an OP-CABG procedure (Table 2). As shown in Table 3, fewer patients had signs of persistent pain after the regional block. Moreover, acute pain severity and oxycodone consumption were minor in patients following the regional block. The regional block group also had shorter postoperative mechanical ventilation and hospital length of stay times. The results of the logistic regression could suggest that CPSP occurrence at month 6 was associated with incidences of breakthrough pain in the postoperative period, which required additional doses of opioids.

We showed in the present study that bilateral ESPB could reduce CPSP severity and incidence. According to the results of previous research, regional anesthesia procedures might prevent the occurrence of CPSP [4,15]. The effectiveness of TEA in reducing the incidence of CPSP in patients following thoracic surgery was presented in a study by Lu et al. [16]. Kairaluoma et al. showed a reduction of CPSP intensity by preemptive paravertebral block in breast surgery patients [17]. The authors of this trial performed a single preemptive injection of a local anesthetic. We reported a reduction in the incidence and intensity of CPSP in patients following thoracotomy [5]. However, in this study, continuous paravertebral block was used. In our recent study, we presented that quadratus lumborum block can reduce CPSP severity in patients undergoing nephrectomy [18]. However, the effect of new regional anesthesia techniques on preventing CPSP development requires further studies.

Limited treatment modalities can prevent CPSP development following cardiac surgery procedures [19]. In a meta-analysis by Carley et al. concerning prophylaxis of CPSP with drugs following surgeries, only gabapentoids were showed to prevent persistent pain three months after cardiac surgery [20]. However, as stated by the authors of this meta-analysis, the results should be interpreted cautiously due to the small study sizes.

New regional anesthesia techniques have been explored extensively in acute postoperative pain treatment [21,22]. We confirmed in the present study that ESPB could reduce acute pain intensity and opioid demands in patients undergoing OP-CABG. In a trial by Krishna et al., bilateral ESPB reduced pain intensity in patients undergoing cardiac surgery procedures requiring cardiopulmonary bypass [7]. Nagaraja and colleagues showed that ESPB was comparable to continuous TEA in the reduction of acute pain severity in patients following a cardiac surgery procedure [8]. Macaire et al. presented that continuous ESPB improved patient postoperative rehabilitation after open cardiac surgery and reduced opioid consumption [23].

Our study has some limitations. It was an observational study. Thus, selection bias is possible. In addition, we enrolled a relatively small group of patients, and we did not examine the quality of regional block with the pinprick technique. Patients in the CON group did not receive a sham block with saline. There was no blinding in our study.

To conclude, our results suggest that preemptive ESPB can decrease the risk of CPSP development in patients after an OP-CABG procedure. The lower acute pain severity and shorter mechanical ventilation times and hospital stays associated with the procedure should improve patients' satisfaction and reduce hospital costs and perioperative complications.

Author Contributions: Conceptualization, M.B. and M.W.; Methodology, M.B. and B.H.; Formal Analysis, M.B.; Investigation, S.Ż., A.K. and B.H.; Resources, K.W. and B.H.; Data Curation, S.Ż., A.K. and M.C.; Writing—Original Draft Preparation, M.W., M.B. and P.P.; Writing—Review and Editing, M.C. and M.W.; Visualization, M.W.; Supervision, M.B.; Project Administration, K.W. All authors have read and agreed to the published version of the manuscript.

Funding: This research received no external funding.

Institutional Review Board Statement: The study was conducted according to the guidelines of the Declaration of Helsinki and approved by the Ethics Committee of the Medical University of Lublin, Lublin, Poland (permit number KE-0254/219/2018, approved 29 November 2018).

Informed Consent Statement: Informed consent was obtained from all the patients involved in the study.

Data Availability Statement: The data presented in this study are available on request from the corresponding author.

Conflicts of Interest: The authors declare no conflict of interest.

References

1. Head, S.J.; Milojevic, M.; Taggart, D.P.; Puskas, J.D. Current practice of state-of-the-art surgical coronary revascularization. *Circulation* **2017**, *136*, 1331–1345. [CrossRef] [PubMed]
2. Kalso, E.; Mennander, S.; Tasmuth, T. Chronic post-sternotomy pain. *Acta Anaesthesiol. Scand.* **2001**, *45*, 935–939. [CrossRef] [PubMed]
3. Eisenberg, E.; Pultorak, Y.; Pud, D.; Bar-El, Y. Prevalence and characteristics of post coronary artery bypass graft surgery pain (PCP). *Pain* **2001**, *92*, 11–17. [CrossRef]
4. Andreae, M.H.; Andreae, D.A. Regional anaesthesia to prevent chronic pain after surgery: A Cochrane systematic review and meta-analysis. *Br. J. Anaesth.* **2013**, *111*, 711–720. [CrossRef]
5. Borys, M.; Hanych, A.; Czuczwar, M. Paravertebral block versus preemptive ketamine effect on pain intensity after posterolateral thoracotomies: A randomized controlled trial. *J. Clin. Med.* **2020**, *9*, 793. [CrossRef]
6. Forero, M.; Rajarathinam, M.; Adhikary, S.; Chin, J.K. Continuous erector spinae plane block for rescue analgesia in thoracotomy after epidural failure: A case report. *A A Case. Rep.* **2017**, *8*, 254–256. [CrossRef]
7. Nagaraja, P.S.; Ragavendran, S.; Singh, N.G.; Omshubham, A.; Bhavya, G.; Manjunath, N.; Rajesh, K. Comparison of continuous thoracic epidural analgesia with bilateral erector spinae plane block for perioperative pain management in cardiac surgery. *Ann. Card. Anaesth.* **2018**, *21*, 323–327.
8. Krishna, S.N.; Chauhan, S.; Bhoi, D.; Kaushal, B.; Hasija, S.; Sangdup, T.; Bisoi, A.K. Bilateral erector spinae plane block for acute post-surgical pain in adult cardiac surgical patients: A randomized controlled trial. *J. Cardiothorac. Vasc. Anesth.* **2019**, *33*, 368–375. [CrossRef]
9. Borys, M.; Gawęda, B.; Horeczy, B.; Kolowca, M.; Olszówka, P.; Czuczwar, M. Erector spinae-plane block as an analgesic alternative in patients undergoing mitral and/or tricuspid valve repair through a right mini-thoracotomy—An observational cohort study. *Videosurg. Other Miniinvasive Tech.* **2020**, *15*, 208–214. [CrossRef]
10. Gawęda, B.; Borys, M.; Belina, B.; Bąk, J.; Czuczwar, M.; Wołoszczuk-Gębicka, B.; Kolowca, M.; Widenka, K. Postoperative pain treatment with erector spinae plane block and pectoralis nerve blocks in patients undergoing mitral/tricuspid valve repair—A randomized controlled trial. *BMC Anesthesiol.* **2020**, *20*, 51. [CrossRef]
11. Borys, M.; Żurek, S.; Kurowicki, A.; Horeczy, B.; Bielina, B.; Sejboth, J.; Wołoszczuk-Gębicka, B.; Czuczwar, M.; Widenka, K. Implementation of enhanced recovery after surgery (ERAS) protocol in off-pump coronary artery bypass graft surgery. A prospective cohort feasibility study. *Anaesthesiol. Intensive Ther.* **2020**, *52*, 10–14. [CrossRef]
12. Bouhassira, D.; Attal, N.; Fermanian, J.; Alchaar, H.; Gautron, M.; Masquelier, E.; Rostaing, S.; Lanteri-Minet, M.; Collin, E.; Grisart, J.; et al. Development and validation of the neuropathic pain symptom inventory. *Pain* **2004**, *108*, 248–257. [CrossRef]
13. Borys, M.; Potręć-Studzińska, B.; Wiech, M.; Piwowarczyk, P.; Sysiak-Sławecka, J.; Rypulak, E.; Gęca, T.; Kwaśniewska, A.; Czuczwar, M. Transversus abdominis plane block and quadratus lumborum block did not reduce the incidence or severity of chronic postsurgical pain following cesarean section: A prospective, observational study. *Anaesthesiol. Intensive Ther.* **2019**, *51*, 257–261. [CrossRef]
14. Borys, M.; Zamaro, A.; Horeczy, B.; Gęszka, E.; Janiak, M.; Węgrzyn, P.; Czuczwar, M.; Piwowarczyk, P. Quadratus lumborum and transversus abdominis plane blocks and their impact on acute and chronic pain in patients after cesarean section: A randomized controlled Study. *Int. J. Environ. Res. Public Health* **2021**, *18*, 3500. [CrossRef]

15. Weinstein, E.; Levene, J.; Cohen, M.; Andreae, D.; Chao, J.; Johnson, M.; Hall, C.; Andreae, M. Local anaesthetics and regional anaesthesia versus conventional analgesia for preventing persistent postoperative pain in adults and children. *Cochrane Database Syst. Rev.* **2018**. [CrossRef]
16. Lu, Y.; Wang, X.; Lai, R.; Huang, W.; Xu, M. Correlation of acute pain treatment to occurrence of chronic pain in tumor patients after thoracotomy. *Aizheng* **2008**, *27*, 206–209.
17. Kairaluoma, P.; Bachmann, M.; Rosenberg, P.; Pere, P. Preincisional paravertebral block reduces the prevalence of chronic pain after breast surgery. *Anesth. Analg.* **2006**, *103*, 703–708. [CrossRef]
18. Borys, M.; Szajowska, P.; Jednakiewicz, M.; Wita, G.; Czarnik, T.; Mieszkowski, M.; Tuyakov, B.; Gałkin, P.; Rahnama-Hezavah, M.; Czuczwar, M.; et al. Quadratus Lumborum Block Reduces Postoperative Opioid Consumption and Decreases Persistent Postoperative Pain Severity in Patients Undergoing Both Open and Laparoscopic Nephrectomies-A Randomized Controlled Trial. *J. Clin. Med.* **2021**, *10*, 3590. [CrossRef]
19. Kleiman, A.M.; Sanders, D.T.; Nemergut, E.C.; Huffmyer, J.L. Chronic Poststernotomy Pain: Incidence, Risk Factors, Treatment, Prevention, and the Anesthesiologist's Role. *Reg. Anesth. Pain Med.* **2017**, *42*, 698–708. [CrossRef]
20. Carley, M.E.; Chaparro, L.E.; Choinière, M.; Kehlet, H.; Moore, R.A.; Van Den Kerkhof, E.; Gilron, I. Pharmacotherapy for the Prevention of Chronic Pain after Surgery in Adults: An Updated Systematic Review and Meta-analysis. *Anesthesiology* **2021**, *135*, 304–325. [CrossRef]
21. Leong, R.; Tan, E.; Wong, S.; Tan, K.; Liu, C. Efficacy of erector spinae plane block for analgesia in breast surgery: A systematic review and meta-analysis. *Anaesthesia* **2021**, *76*, 404–413. [CrossRef] [PubMed]
22. Uppal, V.; Retter, S.; Kehoe, E.; McKeen, D.M. Quadratus lumborum block for postoperative analgesia: A systematic review and meta-analysis. *Can. J. Anaesth.* **2020**, *67*, 1557–1575. [CrossRef] [PubMed]
23. Macaire, P.; Ho, N.; Nguyen, T.; Nguyen, B.; Vu, V.; Quach, C.; Roques, V.; Capdevila, X. Ultrasound-Guided Continuous Thoracic Erector Spinae Plane Block Within an Enhanced Recovery Program Is Associated with Decreased Opioid Consumption and Improved Patient Postoperative Rehabilitation After Open Cardiac Surgery-A Patient-Matched, Controlled Before-and-After Study. *J. Cardiothorac. Vasc. Anesth.* **2019**, *33*, 1659–1667. [PubMed]

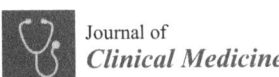

Journal of Clinical Medicine

Article

Real Time Ultrasound-Guided Thoracic Epidural Catheterization with Patients in the Lateral Decubitus Position without Flexion of Knees and Neck: A Preliminary Investigation

Yuexin Huang [1,†], Tingting Li [1,†], Tianhong Wang [1,†], Yanhuan Wei [2], Liulin Xiong [3], Tinghua Wang [1,3,*] and Fei Liu [1,*]

1. Department of Anesthesiology, Institute of Neurological Disease, West China Hospital, Sichuan University, Chengdu 610044, China
2. Graduate School of Education, Beijing Foreign Studies University, Beijing 100039, China
3. Department of Anesthesiology, Affiliated Hospital of Zunyi Medical University, Zunyi 563000, China
* Correspondence: wangth_email@163.com (T.W.); liufei@scu.edu.cn (F.L.)
† These authors contributed equally to this work.

Abstract: Objectives: For some patients, such as pregnant women, it can be difficult to maintain the ideal "forehead to knees" position for several minutes for epidural catheter placement. We conducted this study to investigate the feasibility of real-time ultrasound-guided (US) epidural catheterization under a comfortable lateral position without flexion of knees and neck. **Materials and Methods:** 60 patients aged 18–80 years with a body mass index of 18–30 kg/m^2 after general surgery were included. In a comfortable left lateral position, thoracic epidural catheterization was performed under real-time US for postoperative analgesia. The visibility of the neuraxial structures, procedural time from needle insertion to loss of resistance in the epidural space, the number of needle redirections, success rate of epidural catheter placement and postoperative analgesic effect were recorded. **Results:** In the paramedian oblique sagittal view, the well visible of vertebral lamina, intervertebral space and posterior complex under ultrasound were as high as 93.33%, 81.67% and 70.00%, respectively. The success rate of thoracic epidural catheterization was as high as 91.67%, and the satisfactory postoperative analgesic effect was 98.2% for patients without nausea, pruritus and other discomfort. **Discussion:** Thoracic epidural catheterization with patients in the lateral position without flexion of knees and neck under real time ultrasound guidance has a high success rate and strong feasibility. This visual manipulation makes epidural catheterization not only "easier" to perform, but also reduces the requirements of the procedure.

Keywords: thoracic epidural puncture and catheterization; position; ultrasound image

Citation: Huang, Y.; Li, T.; Wang, T.; Wei, Y.; Xiong, L.; Wang, T.; Liu, F. Real Time Ultrasound-Guided Thoracic Epidural Catheterization with Patients in the Lateral Decubitus Position without Flexion of Knees and Neck: A Preliminary Investigation. *J. Clin. Med.* **2022**, *11*, 6459. https://doi.org/10.3390/jcm11216459

Academic Editor: Marco Cascella

Received: 24 September 2022
Accepted: 27 October 2022
Published: 31 October 2022

Publisher's Note: MDPI stays neutral with regard to jurisdictional claims in published maps and institutional affiliations.

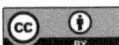

Copyright: © 2022 by the authors. Licensee MDPI, Basel, Switzerland. This article is an open access article distributed under the terms and conditions of the Creative Commons Attribution (CC BY) license (https://creativecommons.org/licenses/by/4.0/).

1. Key Points Summary

Question: To improve patients' comfort, can we perform epidural space puncture and catheterization without maintaining the "ideal position"?

Findings: Thoracic epidural space catheterization (T6-L1) to patients without flexion of knees and neck (comfortable left lateral position) under ultrasound guidance has a high success rate (91.67%, 55/60) and satisfactory postoperative analgesic effect (98.18%, 54/55), and no patients experienced nausea, pruritus and other discomfort.

Meaning: Under a comfortable lateral position, ultrasound-guided epidural space puncture and catheterization is feasible.

2. Introduction

Epidural space puncture and catheterization can be used for intraoperative anesthesia and postoperative analgesia [1]. The lateral position is one of the most commonly used positions for spinal and epidural anesthesia, in which the patients have to flex their thighs on their abdomen and flex their neck to allow the forehead to be as close possible to the knees ("forehead to knees", Figure 1 Left) [2]. This position allows the operator to obtain the presence of palpable spinal apophyses and easy determine the needle puncture space, and this influences the success rate of epidural catheterization [3,4]. However, it is difficult for some patients to maintain this position for several minutes without movement, which has been identified as a risk factor for dural puncture during epidural anesthesia [5]. Ultrasound (US) imaging can now be a valuable tool to view tissue and structures like nerve and spine anatomy, which could improve the clinical efficacy of epidural catheter placement, reduce the risk of failed or traumatic procedures, and decrease the number of attempts and redirections of the needle [6–11]. Until now, there have been no reports on whether the US has an advantage in epidural catheter placement in patients who cannot maintain the "forehead to knees" ideal position. Thus, we planned to do thoracic epidural catheter placement under real time US-guidance for the patients in the lateral decubitus position without flexion of knees and neck in order to explore the possibility of thoracic epidural catheterization under ultrasound in a comfortable position, and to provide the relevant imaging data of thoracic epidural catheterization under ultrasound.

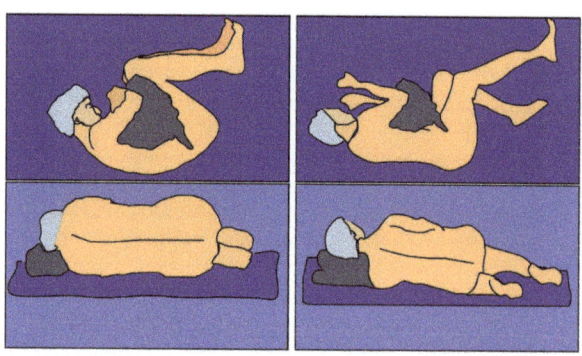

Figure 1. Patient's position during the epidural catheter puncture. (**Left**): Ideal position ("forehead to knee"). (**Right**): Comfortable position (The patient wasn't required to flex their thighs on their abdomen and flex their neck).

3. Materials and Methods

3.1. Ethic

A single-center case series study was performed. Ethical approval for the study was provided by the Ethics Committee of our institution (West China Biomedical Ethics Committee, Sichuan University. No. 2016 (332). 18 February 2019.), and written patient informed consent was obtained from all patients. This study was retrospectively registered on ClinicalTrials.gov (ChiCTR2100054727). All procedures in this study were in accordance with the ethical standards of the Helsinki Declaration and the international ethical guidelines for human biomedical research. This manuscript adheres to the applicable STROBE guidelines.

3.2. Patients

A total 60 patients aged 18–80 with American Society of Anesthesiologists (ASA) classification of I or II, who were scheduled to undergo abdominal surgeries under GA, were enrolled in the study from 1 September to 30 November 2020 at the West China Hospital of Sichuan University. Patients with neurological disorders, seizures, history of spine surgeries or deformities, a history of local anesthetic allergy, local site infection, or coagulopathies were excluded. Epidural catheterization was performed by Fei Liu, the corresponding author of this article, who is skilled in ultrasound guiding epidural puncture.

The level of epidural puncture was determined by the surgical incision. Ultrasound imaging was completed using an M-turbo curved probe of 2–5 MHz (FUJIFILM Sonosite, Inc. Bothell, WA, USA). All of the patients were followed for up to 1 week after surgery. If patients had adverse reactions, patients were observed until recovery.

3.3. Operational Process

Epidural puncture and catheterization were performed preoperatively. Intravenous access and standard ASA monitors (pulse oximetry, electrocardiogram, and noninvasive blood pressure) were established prior to epidural puncture. All of the patients lied in a comfortable position of left lateral decubitus (they were not required to flex their thighs on their abdomen and flex their neck), as shown in Figure 1 right). The paramedian oblique sagittal plane of the target epidural space was identified and marked by applying the probe from the 12th rib in the pre-procedure scanning and using the counting up method [12]. (The scanning procedure could be found in the Video S1). After aseptic skin disinfection, the probe was firmly held in the marked position by the operator's left hand (Figure 2 Left) and applied at the congruent thoracic level to obtain a paramedian longitudinal view of the spine. A 18G Tuohy needle from the caudal of the probe was advanced to the interlaminar space under real-time ultrasound guidance using an in-plane approach until the needle tip reached the posterior part of the ligamentum flavum-dura mater complex by the operator's right hand (Figure 2 Right). The ultrasound probe was then left aside and the two hands of the single operator held the needle to continue the procedure until the epidural space was identified with loss of resistance to air [4] Finally, the epidural catheter was advanced 4–5 cm inside the epidural space and secured at the back with transparent dressings. (The puncturing procedure can be found in the operating Video S1).

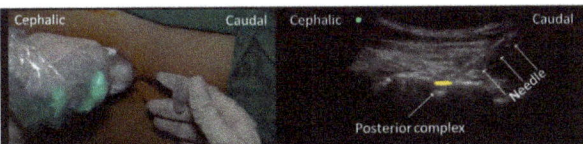

Figure 2. Example of how to hold the probe (**left the probe was firmly held in the marked position by the operator's left hand. A 18G Tuohy needle from the caudal of the probe was advanced to by the operator's right hand**). Ultrasound imaging while operating puncture (**right**) THE needle was seen in the ultrasound image.

3.4. Data Collection

(1) Characteristics of patients, including gender, age, height, weight, and body mass index (BMI), history of hypertension or chronic bronchitis. (2) The operation information. (3) The ultrasound visibility of neuraxial structures at the punctured interlaminar space [13] (including vertebral lamina, intervertebral space, dural sac, anterior complex and posterior complex) were also assessed by an independent observer using a 4-point Likert scale (0-point = not visible, 1-point = hardly visible, 2-point = well visible, 3-point = very well visible), and the total ultrasound visibility score (UVS, maximum score possible = 15) for each patient was determined. (4) Vertical and oblique distances from the skin to the posterior dura (Figure 3A,B) and width of the interlaminar space were measured (Figure 3C). (5) Puncture Outcome, including time for the US pre-procedure scanning and epidural space puncture (from the start of the skin puncture to the confirmation of the needle tip in the epidural space), success rate of epidural puncture and catheterization, analgesia effect, and adverse reaction were recorded. Mild adverse effects included dural puncture, bloody tap, paresthesia during needle insertion or catheterization and severe adverse effects contained total spinal anesthesia, epidural hematoma or abscess related to epidural puncture.

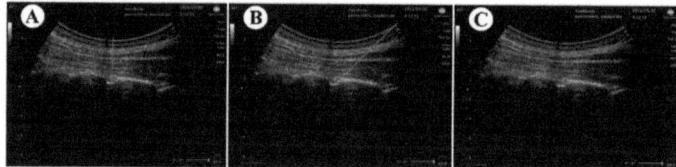

Figure 3. Example of ultrasonic image measurement in comfortable position. Vertical (**A**) and oblique distances (**B**) from the skin to the posterior dura and width of the interlaminar space were also measured (**C**) using the relevant "frozen image" of the ultrasound.

3.5. Statistical Analysis

The data was analyzed using SPSS (Version 21.0, IBM, Chicago, IL, USA). Measurement data were described as mean ± standard deviation (Std), or median (interquaternary interval, IQR). The enumeration data were described by frequency and composition ratio. The correlation between patient characteristics, ultrasonic imaging and epidural puncture time was analyzed. The influence degree of each influencing factor on the epidural puncture time was then analyzed. According to our institution's previous experience with ultrasound-guided catheterization, the success rate is approximately 90%. Thus, when we calculated the sample size, we assumed the success rate to be 90%, the confidence interval width to be 16%, the allowable error range to be 8%, the dropout rate to be 10%, and $\alpha = 0.05$. By using PASS 2021 (Version 21.0.3), a sample size of 54 patients were calculated, and we choose 60 patients as the final sample size.

4. Results

Real-time US-guided epidural space catheters were successfully finished in 55 patients of the 60 patients (41 male and 19 female) under a comfortable left lateral decubitus, with a mean age of 57.44 years and BMI of 21.88 kg/m^2. Time of pre-procedure scanning and puncture was 44.78 ± 24.81 s and 119.37 ± 116.70 s. During the procedure, one epidural puncture was cancelled due to poor visibility of the target interlaminar space during preprocedure scanning; the catheterization in four patients was cancelled because of one catheter expected into the blood vessel, while the other three patients reported transient paresthesia. Of the 55 patients with successful puncture and catheterization, 98.18% reported a satisfactory analgesic effect. No complication related to epidural puncture was found until discharge.

4.1. Basic Characteristics of Patients

Among the 60 patients, 68.33% (41/60) were male and 31.67% (19/60) were female. Patients ranged in age from 29 to 80 years (57.44 ± 11.36 years), in which 29 patients were older than 60 years old (29/59, 49.15%). The height of the patients was 163.91 ± 6.82 cm (cm), and the weight was 59.30 ± 9.26 kilograms (kg). The BMI was between 18.00 and 30.00 kg/m^2 (21.88 ± 3.07 kg/m^2). Among them, patients with overweight body (BMI ≥ 24 kg/m^2) accounted for 21.82% (12/55) (Table 1).

Table 1. Basic characteristics of patients.

Parameter		Numerical Information
Gender	Male, n, %	41, 68.33%
	Female, n, %	19, 31.67%
Age (years-old)	Mean ± Std	57.44 ± 11.36
	Min~Max	29–80
	Md (IQR)	59.00 (18.00)
	≥ 60 years, n, %	29, 49.15%
Height (cm)	Mean ± Std	163.91 ± 6.82
	Min~Max	150.00~180.00
	Md (IQR)	165.00 (11.00)

Table 1. Cont.

Parameter		Numerical Information
Weight (kg)	Mean ± Std	59.30 ± 9.26
	Min~Max	42.00~82.50
	Md (IQR)	58.25 (11.75)
BMI (kg/m^2)	Mean ± Std	21.88 ± 3.07
	Min~Max	18.00~30.00
	Md (IQR)	21.63 (4.17)
	≥24 kg/m^2	12, 21,82%
Hypertension, n, %		4, 6.67%
Abnormal ECG, n, %		2, 3.33%
Chronic bronchitis, n, %		4, 6.67%

Abbreviation: n = number(s), % = percentage, Std = Standard deviation, Min = Minimum value, Max = Maximum value, Md = Median, IQR = Interquartile range, cm = centimeter(s), kg = kilogram(s), m = meter(s), ECG = Electrocardiograph.

4.2. Complicated Diseases of Patients

Among the 60 included patients, there were four patients who had complications of hypertension (6.67%), four patients who experienced chronic bronchitis (6.67%), and two patients who showed abnormal ECGs in their preoperative examination (3.33%) (Table 1). In the two patients with abnormal ECG, one patient had sinus bradycardia, and the other patient reported premature ventricular beats.

4.3. Information on Surgical Treatment of Patients

Among the 60 cases, four cases underwent chest surgery (6.67%, all of which were via lobotomy) and 56 cases underwent abdominal or pelvic surgery (93.33%) (stomach or jejunum: 31/56, 55.36%; colorectum: 15/56, 26.79%; others: 10/56, 17.86%). Among the 60 cases, 50 cases underwent laparoscopic or thoracoscopic surgery (83.33%), and 10 cases underwent open surgery (16.67%).

4.4. Ultrasonic Imaging

During this observation period, ultrasound localization required 44.66 ± 25.72 s per case, and all was completed within 2 min (Figure 4A). The vertical distance from skin to dura was 3.75 ± 0.70 cm (a range of 2.09–6.10 cm). The oblique depth was 5.62 ± 0.59 cm (a range of 3.68–6.85 cm). Intervertebral space distance ranged from 0.31 to 1.55 cm (Mean ± Std: 0.70 ± 0.23 cm) (Figure 4B).

According to the visibility of the neuraxial structures (Table 2), the UVS of the included cases was measured to be 10.73 ± 5.58 (95% CI: 9.29–12.18, median 10.00, IQR 9.75, min 1.00, max 25.00) (Figure 4C). Among these structures, the proportion of vertebral lamina imaging visible was the highest (93.33%, well visible: 21/60, 35%; very well visible: 35/60, 58.33%), followed by intervertebral space (81.67%, well visible: 21/60, 35%; very well visible: 28/60, 46.67%) and posterior complex (70.00%, well visible: 27/60, 45%; very well visible: 15/60, 25.00%). The dural sac (45.00%, well visible: 16/60, 26.67%; very well visible: 11/60, 18.33%) and the anterior complex (40.00%, well visible: 13/60, 21.67%; very well visible: 11/60, 18.33%) showed poorly under ultrasound (Figure 4D).

Table 2. Ultrasound Visibility Score of Neuraxial Structures.

	0 Point	1 Point	2 Point	3 Point	Mean	Std	Median	IQR
vertebral lamina	0 (0.00%)	4 (6.67%)	21 (35.00%)	35 (58.33%)	2.52	0.62	3.00	1.00
intervertebral space	2 (3.33%)	9 (15.00%)	21 (35.00%)	28 (46.67%)	2.25	0.84	2.00	1.00

Table 2. Cont.

	0 Point	1 Point	2 Point	3 Point	Mean	Std	Median	IQR
dural sac	26 (43.33%)	7 (11.67%)	16 (26.67%)	11 (18.33%)	1.20	1.19	1.00	2.00
Anterior complex	26 (43.33%)	10 (16.67%)	13 (21.67%)	11 (18.33%)	1.15	1.18	1.00	2.00
Posterior complex	3 (5.00%)	15 (25.00%)	27 (45.00%)	15 (25.00%)	1.90	0.84	2.00	1.25

Abbreviation: % = percentage, Std = Standard deviation, IQR = Interquartile range. Note: 0 point = not visible, 1 point = hardly visible, 2 point = well visible, 3 point = very well visible.

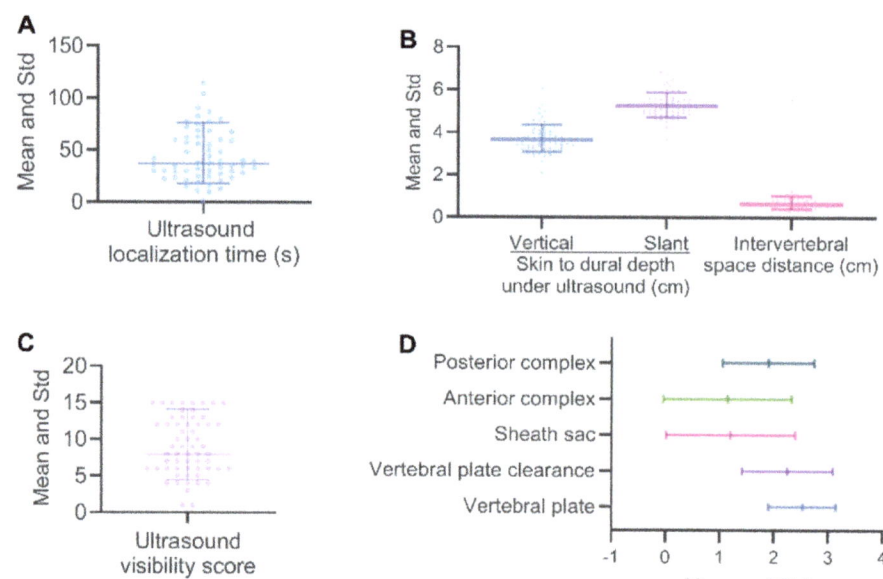

Figure 4. Quantitative measurements and ultrasound visibility score of neuraxial structures. The ultrasound localization time of all patients was under 2 min (120 s) (**A**: ultrasound localization time (s)). The vertical distance from skin to dura measured by ultrasound was about 3.75 cm (**B**, left), and the slope distance was about 5.62 cm (**B**, right). Different transverse nerve structures were shown in different states under ultrasound (**D**), and the total UVS score ranged from 1 to 15 points (**C**). Abbreviation: % = percentage, Std = Standard deviation, s = second(s); cm = centimeter(s).

4.5. Results of Epidural Catheterization

Of the 60 cases observed, only one patient abandoned the epidural puncture due to poor ultrasound imaging results, while the remaining patients successfully completed the epidural needle puncture (59/60, 98.33%). During the procedure, there was one patient that experienced a vascular puncture and three patients who experienced transient paresthesia; therefore, 55 of 60 patients were successfully catheterized (55/60, 91.67%). Under ultrasound guidance, one patient underwent epidural puncture at thoracic vertebra (T) 6-7 (1.67%), two patients at T 7-8 (3.39%), 35 patients at T 8-9 (59.32%), five patients at T 9-10 (8.47%), one patient at T 10-11 (1.69%), four patients at T 11-12 (6.78%), and 11 patients at T 12-lumbar vertebra (L) 1 (18.64%) (Figure 5A). The time to complete an epidural puncture was 71 (70) s (95% CI: 87.82–150.92, mean 119.37, Std 116.70, min 10.56, max 636.00) (Figure 5B). The proportion of epidural puncture time under 90 s was 53.33% (32/55). Among the patients with successful puncture, 47 patients were successfully punctured at the first puncture (47/59, 81.03%), seven patients were punctured by the second attempt (7/59, 12.07%), and five patients were successfully punctured by the third attempt (5/59, 8.47%) (Figure 5C). The puncture depth of the needle ranged from 3.00 to 8.00 (Figure 5D).

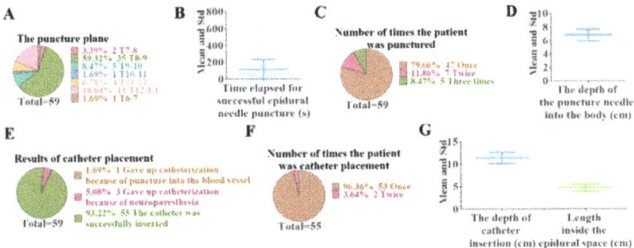

Figure 5. Outcomes of ultrasound-guided epidural catheterization in the absence of specific postures. Of the 60 cases observed, only one patient abandoned epidural puncture due to poor ultrasound imaging results. Among the 59 patients with successful puncture, the patients with puncture plane at T8-9 accounted for the largest proportion (A: Puncture plane distribution of successful epidural puncture), and the average time was 119.37 s (B: Duration of epidural puncture). The majority of patients completed the epidural catheterization procedure successfully the first time (C: Number of epidural punctures performed by the patient), and the average depth of puncture needle placement was 6.83 cm (D: The depth of the epidural puncture needle (cm)). Of the patients with successful puncture, 55 completed epidural catheterization (E: Results of catheter placement), of whom 96.36% completed the catheterization on the first attempt (F). The mean depth of catheter placement (G, Left) and the mean depth in the epidural space (G, Right) were 11.41 cm and 4.72 cm, respectively. Abbreviation: % = percentage, T = Thoracic vertebra, L = lumbar vertebra, Std = Standard deviation, s = second(s); cm = centimeter(s).

Among the 59 patients with successful puncture, one patient gave up catheterization because of puncture into the blood vessel (1.69%), and three patients gave up catheterization because of neuroparesthesia (3/59, 5.08%) (Figure 5E). Among the 55 patients with successful catheterization, 96.36% (53/55) had the catheterization completed successfully in only one attempt, and 3.64% (2/55) needed two attempts (Figure 5F). The distance from catheter tip to skin was 11.41 ± 1.21 cm (95% CI: 11.07–11.75, median 11.50, IQR 1.00, min 7.50, max 13.00), and the depth of the epidural space was between 2 and 8 cm (Mean ± Std: 4.72 ± 0.81cm, 95% CI: 4.49–4.94, Median 5, IQR 0.50) (Figure 5G).

4.6. Analgesic Effect and Complication

Of the 60 patients who underwent ultrasound-guided epidural catheterization, 55 (91.67%) completed the procedure successfully. Only one patient showed poor unilateral analgesic effect (1/55, 1.82%), and the remaining 54 patients reported satisfactory analgesic effect (54/55, 98.18%). No complication (dural puncture, bloody tap, total spinal anesthesia, epidural hematoma or abscess) was found before discharge.

4.7. Correlation Analysis Results

The time of ultrasound-guided epidural catheterization has no correlation with the patients' sex ($p = 0.150$), age ($p = 0.460$), height ($p = 0.096$), weight ($p = 0.834$), BMI ($p = 0.354$), puncture plane ($p = 0.816$), ultrasound localization ($p = 0.956$), vertical distance from skin to dura ($p = 0.195$), UVS ($p = 0.161$), or visibility of several neuraxial structures: vertebral lamina ($p = 0.282$), intervertebral space ($p = 0.160$), and posterior complex ($p = 0.163$).

However, there are correlations among distance to the intervertebral space ($p = 0.010$, $r = -0.358$), oblique distance from skin to dura ($p = 0.012$, $r = 0.338$), and visibility of other neuraxial structures: dural sac ($p = 0.006$, $r = -0.367$), and anterior complex ($p = 0.003$, $r = -0.395$).

5. Discussion

This study is the first study to report that real-time US guidance could facilitate middle and low thoracic epidural puncture for the patients in the left lateral decubitus position without using the forehead to knees position. In this observational study of the 60 patients, 59 patients had a successful epidural puncture. Among them, 55 patients (91.67%) successfully completed epidural catheterization without any related adverse reactions. Except for one patient who had only good unilateral analgesia, the remaining 54 patients had satisfactory bilateral analgesia after surgery. During the process of catheterization, five patients withdrew from the operation due to contact with blood vessels or paresthesia. The visibility of the vertebral lamina, intervertebral space and posterior complex in the paramedian oblique sagittal view were all good at T6-L1 level in the patients without forehead to knees under ultrasound. And epidural catheterization to patients without flexion of knees and neck under ultrasound guidance has a high success rate and strong feasibility. In addition, this study provided detailed ultrasound data for the thoracic epidural puncture.

5.1. Real-Time Ultrasound-Assisted Thoracic Epidural Catheter Placement

Thoracic epidural analgesia provides reliable acute pain relief and reduces morbidity and mortality for patients undergoing abdominal or thoracic surgery. Conventional methods for thoracic epidural puncture relied on the surface anatomy of the spine, which often leads to incorrect identification of the targeted level and high failure rate, which limited the clinical application of epidural analgesia. The success rates of landmark-based lateral epidurals in the thoracic spine in our institution was around 75%. With the widespread use of ultrasound in regional anesthesia, widespread evidence supports neuraxial ultrasound assisting lumbar epidurals with great success, however the use of ultrasound for guidance in thoracic epidurals is still not widespread. David B. Auyong reported the first randomized study to evaluate the value of preprocedure ultrasound in thoracic epidural catheterization [14]. In this study, he found that preprocedural ultrasound did not significantly reduce the time required to identify the thoracic epidural space, but decreased the number of needle skin punctures and mean pain scores after surgery. Furthermore, Daniel J. Pak [12] described the successful real-time ultrasound-guided thoracic epidural technique in a paramedian sagittal oblique view. Recently, Karmakar and his colleagues reported a prospective, randomized superiority trial, which indicates that real-time ultrasound guidance is superior to a conventional anatomic landmark-based technique for first-pass success during TEP [15]. Since 2015, the author Fei Liu started to do ultrasound-guided epidural anesthesia replacing landmark based thoracic epidural anesthesia for postoperative pain in patients after abdominal surgery. A success rate beyond 90% was achieved [16].

5.2. Epidural Catheter Placement Was Achieved in Every Patient

In our center, preprocedure ultrasound scanning or real time ultrasound guidance has been a routine procedure for thoracic and lumbar epidural analgesia for 7 years. The author (the leader of the acute pain service) is skilled in real time ultrasound-guided epidural puncture. She found that some patients complained of severe pain postoperatively, which could not be relieved by strong opioids and NSAIDS. Thus, she thought that only epidural analgesia could help them, and after getting consent from the patients, she started to do real-time ultrasound guiding epidural punctures for them. During the procedure, strong pain prevents them from lying in a standard lateral position (neck to knee). Therefore, the author could only do epidural puncture in these patients lying in a comfortable lateral position. We found that although the patient's position was not ideal for the traditional land mark epidural puncture, under ultrasound guidance we still could find the inter laminar space for needle advancement. Therefore, we started this preliminary study and tried to prove that ultrasound-guided epidural puncture could also be done for patients who could not use the standard knee to head position.

5.3. Under Ultrasound, the Vertebral Lamina, Intervertebral Space and Posterior Complex in the Paramedian Oblique Sagittal View Were All Good at the T6-L1 Level in the Patients without "Forehead to Knees"

In the 60 patients in this study, in the paramedian oblique sagittal view, the visibility of the vertebral lamina, intervertebral space and posterior complex under ultrasound were as high as 93.33%, 81.67% and 70.00%, respectively. The anterior complex and dural sac were poorly visible because of the extreme caudad angulation of the spinous processes and the overlapping laminae. However, we measured the width of the interlaminar space, which was 0.70 ± 0.23 cm at T6-L1, which was much narrower compared to the lumbar spine interlaminar space. Although it was very narrow, the good visibility of the intervertebral space provided an ideal route for epidural needle trajectory. This is consistent with the results of previous literature [8,17–19]. However, it is important to note that all of the articles presented were lumbar epidural punctures. Only ShengJin Ge et al. reported one case of an ultrasound-assisted paramedial-lateral approach of thoracic epidural puncture (T 7-8) [20]. However, this report could not provide information on the success rate of the puncture, catheterization, and adverse reactions. T Grau also showed that, despite the limited capacity of US to depict the thoracic epidural space, US proved to be of better value than MRI in the depiction of the dura mater [21]. These studies suggest that ultrasound-assisted thoracic epidural puncture is acceptable. This study not only provides a series of information about thoracic epidural puncture under ultrasound, but also puts forward the concept of comfort. It aims to provide patients with sufficient therapeutic effects and comfortable care at the same time.

5.4. Epidural Catheterization to Patients without Flexion of Knees and Neck under Ultrasound-Guided Has a High Success Rate and Accurate Analgesic Effect

Among the 60 patients observed, epidural puncture was performed in 59 patients with good visibility, except for one patient with had poor epidural visibility. A total of 55 patients completed the epidural catheterization successfully, with the exception of four patients who experienced puncture into the blood vessel or neuroparesthesia. The success rate of epidural catheterization was as high as 91.67%, and the postoperative analgesic effect was satisfactory for 98.18% of patients without nausea, pruritus and other discomfort. Thoracic epidural analgesia is a common method of pain relief for major thoracic and abdominal surgery [22]. However, due to the difficulty of the puncture in the past, the possible complications such as spinal cord injury and pneumothorax have limited its use [23]. T Grau et al. compared the ultrasound method with the traditional puncture method, and the results showed that the visualization procedure was very effective and reduced the injury caused by repeated puncture [24]. In addition, based on the visualization characteristics of ultrasound, the occurrence of the above complications can be avoided to a certain extent. Although previous studies showed that ultrasound guided epidural puncture in real time was feasible, it was still done when the patient was in an "ideal" position. Interestingly, Ban Tsui et al. performed on epidural space of male adult cadavers and found that ultrasound imaging and real-time ultrasound needle guidance for nerve blocks at the trunk and epidural space can be used in "stiff" cadavers [25]. This provides strong evidence for conducting epidural puncture in the comfortable position. Thus, our study suggests that visual manipulation makes epidural catheterization not only easier to perform, but also reduces the requirements of the procedure. This allows for epidural catheterization in a comfortable position for patients who are unable to provide a strict knee and neck flexion position.

5.5. Limitations

This study was only an observational one, and there was a lack of a control variable. In addition, there were certain limitations in the selection of patients. In the next step, we plan to include a wider range of people (such as patients with obesity, the elderly, and pregnant women), to start a prospective randomized controlled study to compare the success rate between the comfortable position and the strict knee and neck flexion position.

6. Conclusions

Under the comfortable position on the left lateral decubitus, the success rate of epidural catheterization under the guidance of real-time ultrasound was as high as 91.67%, and the analgesic efficiency was 98.18%. This technique is feasible for patients who are unable to achieve the forehead to knees position, while improving the comfort of patients during treatment.

Supplementary Materials: The following supporting information can be downloaded at: https://www.mdpi.com/article/10.3390/jcm11216459/s1, Video S1: The puncturing procedure video.

Author Contributions: F.L.: this author participated in the relevant diagnosis and treatment procedures involved in the study, and helped design of the study. TW. (Tinghua Wang): this author helped design of the study, guidance of the study and writing. T.L.: this author was responsible for data collection, completed the figures and tables summary and the first draft. Y.H.: this author was responsible for data collection and helped completed the figures and tables summary of the results. L.X.: this author was responsible for the manuscript writing. Y.W.: this author was responsible for the manuscript writing. T.W. (Tianhong Wang): this author was responsible for the data curation and software. All authors have read and agreed to the published version of the manuscript.

Funding: This research received no external funding.

Institutional Review Board Statement: The study was conducted in accordance with the Declaration of Helsinki, and approved by the West China Biomedical Ethics Committee, Sichuan University (No. 2016 (332). 18 February 2019).

Informed Consent Statement: All authors agreed to the publication of this article.

Data Availability Statement: The data presented in this study are available on request from the corresponding author.

Conflicts of Interest: The authors declare that they have no conflict of interest.

Glossary

US	Ultrasound imaging
ASA	American Society of Anesthesiologists
BMI	Body mass index
UVS	Ultrasound visibility score
CI	Confidence interval
Std	Standard deviation
IQR	Interquartile range
Min	Minimum
Max	Maximum
T	Thoracic vertebra
L	Lumbar vertebra

References

1. Gerheuser, F.; Roth, A. [Epidural anesthesia]. *Der Anaesthesist* **2007**, *56*, 499–523. [CrossRef] [PubMed]
2. Tran, D.; Kamani, A.A.; Lessoway, V.A.; Peterson, C.; Hor, K.W.; Rohling, R.N. Preinsertion paramedian ultrasound guidance for epidural anesthesia. *Anesth. Analg.* **2009**, *109*, 661–667. [CrossRef] [PubMed]
3. Hermanides, J.; Hollmann, M.W.; Stevens, M.F.; Lirk, P. Failed epidural: Causes and management. *Br. J. Anaesth.* **2012**, *109*, 144–154. [CrossRef] [PubMed]
4. Miller, R.D. *Miller's Anesthesia*, 7th ed.; Churchill Livingstone: New York, NY, USA, 2009.
5. Karmakar, M.K.; Li, X.; Ho, A.M.; Kwok, W.H.; Chui, P.T. Real-time ultrasound-guided paramedian epidural access: Evaluation of a novel in-plane technique. *Br. J. Anaesth.* **2009**, *102*, 845–854. [CrossRef] [PubMed]
6. Shaikh, F.; Brzezinski, J.; Alexander, S.; Arzola, C.; Carvalho, J.C.; Beyene, J.; Sung, L. Ultrasound imaging for lumbar punctures and epidural catheterisations: Systematic review and meta-analysis. *BMJ* **2013**, *346*, f1720. [CrossRef]
7. Perlas, A.; Chaparro, L.E.; Chin, K.J. Lumbar Neuraxial Ultrasound for Spinal and Epidural Anesthesia: A Systematic Review and Meta-Analysis. *Reg. Anesth. Pain Med.* **2016**, *41*, 251–260. [CrossRef]

8. Gnaho, A.; Nau, A.; Gentil, M.E. Real-time ultrasound-guided epidural catheter insertion in obese parturients. *Can. J. Anaesth.* **2015**, *62*, 1226–1227. [CrossRef]
9. Tran, D.; Kamani, A.A.; Al-Attas, E.; Lessoway, V.A.; Massey, S.; Rohling, R.N. Single-operator real-time ultrasound-guidance to aim and insert a lumbar epidural needle. *Can. J. Anaesth.* **2010**, *57*, 313–321. [CrossRef]
10. Zhang, G.T.; Wang, F.L.; Ran, Y.; Liu, D.X. Applications of the ultrasound-guided nerve block technique for nonanalgesic effects. *Ibrain* **2022**, *8*, 389–400. [CrossRef]
11. Ye, M.; Zhou, H.S.; Wei, Y.; Liu, F. Inadvertent mental excitement after ultrasound-guided bilateral thoracic paravertebral block: A case report. *Ibrain* **2021**, *7*, 29–33. [CrossRef]
12. Pak, D.J.; Gulati, A. Real-Time Ultrasound-Assisted Thoracic Epidural Placement: A Feasibility Study of a Novel Technique. *Reg. Anesth. Pain Med.* **2018**, *43*, 613–615. [CrossRef] [PubMed]
13. Karmakar, M.K.; Li, X.; Kwok, W.H.; Ho, A.M.; Ngan Kee, W.D. Sonoanatomy relevant for ultrasound-guided central neuraxial blocks via the paramedian approach in the lumbar region. *Br. J. Radiol.* **2012**, *85*, e262–e269. [CrossRef]
14. Auyong, D.B.; Hostetter, L.; Yuan, S.C.; Slee, A.E.; Hanson, N.A. Evaluation of Ultrasound-Assisted Thoracic Epidural Placement in Patients Undergoing Upper Abdominal and Thoracic Surgery: A Randomized, Double-Blind Study. *Reg. Anesth. Pain Med.* **2017**, *42*, 204–209. [CrossRef] [PubMed]
15. Pakpirom, J.; Thatsanapornsathit, K.; Kovitwanawong, N.; Petsakul, S.; Benjhawaleemas, P.; Narunart, K.; Boonchuduang, S.; Karmakar, M.K. Real-time ultrasound-guided versus anatomic landmark-based thoracic epidural placement: A prospective, randomized, superiority trial. *BMC Anesth.* **2022**, *22*, 198. [CrossRef] [PubMed]
16. Liu, F.; Zhang, J.; Zeng, X.Q.; Zhao, Y.Q.; Zuo, Y.X. Application of general anesthesia combined with epidural anesthesia/analgesia in rehabilitation after gastric cancer resection. *Natl. Med. J. China* **2017**, *97*, 1089–1092.
17. Geng, J.; Li, M. Ultrasound-assisted neuraxial anesthesia in a patient with previous lumbar laminectomy and fusion: A case report. *Beijing Da Xue Xue Bao Yi Xue Ban = J. Peking Univ. Health Sci.* **2016**, *48*, 747–750.
18. Luo, L.; Ni, J.; Wu, L.; Luo, D. Ultrasound-guided epidural anesthesia for a parturient with severe malformations of the skeletal system undergoing cesarean delivery: A case report. *Local Reg. Anesth.* **2015**, *8*, 7–10. [CrossRef]
19. Goyal, R.; Singh, S.; Shukla, R.N.; Singhal, A. Management of a case of ankylosing spondylitis for total hip replacement surgery with the use of ultrasound-assisted central neuraxial blockade. *Indian J. Anaesth.* **2013**, *57*, 69–71. [CrossRef]
20. Ge, S.; Ma, Y.; Yang, Y. Ultrasound-assisted thoracic epidural puncture: A paramedial-lateral approach. *J. Clin. Anesth.* **2020**, *59*, 69–71. [CrossRef]
21. Grau, T.; Leipold, R.W.; Delorme, S.; Martin, E.; Motsch, J. Ultrasound imaging of the thoracic epidural space. *Reg. Anesth. Pain Med.* **2002**, *27*, 200–206. [CrossRef]
22. Grieve, P.P.; Whitta, R.K. Pleural puncture: An unusual complication of a thoracic epidural. *Anaesth. Intensive Care* **2004**, *32*, 113–116. [CrossRef]
23. Wadhwa, R.; Sharma, S.; Poddar, D.; Sharma, S. Pleural puncture with thoracic epidural: A rare complication? *Indian J. Anaesth.* **2011**, *55*, 163–166. [CrossRef] [PubMed]
24. Grau, T.; Leipold, R.W.; Fatehi, S.; Martin, E.; Motsch, J. Real-time ultrasonic observation of combined spinal-epidural anaesthesia. *Eur. J. Anaesthesiol.* **2004**, *21*, 25–31. [CrossRef] [PubMed]
25. Tsui, B.; Dillane, D.; Pillay, J.; Walji, A. Ultrasound imaging in cadavers: Training in imaging for regional blockade at the trunk. *Can. J. Anaesth.* **2008**, *55*, 105–111. [CrossRef] [PubMed]

Article

Sublingual Sufentanil Tablet System (SSTS-Zalviso®) for Postoperative Analgesia after Orthopedic Surgery: A Retrospective Study

Andrea Angelini [1,*], Gian Mario Parise [2], Mariachiara Cerchiaro [1], Francesco Ambrosio [2], Paolo Navalesi [2] and Pietro Ruggieri [1]

1. Department of Orthopedics and Orthopedic Oncology, University of Padova, 35128 Padova, Italy
2. Institute of Anesthesiology and Critical Care, Department of Medicine-DIED, University of Padova, 35128 Padova, Italy
* Correspondence: andrea.angelini@unipd.it; Tel.: +39-04-9821-3311 or +39-33-3442-0795

Abstract: Background: The aim of this study is to compare sublingual sufentanil and the administration device for its delivery (SSST-Zalviso®) with the traditional strategies used for the control of postoperative pain to establish if there is an actual benefit for the patient and healthcare personnel. Materials and Methods: A retrospective study was conducted to compare the efficacy of SSTS in the management of postoperative pain after orthopedic surgery between October 2018 and June 2020. We analyzed 50 patients who underwent a total knee arthroplasty (TKA). The control group consisted of 21 patients who underwent TKA and during the hospitalized recovery received a continuous femoral nerve block (cFNB). The statistical study was conducted with a level of significance $p = 0.05$ using "U" test, Mann–Whitney, to verify if patients had a better control of pain and fewer calls for rescue analgesia. Results: Patients involved in the study showed a significant reduction in pain intensity with the use of SSTS in the 24 h following surgery ($p = 0.0568$), also a drastic drop of the calls for rescue analgesia ($p < 0.0001$) reduces the number of calls for its control. Conclusions: This study demonstrates how SSTS might reduce pain intensity in the first 24 h after surgery and reduce the number of calls for its control, indicating better analgesic coverage and implying reduced interventions from healthcare personnel. This could allow a redistribution of resources and a reduction in the use of analgesic drugs in wards where the SSTS is used.

Keywords: sublingual sufentanil tablet system (SSTS–Zalviso®); total knee arthroplasty; retrospective study; postoperative pain; continuous femoral nerve block

1. Introduction

Postoperative pain after orthopaedic procedures, such as total knee arthroplasty (TKA), is a major problem and represents a challenge. Pain control following TKA is a prerequisite for good outcomes because rehabilitation requires early mobilization and enhanced recovery [1]. TKA has become a fast-track approach, where early rehabilitation is a key factor in reducing morbidity and decreasing the length of hospital stay [2]. Despite the increasing knowledge about postoperative pain management and the implementation of new pain management techniques, an adequate protocol is still debated in the literature [3–7].

The number of total knee arthroplasty procedures has increased over the last 2–3 decades and is projected to increase even further due to population aging and longevity; however, these patients are affected by significant postoperative pain [8,9]. This pain, if uncontrolled, can hinder the recovery process by setting in motion-detrimental pathophysiological processes that increase the risk of postoperative complications. Ineffective pain control can result in low limb mobility, which can result in several medical morbidities, such as venous thrombosis, coronary ischemia, myocardial infarction, and pneumonia [10]. Inefficient pain control can also hinder mobilization and rehabilitation, disrupt sleep, cause cognitive dysfunction, and increase patient anxiety. Therefore, focusing on effective pain control among total knee arthroplasty patients is crucial, as it influences recovery time, cost of healthcare, and overall patient satisfaction [11,12]. The Enhanced Recovery After Surgery (ERAS) protocols make it possible to achieve these objectives thanks to a specific multidisciplinary approach. The advantages include the reduction in the average hospital stay and a low rate of complications, resulting in greater patient satisfaction [13,14]. Early mobilization represents one of the main aspects of ERAS and is closely linked to the use of short-acting anesthetic techniques aimed at minimizing side effects despite multimodal analgesic coverage [13,15]. There is wide debate on the best postoperative analgesia technique after TKA, with the choice of peripheral nerve blocks, epidural analgesia, and local infiltration analgesia (LIA) or (systemic) opioids. [1,16–20]. Sufentanil is a potent synthetic μ-opioid receptor specific agonist primarily used for intraoperative surgical analgesia. Sufentanil can be administered via sublingual route, demonstrating a good bioavailability (60%) and a prolonged duration of action compared to IV-Sufentanil, thanks to its high lipophilicity. For these reasons, sublingual sufentanil has recently been used for postoperative pain management and marketed as a pre-programmed, non-invasive handheld device (The Sufentanil Sublingual Tablet System (SSTS)—Zalviso®, Grünenthal GmbH, Aachen, Germany) [13,21,22]. This system combines the advantages of the non-IV route with self-administration (Figure 1).

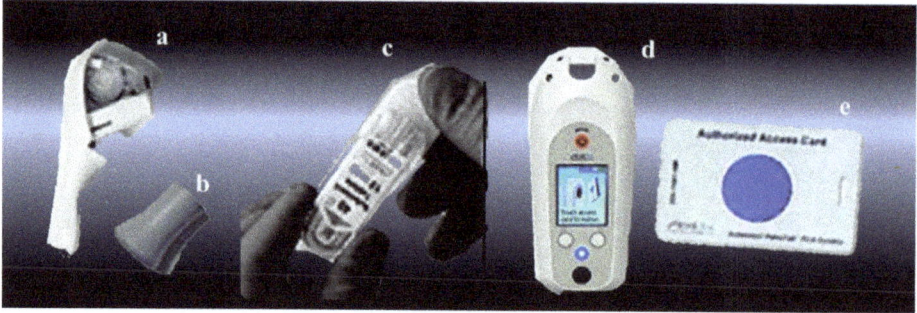

Figure 1. The Zalviso® system consists of a disposable dispenser tip (**a**) and dispenser cap (**b**); a cartridge of Sufentanil sublingual 15 mcg tablets in a disposable bar-coded cartridge (**c**); a reusable handheld controller (**d**) and an authorized access card (**e**).

The purpose of this study is to compare sublingual sufentanil and the administration device for its delivery (SSTS) with the traditional strategies used for the control of postoperative pain to establish if there is an actual benefit for the patient and healthcare personnel [23–25]. Therefore, we compared the efficacy of SSTS and continuous femoral nerve block (CFNB) in the postoperative pain control in patients treated with TKA. We propose that SSTS could show a better profile of pain control, tolerability, and patient and staff satisfaction, reducing the intensity of pain and side effects [25,26]. The primary objectives were to assess the efficacy of SSTS in controlling postoperative pain and its safety in comparison with cFNB. The secondary aim of the study was to analyze the ease of use with the STTS system for the administration of analgesics by physicians, nurses and patients, using feedback analysis [19,20].

2. Materials and Methods

This was a retrospective observational monocentric study on a representative group of 50 patients (30 (60%) women; 20 (40%) men) treated with TKA at a mean age of 66 (min 22–max 83 years) between October 2018 and June 2020. All the patients were treated with perioperative multimodal analgesia. We compared a group of patients receiving the SSTS postoperative analgesia (SSTS group, 50 patients) versus a control group of patients who were treated according to our standard pain management with continuous femoral nerve block (cFNB group, 21 patients). The inclusion criteria were age >18 years and patients' ability to describe and report pain. Exclusion criteria were administration of general anesthesia, postoperative admission to the intensive care unit, and previous history of chronic pain. All data used in this study were obtained from the patients' hospital records and included patient demographic data and all data regarding intraoperative management, postoperative analgesia, and pain scores. All relevant data are within this paper.

2.1. Perioperative Management

All patients received IV midazolam as an anxiolytic premedication. Antibiotic prophylaxis was administered with 2 g of cefazolin. In our ERAS protocol, spinal anesthesia was performed with 10 mg of hyperbaric bupivacaine 0.5% without adjuvant or 7.5 mg/mL (from 1.5 to 2 mL) isobaric levobupivacaine. Both groups received subarachnoid anesthesia and 68 patients (95.8%) underwent one shot single femoral nerve block (FNB) (Ropivacaina 0.5% 20 mL one shot). In case of pain not properly controlled (NRS $\geq$ 4), patients of both groups received a "rescue dose" with ketoprofene 160 mg ev, i.m 2/24 h or toradol 30 mg (max $\times$ 2/die); in the case of intolerance to FANS, paracetamol 1 g ev three times a day, Tramadol 50 mg max 3/die or morphine 5 mg subcutaneous were chosen.

After surgery, the patients in the SSTS group received sufentanil 15 μg upon need plus paracetamol (1 g) three times a day. The SSTS in our population was typically prepared by an anesthetist with a mean set up time 2.7 min ($\pm$1.8). Conversely, patients treated according to our standard protocol (cFNB group/control) underwent continuous femoral nerve block (cFNB) with continuous infusion of local anesthetic (ropivacaine 0.2% 7 mL/h plus paracetamol 1 g (ev) four times a day). The reasons for choosing the analgesic technique were not completely at the patient's discretion, but we consider the ability in terms of drug administration device as a discriminating factor. However, the good preliminary results and the controlled self-administration modality have directed the choice of many patients towards this modality of pain management.

The endpoints measured were pain intensity at rest, number of adverse events, number of rescue doses, length of hospital stay, and usability scores. Pain was measured using the numeric rating scale (NRS) (range: 0 = no pain to 10 = worst pain possible). Pain perception during the postoperative period was calculated using the NRS scale at 24 h (T1), 48 h (T2), and 72 h (T3) for both groups. Pain was evaluated in both groups as the mean scores for T1 throughout T3 (T1 to T3 are the three postoperative days). For the SSTS group, pain scores were collected for the day prior to surgery (T-1), the day of surgery at delivery of the SSTS device to the patient (T0), the first administration, and 2-4-8- and 16 h after the first nanotablet. The practicality and manageability of the drug administration device by the staff (nurses) was analyzed through semi-quantitative data (time for preparation, number of doses administered, and subjective evaluation scales) that measure the usability of the device by the staff, and the understanding of how it works by the patient.

2.2. Statistical Analysis

All data reported in this study are expressed as the mean, standard deviation (SD), range, and median for each value. Continuous variables were compared between two groups using the two-sample t-test and among three groups using one-way analysis of variance (ANOVA). The chi-squared test was used for categorical variables. Pain intensity between the groups was also evaluated using the "U" test (Mann–Whitney), comparing the observation at baseline and final follow-up. Statistical significance was set at a p-value of less than 0.05. The data were analyzed using Minitab v.18® (Minitab 18 Statistical Software (2019). Minitab, Inc.: State College, PA, USA).

3. Results

The study compared 50 patients in the SSTS drug group and 21 patients in the cFNB group presenting similar characteristics (age, comorbidities, type of surgery) and differing limitedly to the analgesic technique received.

Pain scores. In the SSTS group, the NRS scores were: 2.38 (T1), 3.28 (T2), and 2.34 (T3). The NRS scores for the control group were: 3.81 (T1); 3.43 (T2); and 2.57 (T3). The overall differences in pain intensity and the difference in time point T1 between the groups were significantly different ($p = 0.008$) (Figure 2).

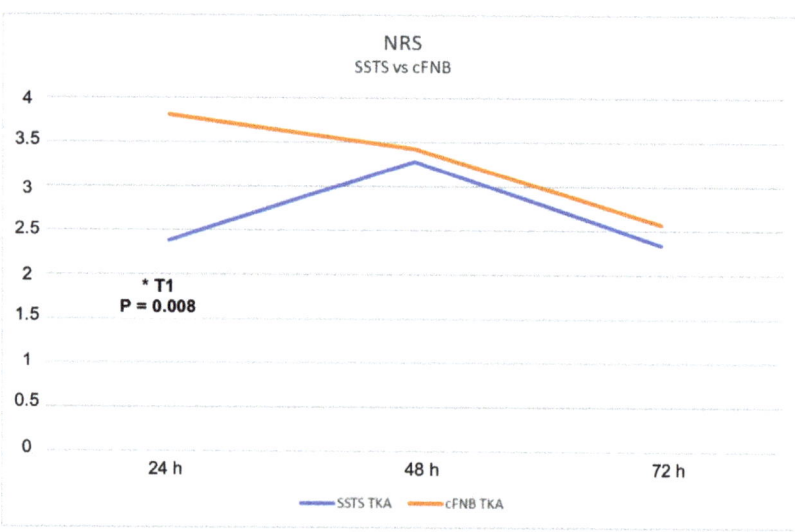

Figure 2. NRS were lower in the SSTS group compared to cFNB group at each time points measured with significant different in T1 ($p = 0.008$) *.

The NRS evaluated at T2 and T3 and compared between the two groups was not statistically significant (Figure 3).

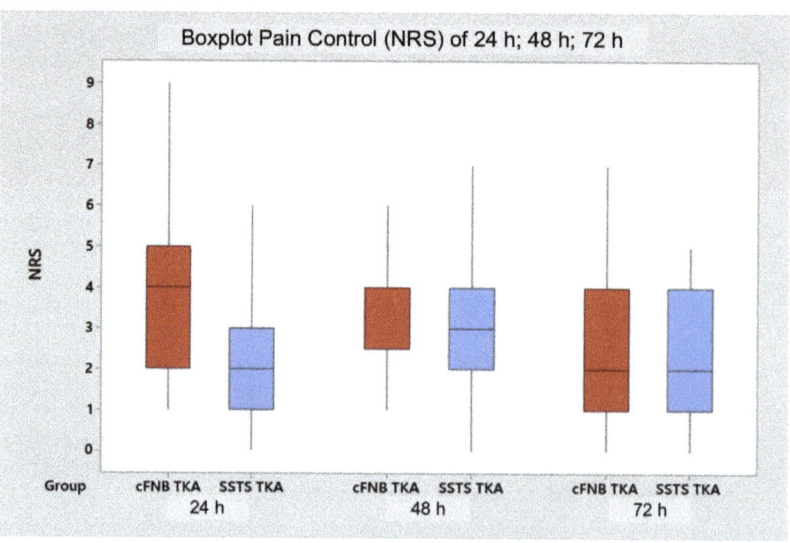

Figure 3. Boxplot analysis of pain control at 24 h, 48 h, and 72 h between the two groups. Horizontal line represents mean value, and the square box represents interquartile range.

3.1. Rescue Analgesic Dose and Patient Satisfaction

Patients treated in the SSTS group required significantly less rescue doses than those in cFNB control (5% of SSTS patients vs. 60% patients, of which 25% on T1, 15% on T2, 10% on T3, and 10% on T4). The mean duration of treatment with SSTS from the first to the last nanotablet received was less than 48 h (no patients used STSS for more than 72 h). Rescue doses were required less often in the SSTS group (66% of SSTS patients) than the cFNB control (100% patients), which resulted in fewer calls and satisfaction of the nursing staff (Figure 4).

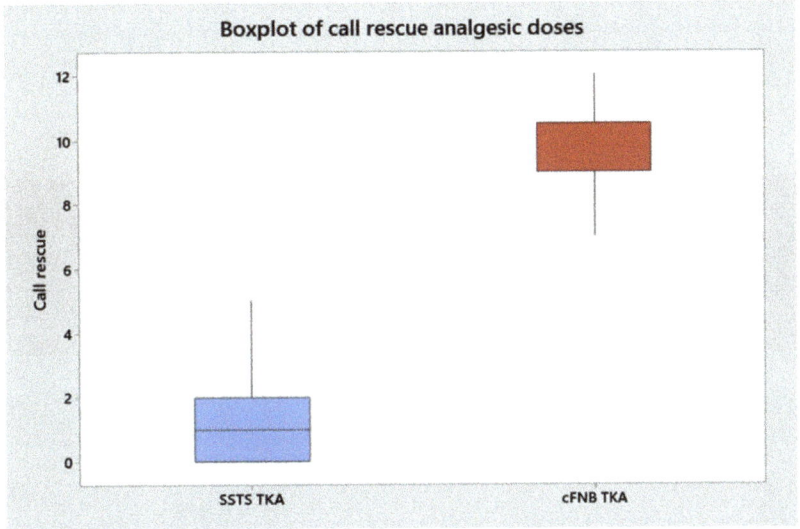

Figure 4. Boxplot analysis rescue doses between the two groups. Horizontal line represents mean value and the square box represents interquartile range.

3.2. Adverse Events

Adverse events reported in the SSTS group were postoperative nausea and vomiting (PONV 6%), nausea (10%), vomiting (2%), constipation (24%), bladder globe (4%), somnolence (2%), headache (2%), and hypertension (2%) disorientation (6%) (Table 1). The adverse events in the SSTS group are shown in Table 1.

Table 1. Adverse events reported in the SSTS group vs. cFNB group.

	SSTS (50)	CFNB (21)
PONV	(3) 6%	(3) 15%
Nausea	(5) 10%	(6) 30%
Vomiting	(1) 2%	(3) 15%
constipation	(12) 24%	(4) 20%
Bladder globe	(2) 4%	(1) 5%
somnolence	(1) 2%	(2) 10%
headache	(1) 2%	(1) 5%
hypertension	(1) 2%	(3) 15%
disorientation	(3) 6%	(1) 5%

3.3. Hospitalization

Patients were dismissed from the hospital for a mean of 7.06 days in the SSTS group vs. 8.62 of the control group. There was a significant difference in the time to hospitalization, with fewer days in the SSTS group ($p = 0.039$) (Figure 5).

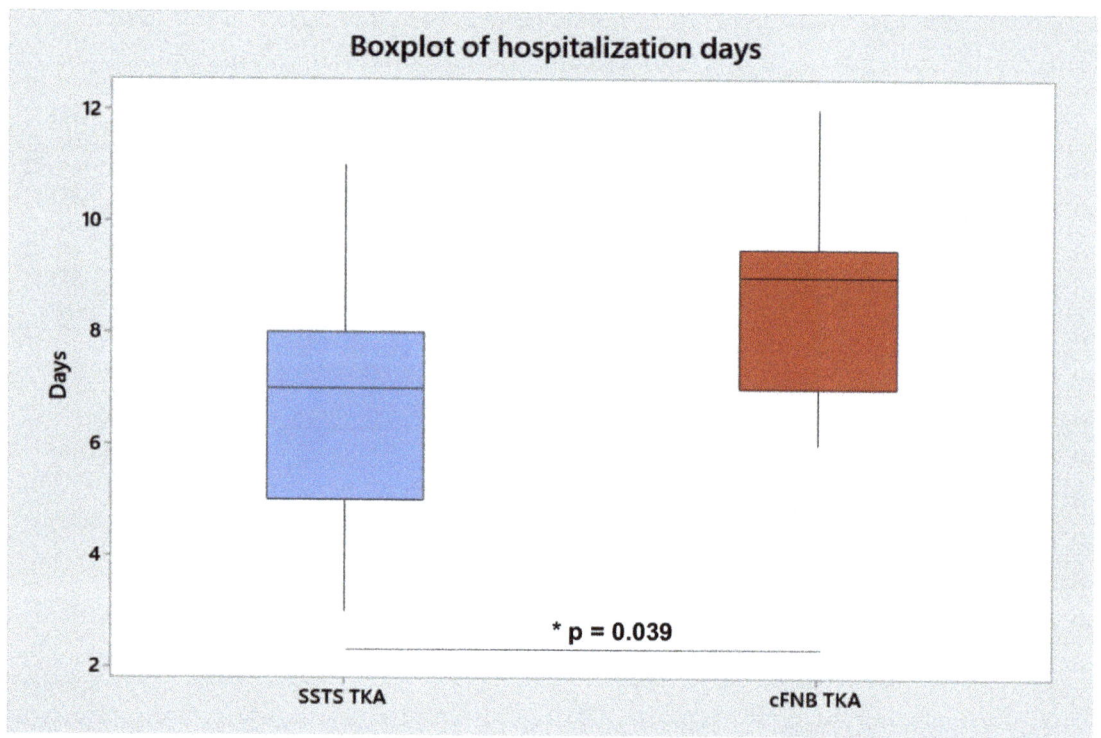

Figure 5. Boxplot analysis hospitalization between the two groups. Horizontal line represents mean value, and the square box represents interquartile range. ($p = 0.039$) *.

3.4. Usability

Most patients confirmed that the SSTS was easy to use and did not report any difficulties in using the device. Most patients report no motor discomfort and 86% of patients reported complete pain relief. Three patients (6%) discontinued SSTS due to ineffective pain relief after T3, and four (8%) due to the malfunctioning of the device (these were excluded from the statistical analysis at the T2 and T3 evaluation).

4. Discussion

This study evaluated the efficacy and safety of the SSTS in comparison with a classic multimodal analgesic approach associated with cFNB for pain control in patients treated with TKA. Our results confirmed the efficacy and safety of SSTS in TKA, in agreement with previous studies [22,27,28]. However, we used a different approach than the other studies: Melson et al. compared SSTS to Intravenous patient-controlled analgesia morphine sulfate enrolling patients scheduled for elective major open abdominal or orthopedic (hip or knee replacement) surgery [22]. Jove et al. evaluated the efficacy SSTS 15 μg vs. an identical placebo system for the management of pain after knee or hip arthroplasty [27]. Minkowitz et al. performed another placebo-controlled trial evaluating sufentanil sublingual tablet 30 mcg [28]. This study reflects the clinical experience of a ward in which patients who used the SSTS were rationally selected from a larger group and therefore cannot claim the authority of a randomized trial. These results must be considered evidence for real-life clinical practice.

There are two main limitations of the study: (1) as a consequence of the relative small number of patients, it was not possible to conduct a comparative statistical analysis for all possible variables, but only for the main aspects (pain score, rescue, nursing assistance, adverse effects, and hospitalization) considered in the study; (2) cFNB provided better analgesia compared with single-shot FNB, however, our control group received only a cFNB plus paracetamol whereby it is well-known that it does not cover the whole pain receptions [29,30]. For sufficient pain control, a sciatic nerve block (SNB) would have to be added. Continuous SNB has been reported to improves analgesia and decreases morphine request compared with single-injection sciatic nerve block in patients undergoing TKA, but it influences the possibility of an early rehabilitation in these patients whereas is not observed in cFNB [31]. This is the main reason that limited its use in our cohort in the period of analysis. A recent metanalysis analyzed the analgesic benefits of adding sciatic nerve block (SNB) to FNB following TKA and authors concluded that SNB can seems to reduce postoperative opioid consumption in these patients, even if the available evidence is marked by significant heterogeneity [32]. Other studies provide evidence-based supports to the benefits of SNB as a complement to FNB in TKA [Zorrilla]. Furthermore, the FNB group did not receive planned doses of stronger analgesics, such as retarded opioids, to cover up for the incomplete pain control by the FNB. Thus, it is natural that the FNB group needed more rescue analgesics. This uncontrolled bias of our series may support that the positive analgesic effect with SSTS might not only be due to superior pain control, but also due to an optimizable current standard pain management in the control group.

Few RCTs have specifically addressed the role of SSTS in postoperative pain. We observed a significant difference in postoperative pain intensity between the two groups, with better control using the SSTS protocol, as reported in other studies. Scardino et al. reported lower pain upon movement in the SSTS group (95 patients) than in the cFNB group (87 patients, control group) at all time points, and pain was properly managed when local infiltration anesthesia (LIA) was worn off [33]. The efficacy of the treatment adopted on pain relief was also suggested by the lower request of rescue doses (60% of patients on cFNB vs. 5% of those using SSTS) [33]. Jove et al. showed that STSS 15 mcg could improve the summed pain intensity difference (SPID) 48 h after TKA or total hip arthroplasty (SSTS 76 vs placebo −11) [27]. They also reported a mean NRS pain scores at 24 h of 3.9 ($\pm$0.2) for SSTS versus 5.1 ($\pm$0.4) for placebo ($p = 0.002$) [27]. However, in both studies, the significant and pronounced effect of SSTS should be analyzed considering that the patients in control group were treated with placebo [27]. Other authors did not find a clinically significant pain improvement analyzing a series of patients treated with TKA in multimodal analgesia under an enhanced recovery protocol, comparing sublingual sufentanil 15 mcg tablet system and oral oxycodone [13]. Different investigators confirmed these results on different scales and at different intervals. We normalized all NRS to a 0–10 range. Most of the authors considered pain intensity between 12 and 24 h after surgery, whereas pain intensity over the first 24 h was reported in 12 studies (including 2327 patients with 1844 in the SSTS group). All participants in SSTS group reported NRS ″4 within 24 h after surgery, [34] and only one trial recorded NRS at 12 h of 5 and at 24 h of 4.5 [2]. It is important to point out that this was the highest pain score recorded among patients treated with SSTS [34]. Numerous studies reported the use of rescue medication medication, IV morphine, oral morphine, oral oxycodone, and acetaminophen, ketorolac) if analgesia with SSTS is insufficient [22,24,27,28,33–37]. In our study, we found a clear reduction in calls for rescue analgesia ($p < 0.0001$), even if it appeared that the pain intensity was not significantly reduced, except for the mean value of NRS in the first 24 h.

Our hypothesis is that SSTS offers a more stable analgesic coverage, distinguishing itself from the strategy used for the controls (ropivacaine + paracetamol), which instead requires continuous rescue intervention to ensure adequate pain control. Furthermore, comparable NRS values but with a higher number of calls suggest that NRS values were not detected every time the patient required rescue intervention but after the therapy had taken effect. This is explained by the fact that in real life, patients complaining of pain are treated without necessarily paying attention to its measurement using appropriate scales. However, we think that a RCT with the combined use of both techniques (SSTS + cFNB) should be carefully evaluated due to promising results. The SSTS system allows the patient to sufficiently control for any pain not being covered by regional analgesia or particularly in case of a failed block, but still, additional regional analgesia may save opioids and thus reduce opioid-related side effects. In addition, a saphenous nerve block may have some advantages over the cFNB regarding motor function and early mobilization.

A clear advantage of SSTS is the administration modality, without the need for additional venous access, which reduces the intrinsic risk of infections linked to invasive routes of administration in selected patients (e.g., oncologic patients). Regarding usability, SSTS was well accepted by both patients and care providers, and Turnbull et al. described SSTS as easy and quick (approximately 4 min per patient), and its functioning is easy to explain to patients. A further advantage of SSTS with sublingual tablets is the oral administration, reducing the risk of infection, analgesic gaps, or conduct obstruction related to the classic pump or IV catheter infusion [27,35,38,39].

We reported an extremely significant reduction in calls to nurses ($p < 0.0001$). This in the SSTS group supports the managerial superiority of the SSTS, both in terms of analgesic therapy (self-administered) and the ward, allowing a redistribution of human resources. In fact, nursing staff are not employed in the preparation and administration of analgesic therapy, which increases patient comfort. The second aspect concerns the intrinsic risk, linked to human factors, of possible mistakes in the administration of analgesic therapy. This risk is eliminated by delegating dosage control of analgesia to the device.

The incidence of adverse effects reported in our study were line with the literature: PONV (6%), with nausea (10%), constipation (24%), disorientation (6%), and bladder globe (4%) the most frequently observed. In a study of 100 patients treated with SSTS after knee or hip arthroplasty, the adverse events reported were nausea (34.9%), vomiting (10.8%), desaturation (7.0%), constipation (4.8%), pruritus (4.8%), headache (4.1%), dizziness (5.1%), and confusion state (2.5%) [27]. Similar results have been reported by Melson et al., with nausea (42.9%), vomiting (13.8%), desaturation (9.6 %), and constipation (11.3%) the most frequent [22]. Although studies have shown that SSTS could save time in the ward, the most interesting advantage we observed from the use of SSTS was the patient's satisfaction rate, as reported in previous papers [13,21,35,40–42].

The mean hospitalization duration was significantly lower in the SSTS group than in the control group (7.06 days vs. 8.62 days; $p = 0.039$). Scardino et al. described how patients in the SSTS group were able to ambulate earlier after surgery and achieve the goals set by the fast-track protocol. Moreover, patients in the SSTS group were all discharged from the hospital within three days of surgery compared to only 36% of the cFNB patients [29]. This study reported similar results but differed from ours in the combined use of cFNB with multimodal drug therapy which included oxycodone/nalaxone 10 mg/5 mg tablets twice daily plus ketoprofen 100 mg 2 capsules/24 h or, in case of NSAID intolerance, paracetamol 1 g three times a day [29].

5. Conclusions

The sublingual sufentanil system (SSTS system, Zalviso®) is an investigational patient-controlled system that utilizes the SST system to treat moderate-to-severe acute pain in the hospital setting. This system has advantages over IV PCA and has been demonstrated to provide rapid analgesia and achieve high patient and nurse satisfaction ratings in clinical use. Our data confirm the safety and tolerability of SSTS in the management of postoperative pain, resulting in a high level of patient satisfaction and acceptance of pain control. This study demonstrates how the SSTS reduces the need for interventions by healthcare personnel, allowing a redistribution of resources and a reduction in the use of analgesic drugs. A randomized controlled trial is required to provide a conclusive answer. Since this study only evaluated results directly after surgery, future studies could be expanded with long-term results, preoperative pain scores, and the inclusion of more patients could help obtain significant results.

Author Contributions: Conceptualization, project administration: A.A. and G.M.P.; data curation and formal analysis: G.M.P. and M.C.; supervision: P.N. and P.R.; writing—original draft: A.A. and M.C.; writing—review and editing: A.A., G.M.P. and F.A. All authors have read and agreed to the published version of the manuscript.

Funding: This research received no external funding.

Institutional Review Board Statement: The study was conducted in accordance with the Declaration of Helsinki approved by the Ethics Committee of University-Hospital of Padova (protocol code 266n/AO/22 and 30 June 2022).

Informed Consent Statement: Informed consent was obtained from all subjects involved in the study.

Data Availability Statement: The dataset supporting the conclusions of this review is available upon request to the corresponding author.

Conflicts of Interest: Ruggieri reports he is a consultant and designer for Stryker and Exactech (no relationship with the present work). The other authors declare that there are no relationships/conditions/circumstances that present a potential conflict of interest with the present manuscript.

References

1. Berninger, M.T.; Friederichs, J.; Leidinger, W.; Augat, P.; Bühren, V.; Fulghum, C.; Reng, W. Effect of local infiltration analgesia, peripheral nerve blocks, general and spinal anesthesia on early functional recovery and pain control in total knee arthroplasty. *BMC Musculoskelet. Disord.* **2018**, *19*, 232. [CrossRef]
2. van Veen, D.E.; Verhelst, C.C.; van Dellen, R.T.; Koopman, J. Sublingual sufentanil (Zalviso) patient-controlled analgesia after total knee arthroplasty: A retrospective comparison with oxycodone with or without dexamethasone. *J. Pain Res.* **2018**, *11*, 3205–3210. [CrossRef] [PubMed]
3. Karlsen, A.P.H.; Wetterslev, M.; Hansen, S.E.; Hansen, M.S.; Mathiesen, O.; Dahl, J.B. Postoperative pain treatment after total knee arthroplasty: A systematic review. *PLoS ONE* **2017**, *12*, e0173107. [CrossRef] [PubMed]
4. Ma, H.-H.; Chou, T.-F.A.; Tsai, S.-W.; Chen, C.-F.; Wu, P.-K.; Chen, W.-M. The efficacy of continuous versus single-injection femoral nerve block in Total knee Arthroplasty: A systematic review and meta-analysis. *BMC Musculoskelet. Disord.* **2020**, *21*, 121. [CrossRef]
5. Dennis, D.A. Evaluation of painful total knee arthroplasty. *J. Arthroplast.* **2004**, *19*, 35–40. [CrossRef]
6. Li, J.; Ma, Y.; Xiao, L. Postoperative Pain Management in Total Knee Arthroplasty. *Orthop. Surg.* **2019**, *11*, 755–761. [CrossRef] [PubMed]
7. Elmallah, R.K.; Chughtai, M.; Khlopas, A.; Newman, J.M.; Stearns, K.L.; Roche, M.; Kelly, M.A.; Harwin, S.F.; Mont, M.A. Pain Control in Total Knee Arthroplasty. *J. Knee Surg.* **2018**, *31*, 504–513. [CrossRef]
8. Zhao, J.; Davis, S.P. An integrative review of multimodal pain management on patient recovery after total hip and knee arthroplasty. *Int. J. Nurs. Stud.* **2019**, *98*, 94–106. [CrossRef] [PubMed]
9. Kaur, M.; Katyal, S.; Kathuria, S.; Singh, P. A comparative evaluation of intrathecal bupivacaine alone, sufentanil or butorphanol in combination with bupivacaine for endoscopic urological surgery. *Saudi J. Anaesth.* **2011**, *5*, 202–227. [CrossRef]
10. Gaffney, C.J.; Pelt, C.E.; Gililland, J.M.; Peters, C.L. Perioperative Pain Management in Hip and Knee Arthroplasty. *Orthop. Clin. North Am.* **2017**, *48*, 407–419. [CrossRef]
11. Kehlet, H.; Thienpont, E. Fast-track knee arthroplasty–status and future challenges. *Knee* **2013**, *20*, S29–S33. [CrossRef]
12. Flierl, M.A.; Sobh, A.H.; Culp, B.M.; Baker, E.A.; Sporer, S.M. Evaluation of the Painful Total Knee Arthroplasty. *J. Am. Acad. Orthop. Surg.* **2019**, *27*, 743–751. [CrossRef] [PubMed]
13. Noel, E.; Miglionico, L.; Leclercq, M.; Jennart, H.; Fils, J.-F.; Van Rompaey, N. Sufentanil sublingual tablet system versus oral oxycodone for management of postoperative pain in enhanced recovery after surgery pathway for total knee arthroplasty: A randomized controlled study. *J. Exp. Orthop.* **2020**, *7*, 92. [CrossRef] [PubMed]
14. Turnbull, Z.A.; Sastow, D.; Giambrone, G.P.; Tedore, T. Anesthesia for the patient undergoing total knee replacement: Current status and future prospects. *Local Reg. Anesth.* **2017**, *10*, 1–7. [CrossRef]
15. Andersen, K.V.; Bak, M.; Christensen, B.V.; Harazuk, J.; Pedersen, N.A.; Søballe, K. A randomized, controlled trial comparing local infiltration analgesia with epidural infusion for total knee arthroplasty. *Acta Orthop.* **2010**, *81*, 606–610. [CrossRef]
16. Bauer, M.C.; Pogatzki-Zahn, E.M.; Zahn, P.K. Regional analgesia techniques for total knee replacement. *Curr. Opin. Anaesthesiol.* **2014**, *27*, 501–506. [CrossRef] [PubMed]

17. Yang, X.; Kang, W.; Xiong, W.; Lu, D.; Zhou, Z.; Chen, X.; Zhou, X.; Feng, X. The Effect of Dexmedetomidine as Adjuvant to Ropivacaine 0.1% for Femoral Nerve Block on Strength of Quadriceps Muscle in Patients Undergoing Total Knee Arthroplasty: A Double-Blinded Randomized Controlled Trial. *J. Pain Res.* 2019, *12*, 3355–3363. [CrossRef]
18. Tian, Y.; Tang, S.; Sun, S.; Zhang, Y.; Chen, L.; Xia, D.; Wang, Y.; Ren, L.; Huang, Y. Comparison between local infiltration analgesia with combined femoral and sciatic nerve block for pain management after total knee arthroplasty. *J. Orthop. Surg. Res.* 2020, *15*, 41. [CrossRef]
19. Zhang, Z.; Yang, Q.; Xin, W.; Zhang, Y. Comparison of local infiltration analgesia and sciatic nerve block as an adjunct to femoral nerve block for pain control after total knee arthroplasty. *Medicine* 2017, *96*, e6829. [CrossRef]
20. Tang, Q.-F.; Li, X.-L.; Yu, L.-X.; Hao, Y.-F.; Lu, G.-H. Preoperative Ropivacaine with or without Tramadol for Femoral Nerve Block in Total Knee Arthroplasty. *J. Orthop. Surg.* 2016, *24*, 183–187. [CrossRef]
21. Van De Donk, T.; Ward, S.; Langford, R.; Dahan, A. Pharmacokinetics and pharmacodynamics of sublingual sufentanil for postoperative pain management. *Anaesthesia* 2018, *73*, 231–237. [CrossRef] [PubMed]
22. Melson, T.I.; Boyer, D.L.; Minkowitz, H.S.; Turan, A.; Chiang, Y.; Evashenk, M.A.; Palmer, P.P. Sufentanil Sublingual Tablet System vs. Intravenous Patient-Controlled Analgesia with Morphine for Postoperative Pain Control: A Randomized, Active-Comparator Trial. *Pain Pract.* 2014, *14*, 679–688. [CrossRef] [PubMed]
23. Kizilkaya, M.; Yildirim, O.S.; Dogan, N.; Kursad, H.; Okur, A. Analgesic Effects of Intraarticular Sufentanil and Sufentanil Plus Methylprednisolone After Arthroscopic Knee Surgery. *Anesth. Analg.* 2004, *98*, 1062–1065. [CrossRef] [PubMed]
24. Rispoli, M.; Fiorelli, A.; Nespoli, M.R.; Esposito, M.; Corcione, A.; Buono, S. Sufentanil Sublingual Tablet System for theManagement of Postoperative Pain afterVideo-Assisted Thoracic Surgery: APreliminary Clinical Experience. *J. Cardiothorac. Vasc. Anesth.* 2018, *32*, e61–e63. [CrossRef] [PubMed]
25. Albrecht, E.; Guyen, O.; Jacot-Guillarmod, A.; Kirkham, K. The analgesic efficacy of local infiltration analgesia vs femoral nerve block after total knee arthroplasty: A systematic review and meta-analysis. *Br. J. Anaesth.* 2016, *116*, 597–609. [CrossRef] [PubMed]
26. Bauer, C.; Pavlakovic, I.; Mercier, C.; Maury, J.-M.; Koffel, C.; Roy, P.; Fellahi, J.-L. Adding sufentanil to ropivacaine in continuous thoracic paravertebral block fails to improve analgesia after video-assisted thoracic surgery. *Eur. J. Anaesthesiol.* 2018, *35*, 766–773. [CrossRef] [PubMed]
27. Jove, M.; Griffin, D.W.; Minkowitz, H.S.; Ben-David, B.; Evashenk, M.A.; Palmer, P.P. Sufentanil Sublingual Tablet System for the Management of Postoperative Pain after Knee or Hip Arthroplasty. *Anesthesiology* 2015, *123*, 434–443. [CrossRef]
28. Minkowitz, H.S.; Leiman, D.; Melson, T.; Singla, N.; DiDonato, K.P.; Palmer, P.P. Sufentanil Sublingual Tablet 30 mcg for the Management of Pain Following Abdominal Surgery: A Randomized, Placebo-Controlled, Phase-3 Study. *Pain Pract.* 2017, *17*, 848–858. [CrossRef]
29. Zorrilla-Vaca, A.; Li, J. The role of sciatic nerve block to complement femoral nerve block in total knee arthroplasty: A meta-analysis of randomized controlled trials. *J. Anesth.* 2018, *32*, 341–350. [CrossRef]
30. Chan, E.-Y.; Fransen, M.; Parker, D.A.; Assam, P.N.; Chua, N. Femoral nerve blocks for acute postoperative pain after knee replacement surgery. *Cochrane Database Syst. Rev.* 2014, *2014*, CD009941. [CrossRef]
31. Beebe, M.J.; Allen, R.; Anderson, M.B.; Swenson, J.D.; Peters, C.L. Continuous Femoral Nerve Block Using 0.125% Bupivacaine Does Not Prevent Early Ambulation After Total Knee Arthroplasty. *Clin. Orthop. Relat. Res.* 2014, *472*, 1394–1399. [CrossRef]
32. Abdallah, F.W.; Madjdpour, C.; Brull, R. Is sciatic nerve block advantageous when combined with femoral nerve block for postoperative analgesia following total knee arthroplasty? a meta-analysis. *Can. J. Anaesth.* 2016, *63*, 552–568. [CrossRef] [PubMed]
33. Scardino, M.; D'Amato, T.; Martorelli, F.; Fenocchio, G.; Simili, V.; Di Matteo, B.; Bugada, D.; Kon, E. Sublingual sufentanil tablet system Zalviso® for postoperative analgesia after knee replacement in fast track surgery: A pilot observational study. *J. Exp. Orthop.* 2018, *5*, 8. [CrossRef] [PubMed]
34. Giaccari, L.G.; Coppolino, F.; Aurilio, C.; Esposito, V.; Pace, M.C.; Paladini, A.; Passavanti, M.B.; Pota, V.; Sansone, P. Sufentanil Sublingual for Acute Post-Operative Pain: A Systematic Literature Review Focused on Pain Intensity, Adverse Events, and Patient Satisfaction. *Pain Ther.* 2020, *9*, 217–230. [CrossRef] [PubMed]
35. Meijer, F.; Cornelissen, P.; Sie, C.; Wagemans, M.; Mars, A.; Hobma, T.; Niesters, M.; Dahan, A.; Koopman, J.S.; Steegers, M.A. Sublingual sufentanil for postoperative pain relief: First clinical experiences. *J. Pain Res.* 2018, *11*, 987–992. [CrossRef]
36. Lötsch, J. Pharmacokinetic-pharmacodynamic modeling of opioids. *J. Pain Symptom Manag.* 2005, *29*, S90–S103. [CrossRef]
37. Hudcova, J.; McNicol, E.; Quah, C.; Lau, J.; Carr, D.B. Patient-controlled opioid analgesia *versus* conventional opioid analgesia for postoperative pain. *Cochrane Database Syst. Rev.* 2006, *4*, CD003348.
38. Panchal, S.J.; Damaraju, C.V.; Nelson, W.W.; Hewitt, D.J.; Schein, J.R. System-Related Events and Analgesic Gaps During Postoperative Pain Management with the Fentanyl Iontophoretic Transdermal System and Morphine Intravenous Patient-Controlled Analgesia. *Anesth. Analg.* 2007, *105*, 1437–1441. [CrossRef]
39. Palmer, P.P.; Miller, R.D. Current and Developing Methods of Patient-Controlled Analgesia. *Anesthesiol. Clin.* 2010, *28*, 587–599. [CrossRef]
40. Scardino, M.; Tartarelli, A.; Coluzzi, F.; Corcione, A.; Lorini, F.L.; Torrano, V.; Martorano, P.P.; Quaini, S. Sublingual sufentanil tablet system for the management of acute postoperative pain in a hospital setting: An observational study. *Minerva Anestesiol.* 2021, *87*, 156–164. [CrossRef]

41. Vergari, A.; Cortegiani, A.; Rispoli, M.; Coluzzi, F.; Deni, F.; Leykin, Y.; Lorini, F.L.; Martorano, P.P.; Paolicchi, A.; Polati, E.; et al. Sufentanil Sublingual Tablet System: From rationale of use to clinical practice. *Eur. Rev. Med. Pharmacol. Sci.* **2020**, *24*, 11891–11899. [CrossRef] [PubMed]
42. Pogatzki-Zahn, E.; Kranke, P.; Winner, J.; Weyland, W.; Reich, A.; Vigelius-Rauch, U.; Paland, M.; Löhr, T.; Eberhart, L. Real-world use of the sufentanil sublingual tablet system for patient-controlled management of acute postoperative pain: A prospective noninterventional study. *Curr. Med. Res. Opin.* **2019**, *36*, 277–284. [CrossRef] [PubMed]

MDPI
St. Alban-Anlage 66
4052 Basel
Switzerland
www.mdpi.com

Journal of Clinical Medicine Editorial Office
E-mail: jcm@mdpi.com
www.mdpi.com/journal/jcm

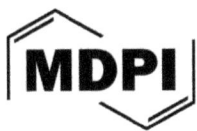

Disclaimer/Publisher's Note: The statements, opinions and data contained in all publications are solely those of the individual author(s) and contributor(s) and not of MDPI and/or the editor(s). MDPI and/or the editor(s) disclaim responsibility for any injury to people or property resulting from any ideas, methods, instructions or products referred to in the content.

www.ingramcontent.com/pod-product-compliance
Lightning Source LLC
LaVergne TN
LVHW070644100526
838202LV00013B/880